Atlas OF

Minor Oral Surgery

Atlas OF

Minor Oral Surgery

HARRY DYM, D.D.S.

Director, Department of Dentistry and
Oral and Maxillofacial Surgery,
Director, Oral and Maxillofacial Surgery
Residency Training Program,
The Brooklyn Hospital Center,
Brooklyn, New York

ORRETT E. OGLE, D.D.S.

Director, Residency Training Program,
Chief, Oral and Maxillofacial Surgery,
Woodhull Medical and Mental Health Center,
Brooklyn, New York

Artwork
Hope L. Wettan, D.D.S.

SAUNDERS

An Imprint of Elsevier

SAUNDERS
An Imprint of Elsevier
The Curtis Center
Independence Square West
Philadelphia, PA 19106

Editor-in-Chief: John Schrefer
Acquisitions Editor: Penny Rudolph
Developmental Editor: Kimberly Frare
Project Manager: Patricia Tannian
Production Editor: Stephen C. Hetager
Book Design Manager: Gail Morey Hudson
Cover Designer: Teresa Breckwoldt

ATLAS OF MINOR ORAL SURGERY

ISBN-13: 978-0-7216-7977-8
ISBN-10: 0-7216-7977-3

Permissions may be sought directly from Elsevier's Health Sciences Rights Department in Philadelphia, USA: phone: (+1)215-238-7869, fax: (+1)215-238-2239, email: healthpermissions@elsevier.com. You may also complete your request on-line via the Elsevier Science homepage (http://www.elsevier.com), by selecting 'Customer Support' and then 'Obtaining Permissions'.

Printed in the United States of America

Last digit is the print number: 9   8   7   6   5   4   3   2

Contributors

RYAZ ANSARI, D.D.S.
Chief Resident,
Division of Oral and Maxillofacial Surgery,
The Brooklyn Hospital Center,
Brooklyn, New York

PAUL R. BAKER, D.D.S.
Assistant Attending Oral and Maxillofacial Surgeon,
Department of Dentistry/Oral and Maxillofacial Surgery,
The Brooklyn Hospital Center and
New York Methodist Hospital,
Brooklyn, New York

FRANCIS CHIONCHIO, D.D.S.
Assistant Attending Oral and Maxillofacial Surgeon,
Department of Dentistry/Oral and Maxillofacial Surgery,
The Brooklyn Hospital Center and
New York Methodist Hospital,
Brooklyn, New York

EARL CLARKSON, D.D.S.
Co-Chairman,
Department of Dentistry,
Interfaith Medical Center;
Associate Director,
Department of Dentistry/Oral and Maxillofacial Surgery,
The Brooklyn Hospital Center;
Associate Director,
Division of Oral and Maxillofacial Surgery,
Woodhull Medical and Mental Health Center;
Brooklyn, New York

HARRY DYM, D.D.S.
Director, Department of Dentistry and Oral and Maxillofacial Surgery,
Director, Oral and Maxillofacial Surgery
Residency Training Program,
The Brooklyn Hospital Center;
Assistant Director,
Department of Dentistry/Oral and Maxillofacial Surgery,
Woodhull Medical and Mental Health Center,
Brooklyn, New York;
Associate Clinical Professor,
Oral and Maxillofacial Surgery,
Columbia University School of Dental and Oral Surgery,
New York, New York

DUDLEY S. JACKMAN, D.M.D.
Clinical Assistant Professor,
Oral and Maxillofacial Surgery, Harlem Hospital,
Columbia University, College of Physicians and Surgeons,
New York, New York;
Private Practice, South Orange, New Jersey;
Attending, Newark Beth Israel Medical Center, Newark,
New Jersey, and Saint Barnabas Medical Center,
Toms River, New Jersey

MICHAEL KLEIN, D.D.S.
Clinical Associate Professor,
Department of Implant Dentistry,
New York University College of Dentistry,
New York, New York;
Clinical Assistant Professor,
Department of Prosthodontics,
University of Medicine and Dentistry of New Jersey,
Newark, New Jersey

WAYNE MAURER, D.D.S.
Assistant Attending Oral and Maxillofacial Surgeon,
Department of Dentistry/Oral and Maxillofacial Surgery,
The Brooklyn Hospital Center,
Brooklyn, New York

ORRETT E. OGLE, D.D.S.
Director, Residency Training Program,
Chief, Oral and Maxillofacial Surgery,
Woodhull Medical and Mental Health Center,
Brooklyn, New York;
Associate Clinical Professor,
Oral and Maxillofacial Surgery,
Columbia University School of Dental and Oral Surgery,
New York, New York;
Adjunct Professor of Pharmacology,
University of Pennsylvania,
School of Dental Medicine,
Philadelphia, Pennsylvania

DARSHAN J. PANCHAL, D.D.S.
Private Practice,
Lindenhurst, New York;
Attending Oral and Maxillofacial Surgeon,
Good Samaritan and Brunswick Medical Centers,
Islip, New York

MANAF SAKER, D.M.D.
Private Practice,
Department of Oral and Maxillofacial Surgery,
South Mountain OMS Center,
South Orange, New Jersey;
Formerly Chief Resident,
Division of Oral and Maxillofacial Surgery,
Woodhull Medical and Mental Health Center,
Brooklyn, New York

STEVEN R. SCHWARTZ, D.D.S.
Attending Oral and Maxillofacial Surgeon,
Department of Dentistry/Oral and Maxillofacial Surgery,
Woodhull Medical and Mental Health Center and
Department of Dentistry/Oral and Maxillofacial Surgery,
The Brooklyn Hospital Center;
Brooklyn, New York

AARON J. VAFAKOS, D.M.D.
Private Practice,
Baltimore, Maryland;
Formerly Chief Resident,
Division of Oral and Maxillofacial Surgery,
Woodhull Medical and Mental Health Center,
Brooklyn, New York

J. HAMIL WILLOUGHBY, D.D.S.
Captain, D.C., U.S.N.R.,
Department of Oral Surgery, Naval Dental Center,
Norfolk, Virginia;
Formerly Chief, Oral and Maxillofacial Surgery,
Department of Dentistry/OMS, Harlem Hospital Center,
New York, New York

This book is dedicated to
my loving wife, partner, and best friend
Freidy
Her constant support, understanding, and encouragement
have made everything possible.
Harry Dym

Dedicated to
God, my family, wife, children,
dearest friends, and all my teachers.
Orrett E. Ogle

Preface

Oral surgical procedures are an integral component of modern-day dentistry, and no clinician can successfully practice his or her profession without a basic understanding of surgical principles and procedures. *Atlas of Minor Oral Surgery* was conceived and written to address and help elucidate the surgical area of dentistry.

The word "minor" in the title of the book is not meant to minimize the degree of importance and complexity of the surgical procedures outlined in the text, but rather only to convey that these are surgical procedures commonly performed in an outpatient office setting with local anesthesia.

The text is heavily and clearly illustrated and divided into nine sections that run the gamut of dental and oral surgical procedures—from endodontic to periodontal surgery, as well as implant and third-molar techniques.

We hope that *Atlas of Minor Oral Surgery* will fill an important niche and become useful not only to the dental student but also to the practicing general dentist as well as the surgical specialist.

The book is designed to provide useful day-to-day clinically applicable information without a great deal of extraneous esoteric knowledge. In addition to acting as a surgical manual and guide, *Atlas of Minor Oral Surgery* provides useful information on antibiotics and sedation techniques and a review of local anesthesia—all clinically relevant and timely information. It is also our hope that *Atlas of Minor Oral Surgery* will be kept in or close to the operatory for "real-time" use and information, so that it becomes the "go-to" book for all things oral surgical in nature.

Finally, and perhaps most important, in addition to developing good technical surgical skills, the clinician must maintain a compassionate, kind, and caring attitude, for that is often all that our anxious patients will remember.

Harry Dym
Orrett E. Ogle

Acknowledgements

The concept of a self-made man is another Madison Avenue mythic creation and one in which I stake no claim. My personal and professional development over the past 25 years was influenced and shaped by many individuals, and I feel it only fitting and proper that I acknowledge them in writing:

Dr. Irwin Mandel, Dr. Charles Barr, and the late Dr. Jerry Stoopack for their guidance and help during my early student and resident years. Mr. Arthur Blutstein, Vice President for Clinical Operations, The Brooklyn Hospital Center, for his early confidence in me and his continued support. Mr. Fred Alley, President and Chief Executive Officer, The Brooklyn Hospital Center, for his dedication to community health care and his continued support of the Department of Dentistry and Oral and Maxillofacial Surgery. Dr. Vincent Tricomi, Medical Director and Executive Vice President, The Brooklyn Hospital Center, for his dedication to resident education and for his ongoing support and counsel. Ms. Cynthia Carrington-Murray, Executive Director, Woodhull Medical and Mental Health Center, for her strong commitment to the dental and oral surgery needs of the community and for her ongoing support.

A special debt is owed to Dr. Peter M. Sherman, Chairman of Dentistry/Oral and Maxillofacial Surgery, The Brooklyn Hospital Center and Woodhull Medical and Mental Health Center, for over two decades of encouragement, advice, and counsel; he has been both a mentor and friend and this text would not have become a reality without his support.

To the secretaries, dental assistants, and nurses at both The Brooklyn Hospital Center and Woodhull Medical and Mental Health Center, Department of Dentistry/OMS, my deepest gratitude for their dedication and hard work.

To my past, present, and future residents, my sincere thanks for you have been and are my greatest teachers. To my colleagues who have contributed to this text, many of whom were my residents, I take great pleasure in your growth and development and look forward to future projects.

Much thanks is owed to the capable editors at Harcourt Health Sciences, for their help and guidance: Penny Rudolph, Kimberly Frare, Judith Fletcher, and Marcia Craig.

Special mention must be made of Dr. Earl I. Clarkson, who contributed to the book, for his quiet strength and vital friendship. He is a surgeon's surgeon who is devoted to patient care and resident education.

To Ms. Luisa Soto, for her preparation of the manuscript and text, my deepest gratitude.

To my parents, Mr. and Mrs. Chaim and Molly Dym, and to my in-laws, Mr. and Mrs. Sol and Heddy Rosner, who in their quiet dignified ways have taught me about courage, ethics, and decency. To my wife Freidy, and children Yehoshua, Hindy, Daniel, and Akiva, who bring me great joy and pride, you have been my inspiration.

I pay tribute to Dr. Hope Wettan for her outstanding illustrations. She is a truly rare individual who combines both science and art in a masterful fashion, and without whom the book would have been greatly diminished.

Dr. Orrett Ogle, who taught me surgery 20 years ago while I was a resident at Greenpoint Hospital, and who continues to be a source of knowledge and guidance, I can truly say that my respect and admiration for him have only been reinforced during the preparation of the *Atlas*.

This is the day the Lord has made. Let us rejoice in it. (Psalms)

Harry Dym

Everyone who is involved in the writing or development of an educational manual draws from several people and relies heavily on the support and cooperation of others. To these special people I wish to express my most sincere thanks. First and foremost, is my co-author, Harry Dym, who has been a friend and confidant for almost 20 years. Special thanks to my colleagues at Woodhull Hospital, Dr. Earl Clarkson, my assistant, and Drs. Steve Wettan, Fred Lifshey, and Steven Schwartz who supported us in the production of this book by giving their time and advice.

The executive director of Woodhull Hospital, Mrs. Cynthia Carrington-Murray, and my departmental Chairman, Dr. Peter Sherman, deserve special mention.

Mrs. Carrington-Murray has always been very supportive of our department and has been a good personal friend. Dr. Peter Sherman, who gave me the opportunity to work and develop, has been the best boss that an employee may ever have.

There are several people from whom I have taken valuable time to develop this book and to whom I wish to say thanks for their understanding and support: my wife, children, family members, my residents, and special friends.

Thanks to Penny Rudolph, our editor, Kimberly Frare, our developmental editor, and all the other people at Harcourt Health Sciences, known and unknown, who worked on this project and to Dr. Hope Wettan, our illustrator, a very gifted lady without whom the quality of this work would not be what it is.

Last, I wish to acknowledge all my teachers, from those in my elementary school in Jamaica to my esteemed professors in universities here in the United States, who contributed to my education, and my clinical attendings at Harlem Hospital and Columbia University, who along with all the patients whom I treated, allowed me to gain the clinical experience that I now pass on.

Orrett E. Ogle

I wish to thank my father, Dr. Steven Wettan, who provided me with technical advice, creative criticism, and endless encouragement. Thank you also to Drs. Harry Dym and Orrett E. Ogle for allowing me to further my education by helping others to do the same.

Hope L. Wettan

Contents

SECTION I
BASIC PRINCIPLES

1 Medical Evaluation of the Patient for Office Oral Surgery, 3
Earl Clarkson

2 Regional Surgical Anatomy, 22
Orrett E. Ogle

3 Local Anesthesia, 30
Orrett E. Ogle

4 Oral and Parenteral Sedation, 41
Steven R. Schwartz

5 Perioperative Hemorrhage, 54
Orrett E. Ogle

SECTION II
EXODONTIA

6 Simple and Surgical Exodontia, 69
Harry Dym

7 Management of Impacted Third Molar Teeth, 80
Harry Dym

8 The Impacted Canine, 93
Harry Dym

SECTION III
ADVANCED PROCEDURES

9 Endodontic Surgery, 103
Orrett E. Ogle

10 Periodontal Surgery, 115
Harry Dym

11 Closure of Oral Antral Communications and Treatment of Sinus Infections, 126
Paul Baker

SECTION IV
INFECTIONS

12 Odontogenic Infections: Anatomy and Surgical Management, 137
Dudley S. Jackman
J. Hamil Willoughby

13 Antibiotics and Their Use in Oral and Maxillofacial Infections, 150
Francis Chionchio

SECTION V
PATHOLOGY

14 Cysts and Their Management, 165
Manaf Saker
Orrett E. Ogle

15 Biopsy Techniques, 177
Orrett E. Ogle

SECTION VI
PROSTHETIC SURGERY

16 Minor Preprosthetic Surgery, 193
Darshan J. Panchal
Orrett E. Ogle

17 Bone Grafting for Implants, 208
Aaron Vafakos

18 The Sinus-Lift Procedure, 219
Harry Dym

SECTION VII
IMPLANTS

19 Evaluation and Treatment Planning for Implants, 225
Michael Klein

20 Principles of Implant Surgery, 231
Harry Dym

SECTION VIII

TRAUMA

21 Evaluation and Treatment of Dentoalveolar Injuries, 245
Wayne Maurer
Ryaz Ansari
Harry Dym

22 Closed Reduction of Mandibular Fractures: Indications and Techniques, 254
Orrett E. Ogle

23 Repair of Lacerations, 262
Orrett E. Ogle

SECTION IX

SALIVARY GLAND DISEASE

24 Management of Commonly Seen Salivary Gland Diseases, 277
Harry Dym

Appendix

Useful Laboratory Information and Common Drug Interactions, 285

BASIC PRINCIPLES

1

Medical Evaluation of the Patient for Office Oral Surgery

EARL CLARKSON, DDS

The health history is an extremely important part of the health assessment. Its performance is the primary vehicle by which rapport is established between the practitioner and the patient requiring ambulatory dentoalveolar surgery. This process differs from that of the patient requiring an in-hospital surgical procedure. The latter would require a comprehensive physical and laboratory exam based on age and existing systemic condition. Most hospitals have laboratory requirements specific for that institution and other factors such as the patient's ASA (American Society of Anesthesiologists) classification. The dentist's approach to the patient will not only determine to a large degree the amount of information that the patient imparts, but, what is more important, may even affect the accuracy of this data. If the patient senses an attitude of sincerity, integrity, and warmth in his dentist, he feels free to relate all matters referable to his health, regardless of how personal they may be.

The dentist must learn to conceal any moral judgement that she may have about the actions and attitude of the patient and must learn more about the origins of her own feelings. The establishment of rapport or lack of it explains why one examiner may elicit a significant history from a patient when another fails to obtain clear-cut information from the same person. Although this may seem obvious, privacy must not be violated in actual practice. The dentist should record any pertinent additional personal information gleaned during the interview process that the patient may have failed to enter into the history form.

In the practice of medicine it is essential that the physician understand the basic mechanisms of disease. The dentist should be prepared and be proficient at being the oral medicine specialist; this means that he should be capable of recognizing and appropriately managing pathologic oral conditions in his patients. Diseases are not abstract quantities; they are various abnormalities, physical and mental, which are part and parcel of human beings. A disease does not exist without a patient, so the dentist must be able to recognize the patient's pathology and observe and consider the patient's feelings and reactions to her disease.

MEDICAL HISTORY

It is mandatory that a medical history be taken for every patient who is to receive dental treatment. The use of a written, patient-completed medical history questionnaire is a legal necessity. This should be reviewed by the dentist who may then discuss selected questions or responses with the patient. The last question should address any issues the patient may prefer to discuss in private. The extent and detail of the history are somewhat dependent on personal preference and type of services to be rendered. However the dentist must be prepared to interpret how a medical problem will alter a patient's response to dental surgery and anesthetic agents.

Regardless of the format used to obtain a health history, a certain amount of essential health information should be known about every patient before examination procedures or treatment are undertaken. This essential information is not all-inclusive by any means but does serve a screening function to protect both patient and dentist. The physical and laboratory examination of a patient plays a relatively minor role in the presurgery evaluation if the history is well taken.

Numerous health questionnaires designed for dental patients are available from sources such as the American Association of Oral and Maxillofacial Surgeons, American Dental Association, dental schools, dental textbooks, and commercial dental supply houses (Fig. 1-1).

The medical interview may have to be abbreviated based on the patient's particular needs, but must be completed in its entirety before the end of the first visit. Certain conditions such as age, language barriers, educational level, pain, and anxiety may affect the medical interview. Patients in severe pain, for example, may

Today's Date ____/____/____ Please Print

PATIENT'S NAME	SEX	AGE	BIRTHDATE	RELATIONSHIP	PHONE HOME: BUS:

RESPONSIBLE PARTY'S NAME	SOC. SEC.#	NAME OF INS PLAN	GROUP#

ADDRESS	EMPLOYER (COMPANY NAME AND ADDRESS)

CITY, STATE, ZIP	SPOUSE'S NAME	SPOUSE'S OCCUPATION

NAME OF RELATIVE (NOT AT SAME ADDRESS)	RELATIVE'S ADDRESS

PHYSICIAN'S NAME	REFERRING DENTIST'S NAME	ORTHODONTIST'S NAME

REASON FOR VISIT HERE	FAMILY MEMBERS WHO HAVE BEEN PATIENTS HERE

In the following questions, circle yes or no, whichever applies. Your answer are for our records only and will be considered confidential.

1. Are you in good health .   Y   N
2. Has there been any change in your general health within the past year?   Y   N
3. My last physical examination was on _____
4. Are you now under the care of a physician?   Y   N
5. The name and address of my physician is _____
6. Have you had any serious illnesses or operation?   Y   N
7. Have you been hospitalized or had a serious illness within the past (5) years?   Y   N
8. Do you have or have you had any of the following diseases or problems?   Y   N
   a. Damaged heart valves or articular heart valves, including heart murmur   Y   N
   b. Congenital heart lesions   Y   N
   c. Cardiovascular disease (heart trouble, heart attack, coronary insufficiency, coronary occlusion, high blood pressure, arteriosclerosis, stroke).   Y   N
      1. Do you have pain in chest upon exertion?   Y   N
      2. Are you short of breath after mild exercise?   Y   N
      3. Do your ankles swell?   Y   N
      4. Do you get short of breath when you lie down, or do you require extra pillows when you sleep   Y   N
      5. Do you have a cardiac pacemaker?.   Y   N
   d. Allergy   Y   N
   e. Sinus trouble   Y   N
   f. Asthma or hay fever   Y   N
   g. Hives or skin rash   Y   N
   h. Fainting spells or seizures   Y   N

FIG. 1-1 Sample of health history form.

		Y	N
i. Diabetes		Y	N
1. Do you have to urinate (pass water) more than six times a day?		Y	N
2. Are you thirsty much of the time?		Y	N
3. Does your mouth frequently become dry?		Y	N
j. Hepatitis, jaundice or liver disease		Y	N
k. Arthritis		Y	N
l. Inflammatory rheumatism (painful swollen joints)		Y	N
m. Stomach ulcers		Y	N
n. Kidney trouble		Y	N
o. Tuberculosis		Y	N
p. Do you have a persistent cough or cough up blood?		Y	N
q. Low blood pressure		Y	N
r. Venereal disease		Y	N
s. Epilepsy		Y	N
t. Psychiatric problems		Y	N
u. Cancer		Y	N
v. AIDS or other immunosuppressive disorders		Y	N

9. Have you had abnormal bleeding associated with previous extractions, surgery, or trauma?   Y   N
   a. Do you bruise easily?   Y   N
   b. Have you ever required a blood transfusion?   Y   N
      If so, explain the circumstances _____

10. Do you have any blood disorder such as anemia?   Y   N

11. Have you had surgery, x-ray or drug treatment for a tumor, growth, or other condition of your head or neck?   Y   N

12. Are you taking any drug or medicine?
   If so, what?_____

13. Are you taking any of the following:

		Y	N
a. Antibiotics or sulfa drugs		Y	N
b. Anticoagulants (blood thinners)		Y	N
c. Medicine for high blood pressure		Y	N
d. Cortisone (steroids)		Y	N
e. Tranquilizers		Y	N
f. Antihistamine		Y	N
g. Aspirin		Y	N
h. Insulin, tolbutamide (Orinase) or similar drug		Y	N
I. Digitalis, or drugs for heart trouble		Y	N
j. Nitroglycerin		Y	N
k. Oral contraceptive or other hormonal therapy		Y	N
l. Other_____			

14. Are you allergic or have you reacted adversely to:

		Y	N
a. Local anesthetics		Y	N
b. Penicillin or other antibiotics		Y	N
c. Sulfa drugs		Y	N
d. Barbiturates, sedatives, or sleeping pills		Y	N
e. Aspirin		Y	N
f. Iodine		Y	N
g. Codeine or other narcotics		Y	N
h. Other _____			

15. Have you had any serious trouble associated with any previous dental treatment?   Y   N
   If so, explain _____
_____

16. Do you have any disease, condition, or problem not listed above that you think I should know about?   Y   N
   If so, explain _____
_____

17. Are you employed in any situation which exposes you regularly to x-rays or other ionizing radiation?   Y   N
18. Are you wearing contact lenses?   Y   N
19. Have you had anything to eat or drink in the last 4 hours?   Y   N
20. Are you wearing removable dental appliances?   Y   N

FIG. 1-1, cont'd   Sample of health history form.   *Continued*

Women

21.	Are you pregnant?	.	.	.	.	.	.	.	Y N
22.	Do you have problems associated with your menstrual period?		.	.	.	.		Y N
23.	Are you nursing?	.	.	.	.	.		Y N
24.	Do you wish to talk to the doctor about anything privately?		.	.	.		Y N

I certify that I have read and understood the above. Knowledge that my questions, if any, about the inquiries set forth have been answered to my satisfaction. I will not hold my dentist, or any other member of his/her staff, responsible for any errors or omissions that I may have made in the completion of this form.

_____
Signature of Patient

_____
Signature of Dentist

FIG. 1-1, cont'd Sample of health history form.

need the painful stimuli attended to before completion of the medical history.[1]

BIOGRAPHIC DATA

At the beginning of any health record, there should be a place to record commonly used and sometimes critically important biographical information. This information should be obtained early during the patient's first visit; on subsequent visits it may be omitted. The following information is to be recorded in the introductory and biographic section of the health history:

A. Full name
B. Gender
C. Age
D. Birthdate
E. Relationship
F. Phone numbers, home and work
G. Information on the insured party
  a. Responsible party's name
  b. Social security number
  c. Name of insurance plan
  d. Group number
  e. Address
  f. Employer's name and address
  g. Spouse's name
  h. Spouse's occupation
H. Name of relative (not at same address)
I. Relative's address
J. Physician's name
K. Referrer's name

The full name is recorded because persons living in an ethnically homogenous geographical area often

have similar names. Precise identification, using first, middle, and last names, assists in assuring accurate information retrieval and coordination.

Gender, age, birthdate, and relationship information are self-explanatory. Many pathologic conditions of the oral cavity are age-, sex-, or race-related and this information might be correlated with problems discovered later in the history.

The patient's phone numbers are recorded, as well as that of a relative or friend, someone with whom he or she is in frequent contact and who would be willing and able to relay a message to the patient in an emergency or if the patient cannot be located.

The insured's information is very important for processing claim forms and obtaining precise information about the patient. The social security number is used to identify each patient. Potential violation of confidentiality is an important concern.

The patient's current physician name, address, and phone number should be recorded. It may become necessary to consult the family physician to clarify or discuss certain aspects of the patient's medical problems. It is not unusual to have patients who are not well-informed or who are unaware of the degree of control of a given disease. The dentist should record the patient's referrer and the reason for the referral. The patient may be in crisis, may be dissatisfied with past care, or may be "shopping."

CHIEF COMPLAINT

The chief complaint (CC) is a short statement, preferably in the patient's own words and recorded in quotation marks, that indicates the patient's purpose for requesting treatment at this time. It includes a notation of the problem's duration. The duration, as stated by the patient, may not be the actual duration of the symptoms; however, it is an indication of the time during which the complaint has become intolerable enough to motivate the patient to seek help.

On occasions, the chief complaint may be a request for an oral screening, health examination, or for promotion. The chief complaint is not a diagnostic statement, and should not be stated in diagnostic terms. It helps the clinician establish priorities during history taking and treatment planning. Also, this is one of the few places where the patient has the opportunity to have recorded his needs in his own words. Too often the dentist loses sight of the patient priorities for care.

HISTORY OF PRESENT ILLNESS

The history of present illness (HPI) section describes the information relevant to the chief complaint. In the case of a patient with a health problem, this portion of the health history challenges the interviewing, clinical knowledge, and written communication skills of the dentist. The dentist should try to chronicle the sequence of the patient's problems. The patient should be asked to describe each symptom's progression since its onset. If the patient complains of pain, the dentist should try to determine what precipitates the painful onset. The patient should also be asked to describe the quality, intensity, duration, location, radiation, and factors that may worsen or relieve the pain. The quality of pain is frequently characterized as dull, aching, sharp, nagging, throbbing, stabbing, or squeezing. The patient should be asked of any accompanying symptoms such as nausea, vomiting, fever, anorexia, chills, weakness, and malaise.

HEALTH HISTORY

The purpose of the patient history section is to identify all the patient's major past health problems. The health questionnaire form used in dental offices is an effective and efficient means of obtaining the patient's history. Office personnel can be trained to scan the questionnaire and to flag all positive responses, thereby bringing them to the attention of the dentist. However, the dentist is responsible for verifying the accuracy of the information. The dentist should always ask the patient of childhood illnesses; although more relevant for a young patient, it is important to know if the adult patient had rheumatic fever, rheumatic heart disease, or heart murmur as a child. Also, the dentist needs to know if the child patient has had the recommended course of immunizations. After a review of the health questionnaire, the dentist should ask the patient of

conditions that specifically may affect or alter the treatment. Conditions such as asthma, tuberculosis, pneumonia, bronchitis, pregnancy, sickle cell disease, venereal disease, hepatomegaly, splenomegaly, myocardial infarction, hypertension, congestive heart failure, diabetes mellitus, HIV, cerebrovascular accident, angina, ulcers, cardiac surgery, seizure disorders, kidney disease, implanted devices, anticoagulants, steroids, and so on can alter the dentist's ability to deliver care on the first visit.

The dentist should review any medications that the patient may be presently taking and also inquire about past medications, such as cortisone, immunosuppressants, or narcotics. Patients should be specifically asked about allergies to medications the dentist prescribes or products that the dentist uses frequently in the office, such as local anesthetics, penicillin, aspirin, ibuprofen, amoxicillin, cephalosporin, clindamycin, codeine, other painkillers, latex, or other rubber products. Female patients should be asked if they are pregnant or currently using oral contraceptives. A pregnancy test should be considered for patients who may be in doubt regarding possible pregnancy. The medical history should be updated periodically dependent on the patient's medical condition, but at the least yearly.

REVIEW OF SYSTEMS

The review of systems (ROS) portion of the history includes a collection of data regarding the past and present health of each of the patient's systems. This review may indicate an undiagnosed medical problem and should be included in a comprehensive health history. Generally the ROS portion of the history is organized from head to toe, from physical to psychosocial. The patient is informed that she will be asked a series of questions, and having a checklist can be helpful. However, the questions are usually guided by responses obtained from the history, and may help the dentist determine if the patient should be referred for consultation or whether the patient can be treated. In the practice of dentistry, anxiety-controlling adjuncts are sometimes used; therefore, the nervous, respiratory, and cardiovascular systems should always be reviewed before administering these agents to patients[2].

DENTAL HISTORY

To offer comprehensive care to the patient, the dentist should inquire into the patient's past experiences with dentistry. It is important to know what has been done in the past, when it was done, and the outcome of treatment. The patient should be asked what kind of treatment he had and about the outcome. Any problems mentioned should be noted.

PHYSICAL EXAM

The dentist should perform an exam of the oral cavity, head and neck region, and obtain vital signs. An assistant should measure the patient's blood pressure, pulse rate, weight, and temperature, if necessary, before the dentist sees the patient. A general survey of the patient's outward appearance can give an indication of her general state of health and well-being. Signs of possible trouble might include a wasted, cachectic appearance; lethargic demeanor; ill-kempt, dirty clothing and hair; staggering or halting gait; extreme thinness or obesity; bent posture; and difficulty breathing. Check the shape and symmetry of the face; it may point to a condition or syndrome. Changes in the skin and nails are often associated with systemic disease. Examine the eyes, especially the lids, sclera, and conjunctiva and also check the nasal bridge and eyelids for lesions suggestive of basal cell carcinomas. The ears are checked for gouti-tophi in the helix or antihelix, along with their shape and size. A thorough inspection of the oral cavity is necessary, including the oropharynx, tongue, floor of mouth, and oral mucosa.[3]

Bimanual palpation of the temporomandibular joints, salivary glands, upper and lower neck, and lymph nodes should be performed. Each salivary gland should be palpated for consistency, color, and flow of saliva.

MANAGEMENT OF PATIENTS WITH UNDERLYING MEDICAL CONDITIONS
Cardiovascular Disease

Infective Endocarditis. Endocarditis ensues when bacteria enters the bloodstream from an oral or other source and lodges on heart valves that may already bear platelet-fibrin thrombi. The frequency of bacteremia is quite high after dental extraction (18% to 85%) or periodontal surgery (32% to 88%) but also is significant following everyday activities such as tooth brushing (0% to 26%) and chewing candy (17% to 51%). The production of extracellular dextran by some strains of streptococcus is responsible for their adherence to dental enamel and also is a factor in the entrapment of circulating organisms on damaged valves and platelet fibrin thrombi. The mitral valve is the most common site of infection. Once infection begins, bacteria proliferate freely within the interstices of the enlarging vegetation. The infection may cause rupture of the valve tissue itself or of the chorda tendineae. Some virulent bacteria (*Staphylococcus aureus* or fungal vegetation) may become large enough to obstruct the valve orifice or create a large embolus. Peripheral septic emboli may occur with left-sided endocarditis and septic pulmonary emboli with right-sided endocarditis.

Some cases of streptococcal endocarditis become manifest clinically within 2 weeks of initiating events such as dental extractions. The most common complaints in patients with infectious endocarditis are fever, chills, weakness, shortness of breath, drenching night sweats, loss of appetite, and weight loss with endocarditis involving the aortic or mitral valve; congestive heart failure occurs in two thirds of patients. Tricuspid valve infection is most common in intravenous drug users.

Serious systemic emboli may cause dramatic findings, at times masking the systemic nature of infectious endocarditis. Embolism to the splenic artery may lead to left upper quadrant pain. Renal, coronary, and mesenteric arteries are frequent alternative sites of clinically important emboli. CNS embolization is one of the most serious complications of infectious endocarditis. The kidney can be the site of abscess formation, multiple infarcts, or immune complex glomerulonephritis.[4]

Dental Management. The dentist's goal is to prevent endocarditis from occurring in susceptible dental patients. Any dental procedure that causes injury to the soft tissue or bone resulting in bleeding can produce a transient bacteremia that, in a susceptible patient, can result in endocarditis (Boxes 1-1 and 1-2). Even minor dental manipulations such as the cleaning of teeth or

---

BOX 1-1 Manifestations of Infective Endocarditis

Weakness	Paralysis
Weight loss	Chest pain
Fatigue	Abdominal pain
Fever, chills, night sweats	Blindness
Arthralgia	Hematuria
Petechiae	Splinter hemorrhages
Murmur	Osler nodes
Clubbing of fingers	Janeway lesions
	Roth's spots

BOX 1-2 Bacteria Causing Infective Endocarditis

Viridans streptococci
Fastidious gram-negative rods
Staphylococcus aureus
Candida species
Bacillus species
Streptococcus pneumoniae
Neisseria gonorrhoeae
Haemophilus
Bacterioides species

the placement of a matrix band can result in a transient bacteremia. In the patient with a heart defect such as rheumatic heart disease the anatomy and function of the affected valve are altered because of scarring following the acute rheumatic fever attack. When bacteremia occurs the altered valvular tissue provides an ideal location for attachment and growth of bacteria. All at-risk patients should be identified and the use of antibiotic prophylaxis before dental procedures followed (Fig. 1-2). Medical consultation should be used to clarify or confirm the patient's current status and the need for antibiotic prophylaxis. Determining whether the patient may be susceptible to endocarditis can be extremely challenging for the dentist. A patient with a history of rheumatic fever has a 66% chance of residual heart damage. Consequently a patient with a single episode of rheumatic fever who needs emergency dental care must be assumed to have residual rheumatic heart disease unless the patient is very clear that the heart was not damaged or if his or her current status can be confirmed by a telephone consultation with the patient's physician. If the patient is not sure of his current status or the medical consultation does not substantiate the absence of a history of rheumatic heart disease, the patient should be given prophylactic antibiotics for the emergency dental procedure. If the patient does not have a physician he should be referred to an internist or cardiologist.

A patient who reports that she has a heart murmur but is not sure if it is functional or pathologic should be prophylaxed. However, as a matter of professional courtesy, consultation with her physician to confirm the patient's status is recommended. Patients needing complete dentures do not require complete antibiotic coverage during denture insertion. Patients with orthodontic appliances and those undergoing exfoliation of their deciduous teeth do not appear to need coverage. Children requiring endocarditis prophylaxis because of conditions such as congenital heart defects should not routinely be given antibiotics for initial or periodic dental work, including examination, radiographic, and fluoride treatment (Box 1-3).

Hypertensive Disease

It is estimated that 1.8 million adults in the United States develop hypertension each year. Hypertension is defined as an average systolic blood pressure on a single occasion of ≥140 mm Hg or a diastolic blood pressure of ≥90 mm Hg. Isolated systolic hypertension is seen mainly in older persons, whereas systolic and diastolic hypertension are more common in men under age 55, African Americans of all ages, women over 55, and persons from lower socioeconomic groups. It is estimated that 95% to 99% of hypertensives do not have an identifiable etiology for their hypertension. Their problem has, therefore, been designated essential hypertension. The patient with essential hypertension has an increase in peripheral arterial resistance, either as a result of inappropriate renal retention of salt and water or increased endogenous pressor activity. The major complication of untreated hypertension is trauma to

1. **Standard general prophylaxis for patients at risk:**
   Amoxicillin: Adults, 2.0 g (Children, 50 mg/kg) given orally 1 hour before procedure.
2. **Unable to take oral medications:**
   Ampicillin: Adults, 2.0 g (Children, 50 mg/kg) given IM or IV within 30 minutes before procedure.
3. **Amoxicillin/Ampicillin/Penicillin – Allergic patients:**
   Clindamycin: Adults, 600 mg (Children, 20 mg/kg) given orally 1 hour before procedure.
   OR
   Cephalexin or cefadroxil: Adults, 20 gm (Children, 50 mg/kg) orally 1 hour before procedure.
   OR
   Azithromycin or clarithromycin: Adults, 500 mg (Children, 15 mg/kg) orally 1 hour before procedure.
4. **Amoxicillin/Ampicillin/Penicillin – Allergic patients unable to take oral medications:**
   Within 30 minutes before the procedure.
   OR
   Cefazolin: Adults, 1.0 g (Children, 25 mg/kg) IM or IV 30 minutes before procedure.

FIG. 1-2 Antibiotic regimen for prophylaxis against bacterial endocarditis.

Dental Procedures and Endocarditis Prophylaxis

ENDOCARDITIS PROPHYLAXIS RECOMMENDED

Dental extractions
Periodontal procedures including surgery, scaling and root planning, probing and recall maintenance
Dental implant placement and reimplantation of avulsed teeth
Endodontic (root canal) instrumentation or surgery only beyond the apex
Subgingival placement of antibiotic fibers or strips
Initial placement of orthodontic band but not brackets
Intraligamentary local anesthetic injections
Prophylactic cleaning of teeth or implants where bleeding is anticipated

ENDOCARDITIS PROPHYLAXIS NOT RECOMMENDED

Restorative dentistry* (operative and prosthodontic) with or without retraction cord†
Local anesthetic injections (nonintraligamentary)
Intracanal endodontic treatment, post placement and buildup
Placement of rubber dams
Postoperative suture removal
Placement of removable prosthodontics or orthodontic appliances
Taking of oral impressions
Fluoride treatments
Taking of oral radiographs
Orthodontic appliance adjustment
Shedding of primary teeth

*This includes restoration of decayed teeth (filling cavities) and replacement of missing teeth.
†Clinical judgement may indicate antibiotic use in selected circumstances that may create significant bleeding.

the vessels in the arterial circulation, leading to accelerated atherosclerosis in large vessels and obliterative changes or thinning and rupture in small vessels. These changes in turn increases the workload of the heart, leading to congestive heart failure and/or angina pectoris. About 1.5% of hypertensives develop an accelerated malignant course characterized by severe blood pressure elevation, papilledema, retinal hemorrhages, exudates, and frequently encephalopathy.[5]

It is important to identify the patient with severe, undiagnosed, or uncontrolled hypertensive disease before starting dental treatment because the stress and anxiety associated with dental procedures may raise the patient's already elevated blood pressure to dangerous levels and may result in a cerebrovascular accident or myocardial infarction. Local anesthesia and gingival retraction cords may contain strong vasopressors that can cause significant increase in blood pressure. From the medical history the dentist should be able to identify the hypertensive patient, ask about current medications, and measure the blood pressure prior to treatment.

Hypertensive patients should be treated in an anxiety-free atmosphere. The dentist should familiarize himself with the side effects and interactions of antihypertensive medications, so that he may be able to use medications that will not interact with the patient's medications. Medications such as diazepam, barbiturates, nitrous oxide/oxygen, fentanyl, and midazolam may be used to reduce anxiety in offices where trained personnel and proper monitoring equipment are available. Office appointments in the morning and short treatment times are beneficial.

The potential danger in administering epinephrine or other vasconstrictors to a patient with hypertension is an untoward increase in the blood pressure from a large quantity of vasoconstrictor injected over a short period of time. The adrenal medulla of a 155-pound adult produces epinephrine at the rate of 0.014 mg per minute. This is approximately equal to the amount of epinephrine contained in one carpule of local anesthetic containing epinephrine 1:100,000. If an individual is stressed from pain and anxiety, the endogeneous production of epinephrine can greatly increase, far in excess of the typical small amounts of exogenously administered epinephrine during dental treatment. Therefore, it becomes clear that the safety and advantages of administering small amounts of epinephrine during dental treatment far outweigh any perceived or potential dangers or disadvantages. Judicious use of local anesthesia with epinephrine in patients on antihypertensives such as adrenergic blockers and monoamine oxidase inhibitors (MAOIs) can be safely recommended. However, phenylephrine should be avoided in patients taking MAOIs, and gingival packing materials with a vasopressor should not be used. Central nervous system depressants like barbiturates, narcotics, and antianxiety drugs should not be given to patients who are taking MAOIs. If it has been at least 2 weeks since a patient has taken an MAOI, the central nervous system depressants can be used. Before using intravenous sedation or general anesthesia, the specific antihypertensive drugs that the patient is taking should be looked up, significant side effects and drug interactions noted, and appropriate action taken, which may include consultation with the patient's physician. Many antihypertensive agents have a tendency to produce nausea and vomiting. Excessive stimulation of the gag reflex during dental treatment in patients taking these drugs may bring on nausea and vomiting and should be avoided. No elective dental procedures should be performed for the patient who has severe uncontrolled hypertension.[6]

Side effects are sometimes seen in patients receiving hypertensive medications. Patients who are receiving diuretics may complain of dry mouth, which may cause oral lesions on an allergic or toxic basis. Facial and oral paresthesia have been reported in patients who take acetazolamide. Lichenoid reactions have been reported with thiazide, methyldopa, propranalol, and labetalol. Lupus-like reactions are only rarely seen with hydralazine. Patients under good medical management can receive any needed emergency dental treatment. Patients who have severe uncontrolled hypertension should receive only conservative treatment, such as antibiotics for infection and analgesics for pain. Surgical procedures should be avoided in these patients. Hypertensive patients should not be given more than 5.4 ml (3 cartridges) of local anesthesia that contains a more than 1:1,000,000 concentration of epinephrine.

Ischemic Heart Disease

Angina Pectoris. Chest pain is one of the most frequent complaints of patients in an ambulatory practice. Ischemic heart disease caused by atherosclerosis is one of the most prevalent ailments in the western world. In the United States it remains the leading nontraumatic cause of disability and death, even though, because of increased public awareness and health education, the mortality from ischemic heart disease has declined over 20% in the last 25 years. However, it is the leading cause of death in American women, ahead of death from cancer.[6]

Normally, the myocardium produces most of its energy by means of aerobic metabolism. When totally deprived of oxygen the heart stops beating within a few minutes. Oxygen supply is dependent on the oxygen content of the blood and on the volume of blood flowing through the coronary arteries. Coronary vascular resistance is determined by the degree of collateralization and the patency of the coronary blood vessels; when the vessels are narrowed by spasm or by an atherosclerotic plaque, coronary resistance increases and oxygen demands may not be satisfied. If the myocardium receives insufficient oxygen to satisfy its metabolic demands, the resultant ischemia usually results in pain, arrhythmia, or left ventricular dysfunction. Transient myocardial ischemia causes transient chest pain, angina pectoris; prolonged ischemia causes more prolonged chest pain, most commonly because of myocardial infarction.

The discomfort of myocardial ischemia is described as squeezing, crushing, burning, or smothering, whereas others describe it as a shortness of breath or simply a feeling of heaviness. Typically the discomfort is midline and substernal; it often radiates to the shoulder, arm, hand, or fingers, usually to the left. Radiation down the inside of the arm into the fingers supplied by the ulnar nerve is classic, and pain may radiate also into the neck, the lower jaw, or the intrascapular region. The atypical pain may be such that the patient may actually consult a dentist because of pain in the lower jaw that is caused by myocardial ischemia but is ascribed to a toothache. The single most important diagnostic feature of the discomfort of myocardial ischemia is its often predictable relationship to exertion, to emotional stress, or to other situations that may either increase myocardial oxygen demand or decrease myocardial oxygen supply. Pain that is experienced at rest, as a result of cardiac ischemia, suggests unstable angina, variant angina, or myocardial infarction. Anxiety is an important provoking factor in many patients. Angina is more likely to occur during cold or windy weather because of increased peripheral vascular resistance, or perhaps because of cold-activated reflexes that produce a decrease in coronary flow. Nocturnal angina may be a consequence of left ventricular failure or may represent unstable angina. Increase in carboxyhemoglobin level that may occur with cigarette smoking or heavy vehicular traffic can be a cause of angina in some persons.

Because angina is due to the result of a discrepancy between oxygen supply and demand, relief of pain is achieved by increasing coronary blood flow or by decreasing oxygen demand. Cessation of effort or relief of anxiety decreases oxygen demand and angina begins to disappear within minutes. Nitroglycerin relieves the chest pain of esophageal spasm, which often presents with similar clinical symptoms as seen in angina patients. For a list by brand name and class of drugs used in the treatment of angina, see Table 1-1.

Dental Management. Patients who have the stable form of angina without a history of infarction generally have a much lower risk of complications while in the dental office than patients who have unstable angina or a history of a recent myocardial infarction. Patients who have had a recent MI should not receive any routine dental care until 6 months after the infarction. This is based on statistical evidence that the risk of reinfarction after an MI drops as low as it will be by about 6 months, particularly if the patient is properly supervised medically. Even after 6 months the dentist should consult with the patient's physician before beginning dental treatment.

The dental management plan that is developed for the patient with a history of MI should include the patient's current status in regard to presence of congestive heart failure, hypertension, and angina, and medications the patient is taking. Patients with a history of coronary atherosclerotic heart disease should be given short morning appointments and may be premedicated with 5 to 10 mg of diazepam before the appointment to reduce anxiety. Nitrous oxide analgesia can be used as

TABLE 1-1 Common Drugs used in the Treatment of Angina

Class	Brand Name
NITRATES	
Nitroglycerin (Sublingual)	Nitrostat
Topical ointment	Nitro-Bid, Nitrol
Patch	Transderm Nitro, Nitro-Dur Nitrodisc
LONG ACTIVE	
Erythritol tetranitrate	Cordilate
Isosorbide dinitrate	Isordil, Sorbitrate
Isosorbate mononitrate	ISMO
ß-ADRENERGIC BLOCKERS	
Propranolol	Inderal
Nadolol	Corgard
Tenormin	Atenolol
Metoprolol	Lopressor
CALCIUM CHANNEL BLOCKERS	
Nifedipine	Procardia
Verapamil	Calan, Isoptin
Diltiazem	Cardiazem
Nicardipine	Cardene
Amlodipine	Norvasc

long as hypoxia is avoided. An effective local anesthetic is a must for these patients. Epinephrine in the concentration of 1:100,000 can be used safely, even if the patient has hypertensive disease. Patients with poorly controlled ischemic heart disease, with labile cardiac rhythms, or with potentially life-threatening arrhythmias should not be given a local anesthetic with vasoconstrictor. These patients should be given 3% mepivacaine or 4% prilocaine. Usually no more than three cartridges of anesthetic with epinephrine should be given per appointment. Vasopressors should not be used to control local bleeding or used in gingival packing material. If the patient is receiving warfarin, it should be discontinued 2 days prior to surgery but only under the advice of the treating physician and restarted before discharge. In an ambulatory or office setting, blood should be drawn the morning of the procedure to check the prothrombin time, to make certain that it is from 1.2 to 2 times normal. For patients taking aspirin, there is little risk of bleeding at low dose (81 mg); however, at higher doses it may be prudent to check the bleeding time. Patients who are receiving antihypertensive agents or digitalis may be prone to nausea and vomiting, thus excessive stimulation of the gag reflex should be avoided. Antisialagogues should not be used in patients with coronary atherosclerotic heart disease unless the patient's physician has been consulted, because the agents tend to cause tachycardia. Antiarrhythmic agents such as quinidine and procainamide may cause nausea and vomiting.

If at any time during the dental appointment a patient with coronary atherosclerotic heart disease becomes fatigued or develops a significant change in pulse rate or rhythm, the appointment should be terminated. Patients who have angina pectoris should bring their nitroglycerin medication with them to every dental appointment. Prophylactic nitroglycerin may be considered for patients who have frequent attacks. If pain develops during the dental appointment in a patient with a history of stable angina, all work should be stopped and the patient should take a nitroglycerin tablet and be allowed to relax, and the blood pressure, pulse rate, and rhythm determined. If the patient is stable but still having pain, then another nitroglycerin tablet should be taken. If the pain persists after 2 to 3 minutes, give another tablet to the patient to a maximum of three nitroglycerin tablets in a 15-minute period. If the patient is stable, the dentist can continue with the dental treatment or reschedule the appointment. If however the patient's vital signs are not stable, the patient should be immediately transferred to the nearest emergency facility.

If emergency dental treatment is required during the 6-month period after an infarction, the patient should be treated in a conservative manner, with pain relief the primary objective. The patient's physician must be consulted and the planned dental approach discussed in detail before any treatment is rendered. Strong analgesics should be used for pain control and antibiotics for infections. Sedative pulpal medications should be considered instead of extractions or endodontic therapy. The same approach is used in patients with unstable angina.

Coronary Artery Bypass Surgery

This surgery is one of the most common surgical procedures performed in this country today. It is accepted generally that patients with incapacitating angina pectoris who have good left ventricular function and who have failed maximal medical therapy should be considered as candidates for coronary arteriography and subsequent surgery. Patients who have had coronary artery bypass surgery are treated in a manner similar to post-MI patients. Before elective surgery is performed 6 months should have elapsed. The patient's physician should be consulted if dental surgery is necessary prior to 6 months. These patients should be managed with the physician's input, because they usually have a history of angina, MI, or both.

Percutaneous Transluminal Coronary Angioplasty (PICA)

This procedure is an important option for the treatment of coronary artery disease that cannot be controlled by the administration of drugs. The coronary orifice is reached with a preshaped guiding catheter through which the balloon catheter with the balloon decompressed is inserted. After successful angioplasty patients are maintained on aspirin. The major limitation of PICA is restenosis, which occurs in 30% to 50% of patients within the first 6 months. After PICA, it is advisable to have patients undergo a stress test within a few weeks. The results are useful in gauging the patient's ability to return to work and whether dental surgery can proceed soon thereafter, usually with the same precautions as those for patients with angina.

Cerebrovascular Disease

Stroke is a major cause of disability and the third leading cause of death in the United States. There are 3 million stroke survivors in this country. About 80% of strokes are caused by thrombotic or embolic cerebral infarction, 12% to cerebral hemorrhage. Seventy-five percent of strokes occur in individuals who are 65 or older. Predisposing factors are history of transient ischemic attacks (TIAs), hypertension, certain cardiac disorders, cigarette smoking, diabetes mellitus, and hyperlipidemia. Patients are usually prescribed the antiplatelet drugs aspirin, and ticlopidine.[4]

If a stroke patient requires dental surgery, it is best to wait until 6 months have passed and any hypertensive tendencies have been controlled. At that time, the patient should be treated following a nonpharmacologic anxiety-reduction protocol, receive supplemental oxygen, and have vital signs carefully monitored during surgery. If pharmacologic sedation is necessary, low concentration of nitrous oxide can be used.

Heart Failure

The amount of blood that the heart pumps per minute is normally precisely adjusted to the metabolic needs of the body. The cardiac output may increase by two or three times as an individual goes from sleep to exercise. The increased cardiac output soon brings about an increase in the amount of blood returning to the right side of the heart; also the heart further increases it output in response to the stretch in the heart muscle that results from the increased volume of venous return. If the heart is unable to pump enough blood to meet the metabolic needs of the body, compensatory mechanisms are brought into play by the heart, kidney, lung, peripheral vascular system, and by neurohormonal responses. These adjustments cause symptoms and signs recognized as the syndrome of heart failure. Symptoms of congestive heart failure include orthopnea, paroxysmal nocturnal dyspnea, and pedal edema. Orthopnea is a respiratory disorder manifest as shortness of breath when a patient is in supine position; it usually occurs as a result of the mobilization of blood pooled in the lower extremities. The heart's ability to handle the increased cardiac preload is overwhelmed, and the blood backs up in the pulmonary circulation, producing pulmonary edema. Patients with orthopnea usually must sleep with their upper body supported on several pillows. Paroxysmal nocturnal dyspnea is a symptom of congestive heart failure similar to orthopnea. The patient has respiratory difficulty 1 to 2 hours after assuming a supine position. The disorder occurs when pooled blood and interstitial fluid is reabsorbed into the vasculature from the legs, overwhelming the heart and producing pulmonary edema. Patients suddenly wake, feeling short of breath and frequently desiring to open a window to breathe cool air.

Fatigue is a common complaint of patients in heart failure. It is frequently described as a general sense of weakness or of lassitude. A history of edema and/or weight gain from retention of salt and water is often elicited from patients in heart failure. Many will also give a history of having taken digitalis, a diuretic, or a converting enzyme inhibitor in the past for a heart problem. Chest pain caused by myocardial ischemia is common in patients in heart failure. Nocturia, a common symptom of heart failure, often occurs early in the illness. It is a result of the redistribution in cardiac output that occurs in the recumbent position. Decreased cardiac output by itself or in association with cerebrovascular disease may lead to impairment in mental function, ranging from mild confusion to overt psychosis. Gastrointestinal systems such as constipation are common in patients with chronic, poorly compensated heart failure.

Patients with congestive heart failure that is well compensated through dietary and drug therapy can safely undergo ambulatory surgery. Supplemental oxygen and anxiety-reduction methods are helpful. Patients with orthopnea must be kept in an upright position during any procedure. Surgery for patients with uncompensated hypertrophic cardiomyopathy is best deferred until compensation is achieved or procedures can be performed in the hospital setting. Dental emergencies in the patient who has untreated congestive heart failure should be dealt with in as conservative a manner as possible. Appropriate analgesic agents for pain control or antibiotics for infection should be given after consultation with the patient's physician.

Arrhythmias

Patients with arrhythmias before dental surgery have significantly increased risks of cardiac morbidity and death. Patients with complete heart block, Mobitz type II second degree block, and a few patients with sick sinus syndrome have a significant risk of complications during anesthesia if a pacemaker is not inserted. On the other hand little or no increased risk is associated with bi- or trifascicular block on ECG in patients who are asymptomatic. Patients with arrhythmia should have the probable etiology delineated. If the arrhythmia is intermittent or control is not certain, 24-hour Holter monitoring should be done. Drug levels of antiarrhythmic drugs that are being administered should be obtained. In general these patients should be referred to an oral surgeon or to a general dentistry program that is hospital-based so the patient can be treated in the hospital. In the hospital setting appropriate consultation can be obtained to optimize the patient prior to dental treatment, which may be performed totally in one setting. Antiarrhythmic drugs should be continued orally through the morning before surgery, after which the following intravenous treatment should be substituted until the patient is able to take oral medications again: intravenous digoxin (75% of oral dose) for patients taking digoxin and intravenous lidocaine or procainamide for patients taking quinidine or disopyramide for ventricular arrhythmias. Limit epinephrine to 0.04 mg. Adjust anticoagulant therapy based on specialist's recommendation. Pacemakers pose no contraindications to dental surgery and no antibiotic prophylaxis is required, but electrical equipment such as electric cautery should not be used.

Pulmonary Problems

Chronic Obstructive Pulmonary Disease (COPD). COPD is a disorder characterized by abnormal tests in expiratory flow that do not change markedly over periods of several months' observation. Specific causes of airflow obstruction such as localized disease of the upper airways, bronchiectasis, and cystic fibrosis are excluded. Bronchial hyperactivity may be present with COPD as measured by an improvement in airflow following the inhalation of beta adrenergic agents or worsening after inhalation of methacholine or histamine. COPD may further be subclassified into emphysema and chronic bronchitis. Emphysema is defined by morphologic criteria as abnormal dilation of the terminal airspaces of the lung with destruction of alveolar septa in the absence of interstitial fibrosis. Chronic bronchitis is a condition of chronic cough and sputum production that excludes other specific disorders such as bronchiectasis, cystic fibrosis, or tuberculosis.

COPD is a chronic disease that has its origins in early adulthood or possibly even childhood, but does not produce symptoms or impairment of activity until it is far advanced, usually in late middle age or in the elderly. The normal aging process causes slowly progressive degeneration of lung function after young adulthood, so a normal person loses about 25% of FEV (forced expiratory volume), between the ages of 25 and 75. These changes are the result of loss of elastic recoil in the lung from the degradation of elastin fibers, similar to the changes that occur in the skin that cause wrinkles. Cigarette smoking is a major risk factor for development of COPD. The mechanism by which cigarettes lead to COPD is thought to be mediated by proinflammatory components of cigarette smoke such as the hydrocarbon compound acrolein. Neutrophils destroy the elastin elements in the alveolar walls, and that induces emphysema. Patients with COPD become dyspneic frequently during mild to moderate exertion; they have chronic cough producing large amounts of thick secretions, frequent respiratory tract infections, and barrel shaped chests; and they may purse their lips to breathe and have audible wheezing during breathing. The components of care in COPD consist of education about the disease, prevention of disease progression, treatment of complications, drug treatment to maximize lung function, and rehabilitation to optimize activity levels. Complications of COPD include tracheobronchial infections, chronic hypoxemia, pulmonary hypertension, cor pulmonale, supraventricular tachyarrythmias, hypercapnia, and malnutrition[5].

Bronchodilator and antiinflammatory agents are used in COPD to reverse bronchospasm and to prevent bronchconstriction in response to provocative agents. The recommended stepped treatment approach is to start with anticholinergic agents (ipratropium bromide), then beta adrenergic agents (albuterol, metaproterenol, isoetharine), followed by theophylline and corticosteroids.

The dentist should place the patient in an upright position for treatment, to avoid orthopnea and respiratory discomfort. There is no contraindication to the usual usage of local anesthetics; however, bilateral mandibular blocks or bilateral palatal blocks are not recommended because of a possible unpleasant choking sensation or difficulty swallowing. With COPD the use of a rubber dam is not advisable, because this may result in a feeling of compromised air supply. A low flow of oxygen during dental procedures may be helpful. If sedative medication is required, the preferred approach is nitrous oxide/oxygen inhalation sedation, because respiration is not depressed with nitrous oxide nor is it a pulmonary irritant. Low dose oral diazepam may also be used. Narcotics and barbiturates are to be avoided because of their respiratory depressant properties. Anticholinergics and antihistamines are contraindicated because of their drying properties and the resultant increase in mucous tenacity. Patients who are taking corticosteroids may require supplemental dosing because of adrenal suppression. Outpatient general anesthesia is contraindicated in patients with COPD.

Asthma. This is a disorder characterized symptomatically by cough, chest tightness, shortness of breath, and wheezing associated with limitation of airflow. The symptoms may be acute and episodic, or may wax and wane over long periods of time. One or more of the symptoms may be dominant, but usually all are present. Between episodes, most asthmatics are symptom-free, but they are susceptible to attacks of wheezing, cough, and chest tightness when exposed to various triggers.

About one in 20 residents of the United States has asthma, and it is even more common in other developing countries. About half of the asthmatics in the United States have onset of the disease during childhood, and about half will have spontaneous resolution of the disease by young adulthood.

The goal of management for asthmatic dental patients must be to prevent an acute asthmatic attack. The patient should be questioned about the type of asthma (allergic versus nonallergic), precipitating substances, frequency and severity of attacks, how attacks are usually managed, and whether it has ever been necessary to receive emergency treatment of an acute attack. For a severe asthmatic, consultation with the patient's physician is advised. The patient should be instructed to bring his inhaler to every appointment. The inhalation of selective beta2 agonist is the preferred treatment for an acute asthmatic attack. Some patients may require theophylline, corticosteroid, cromolyn sodium, or sympathomimetic amines such as epinephrine or metaproterenol.

Because aspirin ingestion is associated with precipitating a small percentage of asthmatic attacks, it is advisable not to administer aspirin-containing medication or other NSAIDs to patients with asthma. Acetaminophen can safely be used for mild to moderate pain. Barbiturates and narcotics should not be administered because of the potential of precipitating an attack. Patients taking theophylline preparations should not be given erythromycin because this may result in an increased blood level of theophylline. Asthmatics who are chronically medicated with corticosteroids may require supplementation for dental procedures. Efforts should be made to make the patient's appointment stress-free. Preoperative and intraoperative sedation may also be desirable. Nitrous oxide/oxygen sedation can be used because nitrous oxide is not a respiratory depressant or irritant. Small oral doses of diazepam can be used. If general anesthesia is required it should be performed in the hospital setting.

Renal Disease

Renal insufficiency, presenting either as a primary renal event or complicating another illness is a common clinical problem. The healthy kidney performs a wide variety of functions that contribute to the maintenance of the internal environment of the body. In addition to its role in maintaining the balance of water and electrolytes, the kidney has important endocrine and metabolic functions. It produces hormones responsible for normal bone formation (1,25-dihydroxyvitamin D3), red blood cell production (erythropoietin), and blood pressure control (renin, prostaglandins). The kidney is responsible for degrading a number of polypeptide hormones, including parathyroid hormone, insulin, gastrin, and prolactin. Also the kidney serves as a major excretory route for many toxic wastes and a wide variety of drugs or their breakdown products.

There are currently over 160,000 patients on dialysis in the United States and many more living with successful kidney transplants. Kidney diseases are often classified according to whether they produce acute or chronic renal failure. Acute renal failure is defined as a deterioration of glomerular filtration that occurs over days or weeks, whereas the course of chronic renal failure often runs from months to years. The course of chronic kidney disease is often characterized by the progressive loss of functioning nephrons. Usually signs and symptoms do not appear until 80% of the original number of nephrons have been lost.

Patients with renal insufficiency requiring periodic dialysis need special consideration during oral surgical care. Chronic dialysis treatment requires the presence of an arteriovenous shunt, which allows easy vascular access, and heparin administration, allowing blood to move through the dialysis equipment without clotting. Patients with shunts should be given prophylactic antibiotics during oral surgery to prevent infection of the shunt. The shunt should not be used by the dentist for venous access, except in an emergency.

Elective oral surgery is best undertaken the day after a dialysis treatment has been performed. This allows the heparin used during dialysis to disappear and the patient to be in the best physiologic state with respect to intravascular volume and metabolic by-products. Drugs that depend on renal metabolism or excretion should be avoided or used in modified doses to prevent systemic toxicity. Relatively nephrotoxic drugs such as NSAIDs also should be avoided in patients with compromised kidneys. Drugs dependent on renal excretion or removed during dialysis will need special dosing regimens. Because of the higher incidence of hepatitis in renal dialysis patients, the treating dentist should take the necessary precautions. In addition, the altered appearance of the bone caused by secondary hyperparathyroidism in patients with renal failure should be noted. Metabolic radiolucencies should not be mistaken for dental disease.

Diseases of the Liver

Hepatitis is an inflammatory condition that may be localized in the liver or may be part of a generalized systemic disease. Acute hepatitis is usually a self-limited disease. The principal causes of acute hepatitis are viruses, drugs, and alcohol. Chronic hepatitis refers to unresolved hepatitis that has persisted for a period longer than 6 months. Cirrhosis is often the principal consequence of chronic hepatitis. Viral hepatitis is a systemic infection whose principal manifestations are hepatic. The six types of viral hepatitis that are well-defined separate entities are designated types A, B, C, D, E, and F.

The production of vitamin K-dependent coagulation factors (II, VII, IX, X) may be depressed in severe liver disease; therefore, obtaining a prothrombin time (PT) or partial thromboplastin time (PTT) may be useful before surgery. Portal hypertension caused by liver disease also may cause hypersplenism, a sequestering of platelets causing thrombocytopenia. This problem is revealed by finding a prolonged bleeding time. Patients with severe liver dysfunction may require hospitalization during dental surgery because of their decreased ability to metabolize the nitrogen in swallowed blood which may cause encephalopathy after dental surgery.

Routine dental care should not be performed for a patient with active hepatitis. For patients with a history of hepatitis, adopt a strict aseptic technique. It is recommended that protective attire and barrier techniques be used by dentist and staff. Proper hand washing, proper use and care of sharp instruments and needles, and the sterilization of instruments and equipment should be as outlined by the U.S. Public Health Service's Centers for Disease Control.

Diabetes Mellitus

Diabetes mellitus is a condition that is characterized by an abnormality of glucose utilization and associated with elevation of blood glucose concentration. The commonest varieties of diabetes mellitus are known to be associated with abnormalities of insulin secretion and concentration, with cellular resistance to insulin action, and with vascular abnormalities such as basement membrane thickening. The diagnosis is based on the finding of persistently abnormal blood glucose concentrations at some time in life. Non–insulin-dependent diabetes mellitus is the commonest form and accounts for about 80% to 90% of patients presenting with an abnormality of glucose metabolism. Pa-

tients with NIDDM are neither absolutely dependent on treatment with insulin nor ketosis-prone. There is a familial pattern of expression in NIDDM.

Insulin-dependent diabetes mellitus accounts for 10% to 12% of cases, and generally has its onset in childhood, often near puberty. The essential characteristic is that insulin dependence is absolute; without insulin therapy, ketosis–acidosis ensues rapidly. Recent studies have focused on IDDM as an autoimmune disease.

Most diagnoses of diabetes mellitus are now made at an asymptomatic stage of the disease as a result of routine blood tests that reveal elevation of blood glucose concentration. Glucose tolerance tests may identify many patients who are symptomatic at the time of diagnosis; most will complain of increased frequency of urination (polyuria), excessive thirst with increased fluid intake (polydipsia), and, if the disease is very severe, increased appetite and increased food consumption (polyphagia) associated with weight loss. All of these symptoms are manifestations of excessive blood sugar and of secondary glucosuria. Other symptomatic manifestations include blurred vision, vaginitis, and skin infections. Some patients present with minimal symptoms resulting from hyperglycemia and glycosuria but have already developed complications of the diabetic state such as neuropathy or vascular disease.

Elevation of blood sugar concentration is the hallmark of diabetes mellitus. Glucosuria alone is not a diagnostic finding, because rare individuals may have a renal tubular glucose leak at normal concentrations of blood sugar. The criteria for diagnosis have been suggested as follows:

1. unequivocal elevation of plasma glucose concentrations associated with classic symptoms of diabetes mellitus, or
2. elevation of fasting plasma glucose on more than one occasion, or
3. elevation of plasma glucose following an oral glucose challenge on more than one occasion.

The patient with diabetes is usually identified in the dental office through the history, and the type of medical treatment they are receiving is established. The type of diabetes should be determined and the presence of complications noted. Patients being treated with insulin should be asked how much insulin they use and how often they inject themselves daily. The patient should be asked of visits to his physician and whether the patient checks his urine for glucose. This information will help assess the severity and control of the diabetes.

Patients with NIDDM who have no evidence of complications and have their disease under good medical control will require little or no special attention when receiving dental treatment, unless they should develop an acute dental or oral infection. Patients with complications such as renal and cardiovascular disease may need to be managed in special ways. Patients receiving insulin and not under good medical management should be referred to their physician for evaluation.

Patients who have not seen their physician for a long time or who have recurrent episodes of insulin shock or whose diabetes is out of control should be optimized by their physician prior to dental surgery.

Short term mild to moderate hyperglycemia usually is not a significant problem for people with diabetes. Therefore when a dentoalveolar procedure is planned, it is best to err on the side of hyperglycemia rather than hypoglycemia. The procedure should be planned early in the day. If intravenous sedation is not being used, the patient should be asked to eat a normal meal and take the usual morning amount of regular insulin and half his dose of NPH insulin. The patient's vital signs should be monitored, and if signs of hypoglycemia occur, such as hypotension, hunger, drowsiness, nausea, diaphoresis, tachycardia, or a mood change, an oral or intravenous supply of glucose should be administered. If the patient will not be able to eat after the surgery, the morning dose of NPH should not be taken before surgery, but can be started when the patient goes back to regular meals. The patient's urine or blood glucose should be monitored the day after surgery.

If the patient will miss the morning meal he should not take any insulin that morning, because insulin can be given after venous access in the office or hospital, where usually one half of the insulin dose and no NPH is given. Following the procedure but before the patient returns to his regular diet, his insulin regimen should be based on the serum glucose levels.

Infection in the diabetic patient is more difficult to control than in people without diabetes. This is caused by altered leukocyte function, as well as by other factors that affect the body's ability to control an infection. Difficulty in containing infections is more significant in people with poorly controlled diabetes. In emergency situations involving diabetic patients with serious infections, hospitalization should be considered where-appropriate doses of intravenous antibiotics can be given and aggressive surgical management of the infection performed. Antibiotics may need to be given to most diabetic patients when dentoalveolar surgery is performed.

Thyroid Disease

Disturbance of thyroid growth and function is a very common endocrine problem. Excessive production of the iodine-containing thyroid hormones thyroxine (T4) and triiodothyronine (T3) results in hyperthyroidism or thyrotoxicosis; decreased hormone production results in hypothyroidism. Generalized enlargement of the thyroid regardless of cause is termed goiter. Focal enlargement of the thyroid is termed a nodule and is usually benign. Either goiter or focal enlargement may be associated with abnormal thyroid function. Goiter can produce anatomical changes ranging from simply cosmetic to obstruction of contiguous structures such as the trachea and esophagus.

The thyroid secretes thyroxine, triiodothyronine, and calcitonin. Calcitonin is secreted by the perifollicular cells. T4 and T3 are controlled by the hypothalamus and pituitary gland by a classic negative feedback mechanism. As the serum levels of the hormones decrease, the anterior pituitary gland releases a thyroid-stimulating hormone (TSH) that stimulates the secretion of T4 and T3 by the thyroid gland. Under normal conditions 10% to 20% of the circulating pool of T3 comes from the thyroid gland, and the rest of the circulating T3 comes from the monodeiodination of T4. In cases of hyperthyroidism 30% to 40% of circulating T3 comes from the thyroid. Fasting, illness, steroids, and certain drugs can inhibit the conversion of T4 to T3. Iodine is needed for the synthesis of T3 and T4; the minimum daily requirement is 75 mg. In circulation T3 and T4 are bound to plasma proteins. Calcitonin is involved along with parathyroid hormone and vitamin D in regulating serum calcium and phosphorus levels as well as skeletal remolding.[4]

The anterior neck should be examined for evidence of thyroid surgery, the tongue for lingual thyroid tissue, and the area of the thyroid cartilage for the presence of a pyramidal lobe. The thyroid gland has a rubbery consistency on palpation and moves in the midline as the patient swallows. A hyperplastic gland (goiter) feels soft, whereas adenomas and tumors feel firmer, as in patients with Hashimoto disease or Riedel thyroiditis. The term thyrotoxicosis refers to an excess of T3 and T4 in circulation either as a result of ectopic thyroid tissue, Graves disease, multinodular goiter, thyroid adenoma, or pituitary disease. The patient with Graves disease has an excess of thyroid hormones; the patient's skin is warm and moist, with a rosy complexion that blushes readily. Palmar erythema may be present, profuse sweating is common, and excessive melanin pigmentation of the skin occurs. The nails are soft and friable, the hair fine, and the eyes proptotic. There may be retrusion of the upper lid, lid lag, a bright-eyed stare, and jerky movement of the lids. Patients may develop optic neuritis, corneal ulceration, and weakness of the eye muscles. Cardiac manifestations include increased stroke volume and heart rate, widenedpulse pressure, supraventricular cardiac dysrhythmias, and congestive heart failure. Even with an increased appetite, patients may complain of weight loss, and may be emotionally labile. Patients with untreated or poorly managed hyperthyroidism may develop a thyrotoxic crisis in the office, which is a medical emergency. To treat this, the dentist should notify the emergency system, cool the patient with cold towels, administer hydrocortisone (100 to 300 mg), start an IV of D5W, and monitor the vital signs. Do not administer epinephrine or other pressor amines to patients with Graves disease unless the patient is euthyroid from a medical standpoint.

Hypothyroidism can be congenital or acquired. Cretinism refers to congenital hypothyroidism and myxedema to acquired hypothyroidism. The congenital form may present with thyroid dysgenesis or thyroid agenesis. The acquired form results from thyroid or pituitary gland failure. Surgical removal, radiation treatment, or drug therapy may cause hypothyroidism. Cretinism is characterized by dwarfism, overweight, broad flat nose, eyes set wide apart, thick lips, large protruding tongue, poor muscle tone, pale skin, stubby hands, retarded bone age, delayed eruption of teeth, umbilical hernia, malocclusion, and mental retardation. If the onset of the disease occurred in older children and adults, they may present with puffy eyes, hair loss, dry rough skin, decreased mental and physical activity, inability to handle cold weather, muscle weakness, and deafness. These patients are usually treated with synthetic thyroid preparations. Narcotics, tranquilizers, and barbiturates should be used with care in these patients. Myxedema coma is characterized by hypothermia, bradycardia, and hypotension.

The hypothyroid patient with mild symptoms can receive the usual treatment. However, when in doubt, contact the patient's physician prior to dental treatments.

Adrenal Insufficiency

This disease is now most commonly caused by autoimmune disease and is associated with the presence of antibodies to adrenal tissue; other cases are secondary to pituitary disease. Many cases of autoimmune adrenocortical insufficiency are associated with autoimmune thyroiditis. The simultaneous occurrence of autoimmune thyroid and adrenal disease is termed Schmidt syndrome. Rarely, autoimmune adrenocortical insufficiency, autoimmune hypothyroidism, and autoimmune gonadal failure occur in the syndrome of polyglandular failure. There is also an association of autoimmune adrenocortical insufficiency with pernicious anemia and Sjogren syndrome and probably with systemic lupus erythematosus. Other rare causes of adrenocortical insufficiency include histoplasmosis and sarcoidosis.

Chronic symptoms include anorexia, weight loss, weakness, and decreased physical endurance. Vomiting may occur with abdominal pain. Other symptoms include mental sluggishness, irritability, postural hypotension, or hypoglycemia. In primary adrenal insufficiency, increasing pigmentation (white patients) or a further darkening of the skin (African-American patients) may be noted. Loss of axillary and pubic hair may occur in women. Pigmentation of buccal mucous membrane in white patients is pathognomonic of the disease. Classically, hyponatremia associated with hyperkalemia and azotemia provide clues to the diagnosis.

It is probably prudent to consult the physician of the patient with adrenal insufficiency prior to dental treatment to discuss the management of the patient. Minor procedures require anxiety-reducing measures, whereas complicated procedures require supplemental steroid treatment.

Usually the patient's daily dosage of steroids is doubled prior to surgery or by administering 60 mg of hydrocortisone presurgically and decreasing the amount to 40 mg the first 2 days after surgery, 20 mg the next 3 days, and the usual dose thereafter. In case of acute adrenal crisis, administer 100 mg of hydrocortisone IV or IM and transport the patient to an emergency facility. When there is doubt about the patient's steroid usage it is better to overtreat than run the risk of an acute adrenal crisis. If the patient has taken more than 20 mg of hydrocortisone, over a 2 week period within the past 2 years, they should receive supplemental steroid therapy.

Headaches and Facial Pain

A significant number of patients, usually females, are referred for treatment of headache or facial pain. Usually the headaches are described as severe or disabling at times and unresponsive to over-the-counter remedies. These headaches are described as tension and migraine headaches; individual patients often suffer from both types of headache. Some patients with frequent tension headache respond to drugs used for migraine, and some with a typical migraine pattern respond to regimens recommended for tension headache. The most useful aspects of the history in determining etiology are the temporal profile, associated symptoms, and family history; the least specific aspects are the character and location of the pain, except in temporomandibular joint disease.

The term tension headaches applies to headaches that present as episodic headache or chronic daily headache. Some of these patients respond to simple over-the-counter analgesics. Patients with continuous daily headaches of many months or years duration usually have depression and/or anxiety states. These patients describe constant headaches that lack any localizing characteristics and are refractory to analgesics and to migraine prophylaxis with the exception of the antide-pressants. Nonpharmacologic therapy such as reassurance that it is not a brain tumor, massage of the scalp and neck muscles, and relaxation techniques usually help. Drugs including codeine sulfate, propoxyphene, and combination products of analgesics, sedatives, and caffeine (such as Fiorinal and Percodan) may help. Patients with migraine headaches usually respond to ergotamine tartrate, sumatriptan, or a nonsteroidal antiinflammatory drug. If the patient develops nausea and vomiting associated with the headache they can be treated with prochlorperazine suppositories (25 mg).

Bleeding Disorders

Most patients with inherited bleeding disorders will notify the dentist before treatment. However, patients who are not sure if a bleeding disorder exists should be questioned about duration of bleeding following minor trauma or surgical procedures. Frequent episodes of nose bleeds, easy bruising, hematuria, or heavy menstrual bleeding may indicate the need for coagulation screening. A test of the intrinsic and extrinsic pathways, PT, and PTT is usually sufficient initially. If the patient has a relative platelet inadequacy, a hematologist should be consulted. Patients with hemophilia A, B, C, or Von Willebrand disease should be given Amicar prior to any oral surgical procedure. Elective surgery should be planned with the hematologist's intervention, because she will be able to suggest the best time for surgical information and whether transfusion of platelets is necessary. Usually no elective procedure should be performed with a platelet count below 50,000. Even in cases above 50,000 but below 100,000, clot promoting substance (that is, Gelfoam, surgical) should be placed in the sockets and every attempt made not to dislodge blood clots.

Patients with prosthetic heart valves may be therapeutically anticoagulated and post-MI patients may be on aspirin and drugs with anticoagulation effects. When elective surgery is planned in these patients, their physician should be consulted. Usually the patient will have to be hospitalized, have warfarin replaced with IV heparin, and treated after a 2 to 3 day delay, then placed on coumadin postoperatively. PT values should be used to gauge the anticoagulant effect of warfarin. Another lab test currently in use to monitor anticoagulation therapy is the INR (International Normalized Ratio).

Seizure Disorder

A review of the health questionnaire will usually identify patients with a seizure disorder. The dentist should inquire about medications used to control the seizures, patient's compliance, and any recent measure of drug levels. If the patient is not able to answer these ques-

tions, the surgery should be postponed and the physician consulted. If the patient is well controlled, no special modifications are necessary. If the patient is not well controlled or if control cannot be attained, the patient should receive intravenous sedation in an ambulatory setting, either an oral surgeon's office or hospital.

Pregnancy

The pregnant patient is at risk of injuring the fetus, so no intervention that can cause genetic damage should be undertaken. Therefore, all elective procedures should be postponed until after delivery. If, however, surgery cannot be postponed, the patient's physician should be consulted prior to treatment. Proper shielding of the patient, including the neck, is a must during dental radiographic exam. Any drug that is prescribed should be discussed with the patient's physician. The patient should be seated in a nearly upright position or turned slightly to one side to prevent compression of the inferior vena cava. Nitrous oxide should not be used in the first trimester, but can be used in the second and third trimester with at least 50% oxygen. Lidocaine, bupivacaine, acetaminophen, codeine, penicillin, and erythromycin can be used in moderate amounts. In the postpartum phase, if the mother is breast-feeding avoid drugs that enter the milk, or ask the patient's physician for guidance; however, avoid corticosteroids, aminoglycosides, and tetracyclines.

Alcoholism

The disease alcoholism is defined as a recurring trouble associated with drinking alcohol. The trouble may occur in one or more of several domains, including interpersonal, educational, legal, financial, medical, or occupational. A predisposition to alcoholism appears to be inherited by at least half of alcoholic patients, and there is some evidence that inherited factors are associated with the inability to control use of alcohol. Alcoholism is the commonest psychosocial disorder in American men between the ages of 18 and 65 and the fourth most common in American women in the age range 18 to 24 years. The various deficiency states involved in a diet composed largely of nutritionally empty alcoholic calories (7 calories/g) as well as the direct toxic actions of alcohol itself, have been implicated in the pathogenesis of many of the medical consequences of alcoholism. Some of the common complications are gastritis, fatty liver, hepatitis or cirrhosis, pancreatitis, cerebellar ataxia, gout, peripheral neuropathy, hypoglycemia, hypokalemia, and hyponatremia.

The dental concerns when treating the alcoholic patient are that of bleeding tendencies and unpredictable metabolism of certain drugs. Unexplained gingival bleeding may be the initial complaint of the alcoholic patient. Oral findings also include glossitis, loss of tongue papillae along with angular or labial cheilosis, which is complicated by concomitant candidal infections. Vitamin C deficiency and hemostasis disorder may lead to spontaneous bleeding, mucosal ecchymosis, and petechiae. A bilateral hypertrophy of the parotid gland is common in patients with cirrhosis. If you must perform surgery on an alcoholic with compromised medical problems, it is best to consult with the patient's physician.

HIV

HIV is a member of the lentivirus subfamily of human retroviruses. These viruses code for an enzyme known as reverse transcriptase, which permits transcription of viral RNA into proviral DNA and subsequent integration into the host's cellular genome, leading to a persistent and latent infection. The retroviruses are associated with disease of long incubation period, involvement with hematopoietic and central nervous systems, and immune suppression. HIV occurs in highest concentrations in blood and semen. It also occurs in lower concentrations in cervical and vaginal secretions, saliva, tears, breast milk, and amniotic fluid. HIV transmission is most commonly through blood and semen, but vaginal secretions and breast milk have been implicated as well in transmission. The percentage of CD4 lymphocytes is the best indicator of disease progression and prognosis. Within a year of seroconversion, CD4 cell counts usually drop 200 to 300 per mm^3 from the normal range of between 800 and 1200. This decline then slows to 85 to 100 cells per year. Individuals with CD4 cell counts greater than 500 are usually asymptomatic and have virtually no risk of developing an AIDS-indicator condition, except for TB, cervical cancer, recurrent bacterial pneumonias, or superficial Kaposi sarcoma, within an 18-month period. Those with CD4 cell counts of 100 are often symptomatic and have a 60% chance of developing an AIDS-indicator disease (Box 1-4). Antibody to HIV usually appears 6 to 12 weeks after infection but may take as long as 6 months to appear. The diagnosis of HIV infection is based on detection of anti-HIV antibodies by the enzyme-linked immunosorbent assay (ELISA), confirmed by the more specific Western blot (Wb) method. A positive Wb test indicates that the individual has been infected with HIV. The processing of a specimen that is positive on initial ELISA testing always includes rerun of the ELISA, to confirm the result, followed by the Wb test.

The major consideration for dentists providing care to AIDS patients is to minimize the possibility of transmission of HIV from an infected patient to themselves, their staff, or other patients. Dental procedures

---

BOX

1-4 AIDS-Indicator Disease

Candidiasis
Invasive cervical cancer
Coccidioidomycosis
Cytomegalovirus disease
HIV-related dementia
Herpes simplex
Histoplasmosis
Kaposi sarcoma
Lymphoma
Tuberculosis
Pneumocystis carinii
Pneumonia
Salmonella septicemia
Toxoplasmosis
Wasting syndrome caused by HIV

---

that result in soft tissue injury allow various amounts of blood to become mixed with saliva. The dentist and his staff should use disposable protective clothing including eye protection, try to minimize the risk of needle sticks, and perform as many procedures as possible in a given appointment. These patients may also be potential bleeders because of severe thrombocytopenia. Five general categories of oral lesions occur in HIV-infected people:

1. Candidiasis
   a. Herpes simplex
   b. CMV infections
2. Aphthous-like ulcerations
3. Hairy leukoplakia
4. Gingivitis and periodontitis
5. Kaposi sarcoma
   a. Non-Hodgkin lymphoma

Patients who are HIV-positive but asymptomatic can receive all indicated dental treatments; however the patient's physician should be consulted regarding degree of immunosuppression and thrombocytopenia. If the consultation will be delayed, the patient can be treated conservatively with pain medication and antibiotics. If the medical consultation reveals significant immunosuppression and thrombocytopenia, bleeding time or platelet count should be performed before any treatment. The patient may require platelet replacement. Approved medications for treatment of HIV include AZT (zidovudine), ddI (dideoxyinosine) and ddc (dideoxycytidine). AZT is eliminated by renal excretion after metabolism in the liver. Toxicity of AZT is mostly hematologic, primarily anemia and neutropenia. Ddl may cause peripheral neuropathy, diarrhea, and pancreatitis. Peripheral neuropathy is the major toxicity of ddl.

Pancreatitis has been noted with ddc, but with much less frequency than with ddl.

REFERENCES

1. Peterson LJ, et al.: *Contemporary oral and maxillofacial surgery*, ed 3, St. Louis, 1998, Mosby.
2. Berg RL, et al.: *Health status indexes*, Chicago, 1973, Hospital Research and Educational Trust.
3. Little JW, et al: *Dental management of the medically compromised patient*, ed 5, St. Louis, 1997, Mosby.
4. Andreoli TE, et al.: *Cecil essentials of medicine*, ed 5, Philadelphia, 2000, WB Saunders.
5. Barker LR, et al.: *Principles of ambulatory medicine*, ed 5, Baltimore, 1998, Lippincott-Williams and Wilkins.
6. Kroenke K, Mangelsdorff D: Common symptoms in ambulatory care: Incidence, evaluation, therapy and outcome, *Am J Med* 86:262, 1989.

2 Regional Surgical Anatomy

ORRETT E. OGLE, DDS

The most important aspect of surgical practice is a detailed knowledge of the regional anatomy. Although emphasis is often placed on surgical techniques, thorough knowledge of the anatomy will make the operator more comfortable with the operation and will avert surgical mishaps.

In this chapter we will present a broad review of surgical anatomy that will be relevant to most of the procedures presented in this atlas. This will not be a rehash of classical anatomy; instead facts will be presented that will be useful to the surgeon. This chapter is not meant to, nor does it, supplant detailed texts on anatomy.

NERVES

The importance of nerves to the surgeon is that inadvertent injury will result in great morbidity to the patient and, in a majority of cases, legal challenges to the surgeon. The second and third divisions of the trigeminal nerve are the ones with which we are mostly concerned in oral surgery. The important aspect of the surgical anatomy of these structures will be reviewed.

Maxillary Nerve

The maxillary nerve consists of three divisions: the pterygopalatine nerve, the infraorbital nerve, and the zygomatic nerve.

Pterygopalatine Nerve. Although this nerve has several divisions, the most significant for us are its two terminal branches. The larger of these two terminal branches, the anterior palatine nerve, enters the oral cavity through the greater palatine foramen. From here it splits into several branches that spread fanwise anteriorly as the greater palatine nerve, to supply the mucosa of the hard palate up to the canine line where they exchange fibers with the nasopalatine nerve.[1] The nerve travels along with the palatine artery within the connective tissue between the periosteum and the palatal mucosa, being in almost intimate contact with the periosteum. Within this neurovascular bundle the ar-

tery will be the largest structure. The closeness to the periosteum allows an area of palatal mucosa from which split thickness grafts may be harvested. Injuries to the nerve endings within the palatal mucosa tend to be self-reparative and patients will usually not be aware of any deficits. The palatal tissue heals rapidly and sensory perception will not be lost.

The smaller branch, the posterior palatine nerve, travels through the lesser palatine foramen and supplies the tonsil with sensory twigs[1] (Fig. 2-1).

Infraorbital Nerve (Fig. 2-2.) The infraorbital nerve releases three branches before it emerges at the infraorbital foramen. These branches are the anterior, middle, and posterior superior alveolar nerves, which supply the upper teeth, their periodontal membranes, and the gingiva on the lateral aspect of the maxilla. In the base of the alveolar process the superior alveolar nerves form a loose plexus called the superior dental plexus. These dental nerves are the ones anesthetized by infiltration of local anesthesia. Surgery on the alveolar process will not lead to any sensory deficits.

The terminal branches of the infraorbital nerve itself spread fanwise from the infraorbital foramen toward the lower eyelid, nose, and upper lip. Three or four superior labial branches enter the lip between its muscles and the mucous membrane. They supply not only the mucous membrane of the upper lip, but also its skin, which they reach by perforating the orbicularis oris muscle. Surgical disruptions of the terminal branches within the lip are of little consequence, as reinnervation will occur. During apicoectomies on the upper canine or premolar teeth, or sinus lift procedures on the atrophic maxilla, care must be taken not to injure the nerve as it emerges from the infraorbital foramen. Injury at this point will lead to a traumatic neuroma and the neurological deficit will be permanent.

Mandibular Nerve (Fig. 2-3)

The mandibular nerve is a mixed nerve containing both motor and sensory fibers. We will be concerned with

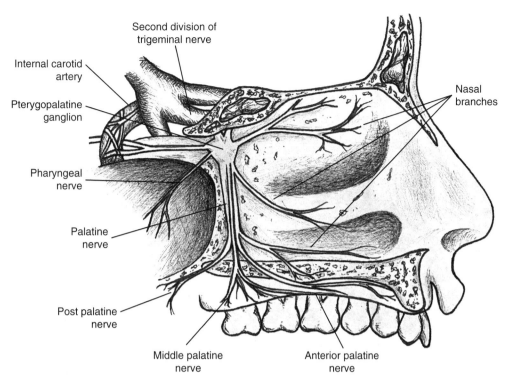

FIG. 2-1 Pterygopalatine nerve: Posterior branch of the maxillary nerve. Cross section shows the sensory distribution to the palatal area of the oral cavity.

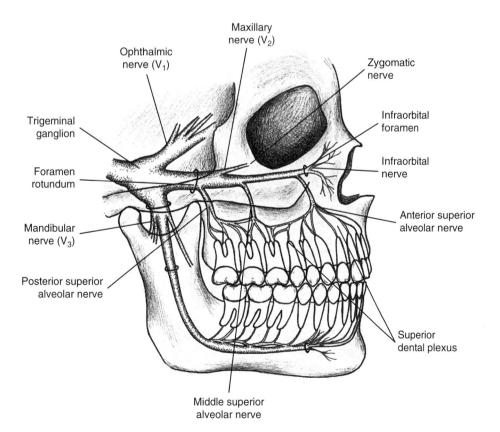

FIG. 2-2 The maxillary nerve showing the infraorbital division. This branch of the maxillary nerve is sensory to the maxillary teeth, periodontal ligament, sinus mucosa, bone, and buccal gingiva of the maxilla.

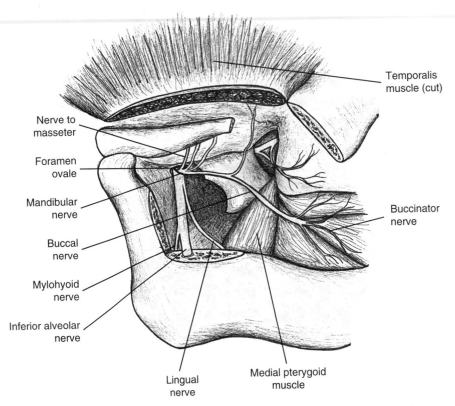

FIG. 2-3 Infratemporal fossa with the mandibular ramus and lateral pterygoid muscle removed to show the mandibular nerve and its sensory divisions.

the sensory fibers. Four sensory branches are organized into internal (two nerves), middle, and external branches. The internal branches are the lingual and buccal branches that supply large areas of the oral mucosa. The middle branch is the inferior alveolar nerve that supplies the mandibular teeth, the skin and mucosal membrane of the lower lip, and the skin of the chin. The external branch is the auriculotemporal nerve, which is never encountered in intraoral procedures.

Buccal Nerve. This nerve enters the oral cavity at the anterior border of the tendon of the temporalis muscle and travels forward and downward within the fascia of the outer portion of the buccinator muscle. Branches perforate the buccinator muscle and supply almost the entire mucosa of the cheek except for a small posterosuperior area, which receives sensory fibers from the gingival branch of the posterior superior alveolar nerves. The buccal nerve will present no surgical challenge. However, it is sometimes a cause of pain perception during retraction when a buccal flap is developed in the third molar area. Local infiltration into the area will suffice to control this problem.

Lingual Nerve. This nerve which carries sensory and taste fibers starts out in close approximation with the inferior alveolar nerve from which it separates at about 5 to 10 mm below the cranial base[1]. It lies anterior and

slightly medial to the inferior alveolar nerve. It follows the lateral surface of the medial pterygoid muscle to the level of the upper end of the mylohyoid line at which point it curves sharply anteriorly to continue horizontally on the upper surface of the mylohyoid muscle into the oral cavity. In the most posterior part of the mouth the lingual nerve is superficial, and may be seen through the lingual mucosa above the mylohyoid line at the level of the third and second molars.

Near the first molar, the nerve turns medially, and goes underneath the submandibular duct, after which point it divides into several branches that enter the substance of the tongue (Fig. 2-4).

The most vulnerable point for injuring the lingual nerve is medial to the retromolar trigone. This usually occurs during the removal of impacted third molars, particularly those in which the patient has had several episodes of pericoronitis. Multiple infections cause tissue contraction that pulls the nerve laterally unto the alveolar crest. The lingual nerve may then become embedded in scar tissue on the superior aspect of the alveolar crest. Further, anatomic studies have shown that an anomalously high position of the lingual nerve relative to the internal oblique ridge occurs in approximately 10% of humans[2]. These two facts make the nerve vulnerable to surgical damage. Recovery of neural

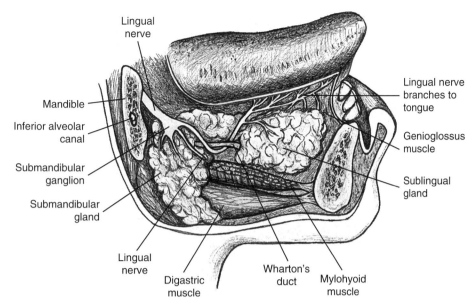

FIG. 2-4 Sagittal section of the floor of the mouth showing the relationship between lingual nerve, Wharton's duct, and other major anatomic structures in the floor of the mouth.

sensation following injury at this location is unlikely. Injuries may also occur during the removal of sialoliths, or any other surgery in the floor of the mouth.

Following injury to the lingual nerve, surgical exploration and surgical repair is indicated when there is no objective evidence of spontaneous signs of recovery 1 month after injury. An 80% success rate of nonpainful sensory return can be expected from microsurgical repairs of the lingual nerve if surgery is performed within the first 3 months following injury.[3]

Inferior Alveolar Nerve (Figs. 2-3 and 2-5). This nerve enters the body of the mandible at the lingula, travels through the length of the mandibular canal and divides in the premolar area into the incisive and mental nerves. The mental nerve leaves the body of the mandible through the mental foramen where it divides into from three to five branches. The incisive branch continues within the bone as a part of the inferior dental plexus. These dental nerves supply the teeth and periodontal ligaments. The organization of these dental nerves is the same as in the upper jaw.

The relative position of the lingula varies with the age of the individual, being more posterior and superior on the ramus in the growing mandible.[4] The relevance of this will be discussed in more detail in the chapter on local anesthesia. The inferior alveolar nerve will be closest to the apex of teeth in the third molar area, and closest to the inferior border of the mandible below the first molar roots (Fig. 2-5). In the premolar area it is midway between the roots and the inferior border of the mandible. In doing apical surgery on lower molars or premolars the position of the nerve should be viewed

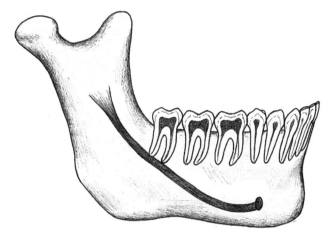

FIG. 2-5 The inferior alveolar canal showing the relationship between the teeth and the inferior border of the mandible.

with a panoramic radiograph or an accurate periapical film. Overall, apical surgery up to the first molar is safe. Second molars should be evaluated carefully. The inferior alveolar canal is located about 4 to 7 mm from the lateral cortical cortex of the mandible.

Injury to the inferior alveolar nerve most often occurs during third molar surgery. Because this nerve is in a bony canal, nerve regrowth is guided, and return of sensation is very likely if the canal is not blocked by an infracturing of the roof of the canal upon the nerve. An observation period of up to 3 months is reasonable before microsurgical repair is considered. It should be noted, however, that a significant association exists between the age of the patient and the permanency of persistent neurosensory deficits.[5] Of patients over the age of 40 who have inferior alveolar nerve injury following oral surgery, 47% will have functionally problematic deficits such as lip biting and drooling more than 50% of the time.[6] Presurgical counseling regarding persistent, functional, neurosensory problems should be stressed to patients over 40. As a matter of fact, age > 40 should be considered as a contraindication to the removal of asymptomatic impacted third molars.

THE MAXILLA

Minor surgical procedures on the maxillary alveolar region are influenced by the two major cavities adjacent to the alveolus. These are the floor of the nasal cavity and the floor of the maxillary sinus (Fig. 2-6). Generally, the incisors are situated below the floor of the nasal cavity, the premolars and molars are below the floor of the maxillary sinus, and the canine occupies a neutral position between the two cavities.

The relationship of the apices of the incisors to the nasal floor will depend on the length of the incisor roots and the height of the alveolar process. In patients with vertical maxillary deficiency (VMD) and long roots, the central incisors may actually reach the floor of the nasal cavity whereas in individuals with vertical maxillary excess (VME), the apex of the central incisor may be 10 mm or more from the nasal floor. The average distance between the nasal floor and the apex of the central incisor is approximately 3 to 5 mm, within the thick bone that forms the inferior portion of the periform rim. The lateral incisor root usually does not have a close relationship to the nasal floor, however, because its root is shorter than the central incisor and the floor of the nose ascends slightly on its lateral aspect.

Cystic lesions, abscess arising from the incisors, or other pathology occurring in the anterior maxilla may bulge into the nasal cavity, and could erode the nasal floor to involve the nasal mucosa. In surgery, the nasal mucosa will appear greyish in color when compared with the oral mucosa. Manipulation, or release of the nasal mucosa from its bony wall, will result in brisk bleeding.

The proximity of the teeth to the maxillary sinus is dependent on the alveolar recess of the maxillary sinus. In cases where the base of the alveolar process is deeply excavated by the maxillary sinus the molars will be in intimate approximation to the floor of the sinus (see Fig. 2-6). The first premolar is usually removed from the sinus floor, because in the anterior the sinus floor rises before continuing into its anterior wall. This anterior junction of floor and anterior wall is well demarcated and presents a convenient area to enter the maxillary sinus either to begin the sinus lift procedure or to remove pathology. The alveolar bone on the lateral sinus wall above the roots is very thin, making entry into the sinus cavity easy.

The Maxillary Sinus

The maxillary sinuses are located within the maxillary bones immediately below the orbits on each side of the lateral walls of the nasal cavity. They are the largest of the paranasal sinuses, and vary considerably in size and shape. The maxillary sinuses are generally

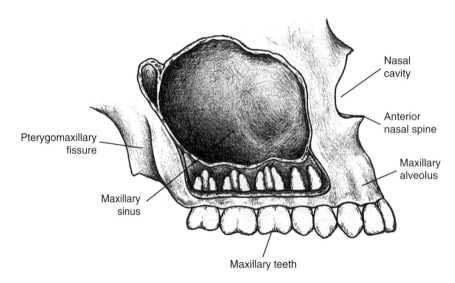

Nasal cavity

Anterior nasal spine

Maxillary alveolus

Pterygomaxillary fissure

Maxillary sinus

Maxillary teeth

FIG. 2-6 A lateral view of the maxilla showing the relationship of the teeth to the maxillary sinus and nasal cavity.

described as pyramidal in shape. The base of this pyramid is the lateral wall of the nasal cavity, with the apex pointing outward to the zygoma; the pterygopalatine fossa forms the posterior wall; and the anterior wall of the maxilla forms the anterior wall of the pyramid. The roof of the sinus is the orbital floor and the floor of the sinus is the alveolar process of the maxilla, which is approximately at the level of the nasal floor or slightly below. (For the size of the maxillary sinus, refer to Table 2-1.)

The maxillary sinuses are frequently asymmetrical, with the sinuses on either side of the head often varying in size and contour in the same individual. Incomplete bony septa, which divide the cavity into irregularly shaped hollows, are sometimes present within the maxillary sinus. A radiographic exam would show this as a multiloculated sinus. The presence of such septa may interfere with the easy retrieval of a root that has been displaced into the sinus. It would also make elevation of the sinus mucosa during the sinus lift procedure impossible to achieve without tearing the mucosa. A Waters view of good quality should be obtained when evaluating a patient for any sinusotomy or grafting of the sinus floor for implants.

Following the loss of teeth, the maxillary sinus may expand into the alveolus from which the teeth were lost. Recess of the sinus may then reach far downward between the remaining teeth, and the floor of the sinus may now become very thin. In very atrophic maxillae it is common to see as little as 3 mm of alveolar bone below the sinus floor (Fig. 2-7).

Palate

The palate is concave, the curvature being greater in the transverse direction. It consists of a skeletal and a muscular portion. The skeletal portion, or hard palate, comprises primarily the bony palatine shelf of the maxilla and its overlying mucosa. Immediately beneath the mucosa are fat globules, along with mucous and mixed glands of varying sizes. This cushion of intervening glands is thickest in the posterior and lateral regions. Beneath the glands of the hard palate, on either side of the palatal vault, lie the greater palatine arteries, nerve, and vein.

Surgical interventions on the hard palate are usually well tolerated and will present little anatomic challenge. Palatine tori are commonly occurring entities. At times they may become pneumatized and be in direct communication with the nasal cavity. Over-aggressive surgical removal of a palatine torus may result in an oronasal fistula.

The Edentulous Maxilla

As bone loss occurs in the maxilla, the palatal vault will become more shallow, and the anterior portion of the alveolar crest will show resorption in an upward and posterior direction. This is because edentulous bone loss in the anterior maxilla occurs mostly on the labial and inferior aspects of the alveolar ridge. In severely atrophic maxillae the nasopalatine neurovascular bundle may end up on the alveolar crest itself, and the anterior nasal spine may be almost level with the alveolar crest. Crestal incisions in the atrophic maxilla should be placed a little toward the buccal so as to avoid the nasopalatine structures.

Upper lip support is progressively lost as the anterior maxilla decreases in size. This, coupled with the relative anterior movement of the mandibular alveolar ridge, tends to give the face a concave or Class III facial appearance and also a Class III ridge relationship.

THE MANDIBLE

The most significant structure that we should consider in mandibular surgery is the inferior alveolar nerve. In this regard, the relationship between the third molar and the inferior alveolar canal, and that between the first premolar and the mental foramen deserve special attention.

The Third Molar

The erupted third molar usually lies close to the lingual cortical plate with a slight lingual inclination of its axis.

TABLE 2-1 Linear Measurements and Volume of the Maxillary Sinus

Gender	Ant-Post Length (mm)	Height (mm)	Width (mm)	Volume (cm³)
Male	30.9	35.9	26.2	11.8
Female	28.9	32.6	24.0	10.6

Data from: Uchida Y, Goto M, Katsuki T, Akioshi T: A cadaveric study of maxillary sinus size as an aid in bone grafting of the maxillary sinus floor, *J Oral Maxillofac Surg* 56:1158-1163, 1998.

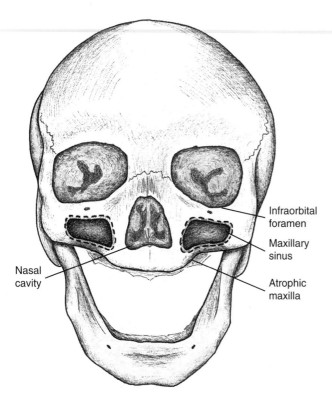

Nasal
cavity

Infraorbital
foramen

Maxillary
sinus

Atrophic
maxilla

FIG. 2-7   The maxillary sinus and nasal cavity in a skull with an atrophic maxilla.

This is because of a medial shift of the alveolar process in relationship to the bulk of the mandible. The external oblique ridge contributes considerable bulk to the outer surface of the mandible in the region of the second and third molars, and there is a thick layer of cancellous bone between the tooth socket and the outer cortical plate. There is also a lateral flair of the vertical ramus in relationship to the horizontal direction of the alveolus.

Impaction of the lower third molar will bring the tooth in very close approximation to the mandibular canal. When this tooth becomes impacted against the distal aspect of the second molar, or by the bone of the ascending ramus, its roots will grow deeper into the bone and will get close to the inferior alveolar canal or may even grow beyond the level of the canal. An actual meeting between roots and canal is rare, however, because in most cases the impacted third molar is usually lingually inclined and its roots pass the canal on its buccal side. Only in a minority of cases are the roots themselves located lingual to the canal.[1] In some cases where the crown is buccally inclined, or in distoangular impactions, the roots may be right above the canal. In an attempt to remove this tooth by applying an instrument that exerts pressure distally, the force may lead to a fracture of the roof of the canal, which may leave

bony fragments impinging on the neurovascular bundle. This type of nerve injury would be persistent if the pressure were not relieved.

The First Premolar

This tooth is in close approximation to the mental nerve. Incision and drainage of an abscess, apicoectomies, buccal flaps, and other procedures done in this area may damage the mental nerve. The mental canal arises from the mandibular canal in the vicinity of the first premolar. This short mental canal runs outward, upward, and backward to open at the mental foramen located between the two premolars, or below the root of the second premolar. If an attempt is made to lower or move the mental nerve, one should understand that its outer end will be at a higher and more posterior plane than its inner end.

The mental nerve is invested with periosteum that is tightly bound to the opening of the mental foramen and forms a thick collar around the nerve. When isolating the mental nerve this periosteal collar must be incised to produce laxity in the nerve, which will make retraction of the nerve easier and will decrease the likelihood of avulsion of the nerve.

THE FLOOR OF THE MOUTH

The floor of the mouth is the area between the lower surface of the tongue and the mylohyoid muscle. It is limited anteriorly and laterally by the mandible, and posteriorly by the glossopalatine arch. It contains a number of important structures, all of which lie above the mylohyoid muscle. Structures in the floor of the mouth in addition to the mylohyoid are the geniohyoid and genioglossus muscle, the sublingual glands and their ducts of Rivinus and Bartholin, the large submandibular duct (Wharton's duct), and the lingual nerves and vessels. These structures are covered by a thin, smooth lining of mucosa that originates from the lingual surface of the mandible. Fig. 2-4 shows the relationship of these structures.

Lingual Frenulum

This is a band of fibrous tissue that is continuous with the under surface of the tongue and the mucosa on the lingual aspect of the mandible. On each side of the frenulum, the ducts of the submandibular and sublingual glands open into the oral cavity through the raised sublingual fold. Near the origins of the frenum at the base of the tongue is an irregularly scalloped fold that can be followed on either side laterally and posteriorly on the inferior surface of the tongue. These folds are called the fimbriated folds. Near these folds, large,

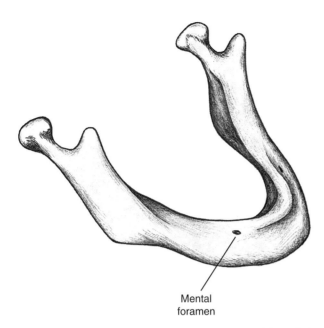

Mental
foramen

FIG. 2-8 The atrophic mandible showing the position of the mental foramen.

torturous veins can almost always be seen through the thin mucosa of the underside of the tongue. These veins sometimes come very close to the origins of the lingual frenum, and are very large in adults.

The Edentulous Mandible

One of the most significant results of edentulous bone loss in the mandible is that the mental foramen becomes closer to the crest as the alveolar process decreases in height. This makes the nerve more vulnerable to injury during any attempted preprosthetic surgery in the area. In severe cases the mandibular nerve, the mental nerve, and the genial tubercle may all be superior to the crest of the mandible (Fig. 2-8).

As bone loss progresses in the mandible, the decrease in height and width of the alveolus occurs so that the crest of the ridge moves slightly to the anterior. Also, autorotation of the mandible moves the entire mandible anteriorly and superiorly as vertical dimension is lost. This results in an increasingly Class III facial form and maxillomandibular jaw relationship.

The mentalis muscle insertion on the mandible may be lost, and this would result in a lifting of the muscle and mucosa above the level of the alveolar ridge. The muscle pull also tends to roll the lower lip toward the alveolar ridge, thus decreasing the amount of alveolar ridge exposed in the mouth.

REFERENCES

1. Sicher H, DuBrul EL: *Oral anatomy*, ed 6, St. Louis, 1975, Mosby.
2. Kiesselbach JE, Chamberlain JG: Clinical and anatomic observations in the relationship of the lingual nerve to the mandibular third molar region, *J Oral Maxillofac Surg* 42:565, 1984.
3. Gregg JM: Surgical management of lingual nerve injuries, *Oral Maxillofac Surg ClinNorth Am* 4(2):417-424, 1992.
4. Kaban LB: Surgical correction of the facial skeleton in childhood. In Kaban LB, editor: *Pediatric oral and maxillofacial surgery*, Philadelphia, 1990, WB Saunders, p. 425.
5. Upton LG, Rajvanakarn M, Hayward JR: Evaluation of the regenerative capacity of the inferior alveolar nerve following surgical trauma, *J Oral Maxillofac Surg* 45:212, 1987.
6. August M, Marchena J, Donady J, Kaban L: Neurosensory deficit and functional impairment after sagittal ramus osteotomy: A long-term follow-up study, *J Oral Maxillofac Surg* 56:1231-1235, 1998.

CHAPTER 3

Local Anesthesia

ORRETT E. OGLE, DDS

Pain control is essential in the surgical practice of dentistry. Good pain control will permit the operator to perform the surgery in a careful, unhurried fashion, and the entire experience will be less strenuous for both the surgeon and the patient. In addition, a comfortable patient will become a great advocate for the dentist. Dentoalveolar surgery and other minor oral surgical procedures performed in the ambulatory setting rely very heavily on good local anesthesia. This is true even when IV sedation is being used. The achievement of good local anesthesia requires a thorough knowledge of the anatomy along with good techniques. This chapter will present a review of the neuroanatomy, some of the agents used, and the technical details of administering selected regional anesthesia.

Local anesthesia is a reversible blockade of nerve conduction in a circumscribed area that produces loss of sensation and motor activity. Local anesthetic agents stabilize neural membranes by inhibiting the ionic fluxes required for the propagation of neural impulses. The site of local anesthetic action is the sodium channel membrane pore that permits ion influx.[1]

Current chemical agents used to produce local anesthesia are classified as either an ester or an amide. They are further classified according to their duration of action as short-, moderate-, and long-acting drugs:

Short-acting	< 2 hours
Moderate-acting	2 to 4 hours
Long-acting	4 to 18 hours

The duration of the planned surgical procedure, along with the anticipated need for postoperative pain control should guide the dentist on which agent to select. Long-acting anesthetic agents offer the doctor the option of long-term control to obliterate postoperative pain. This would be desirable, for example, for the removal of full bony impacted third molars.

ANATOMY OF LOCAL ANESTHESIA

The technique for local anesthesia must be based on exact anatomic knowledge. Local anesthesia can be achieved by infiltration (field anesthesia) or by conduc-

tion (nerve-block) anesthesia. The anatomic basis of infiltration anesthesia is simple, and the main consideration is the density of the tissue into which the anesthetic fluid is to be injected. In oral surgery, infiltration anesthesia is commonly used in the maxilla or for small soft tissue procedures in the lower jaw (Table 3-1 and Box 3-1).

In the maxilla it is the network of nerves in the spongy bone that is anesthetized, along with nerve endings in the adjacent soft tissues. This network is a part of the dental plexus, which is derived from the three superior alveolar nerves (see Chapter 2). Sicher refers to this type of anesthesia as "plexus anesthesia."[2] The cortical plate of the alveolus of the upper jaw is almost always thin and porous enough to make infiltration anesthesia successful. In the spongy bone the anesthetic fluid will diffuse uniformly through the marrow spaces to produce anesthesia of the adjacent tooth and its periodontal ligament, the gingiva on the buccal surface, the adjacent soft tissue, and the bone itself. The mucosa of the maxillary sinus will also be anesthetized.

Procedures on the lower jaw will most often require nerve block anesthesia of the inferior alveolar, lingual, and buccal nerves. These nerves are accessible in the pterygomandibular space.

Applied Anatomy of the Pterygomandibular Space (Fig. 3-1, *A*)

This is an inverted triangularly shaped cleft between the pterygoid musculature and the ramus of the mandible. Superiorly, it is roofed by the inferior head of the lateral pterygoid muscle. The medial pterygoid muscle and the sphenomandibular ligament are medial. The sphenomandibular ligament, which is actually a broad sheet of fibrous tissue, extends from the sphenoid bone, spreading downward and outward to attach to the mandible at the lingula, the inferior margin of the mandibular foramen, and above the attachment of the medial pterygoid muscle.[4] Its zone of attachment continues posteriorly and superiorly to the posterior border of the ramus and extends up to the condylar neck where it

TABLE 3-1 Common Local Anesthetics

Local Anesthetic Agent	Duration[a]	Maximum Adult Dose
Lidocaine 2%	30 min-1 hr	300 mg[b] 8 cartridges
Chloroprocaine HCl 2%	30 min-1 hr	800 mg[c]
Procaine HCl 2%	30 min-1.5 hr	200 mg [c] 6 cartridges
Prilocaine HCl 4%	30 min-1.5 hr	600 mg[b] 8 cartridges
Mepivacaine HCl 3%	45 min-1.5 hr	400 mg[d] 7 cartridges
Lidocaine HCl 2% with epi 1/100,000	2-6 hr	500 mg[b] 12 cartridges
Mepivocaine HCl 2% with Neo-cobefrin 1/20,000	2-6 hr	400 mg[d] 11 cartridges
Bupivacaine HCl 0.5% with epi 1/200,000	3-7 hr	90 mg[e] 10 cartridges
Etidocaine HCl 1.5% with epi 1/200,000	3-7 hr	400 mg[b] 14 cartridges

[a]Duration is for nerve block anesthesia.
[b]Product Information, Professional Information Department, Astra Pharmaceutical, 50 Otis Ave., Westborough, MA 01581-4502.
[c]Data from: *Drug Information Handbook for Dentistry,* ed 3, Cleveland, 1997-1998, Lexi-Comp, Inc.
[d]Product Insert, Novocol Pharmaceutical of Canada, Inc., Cambridge, Ont., Canada N1R643.
[e]Product Information Services, Sanofi Winthrop, 90 Park Ave,. New York, NY 10016.

BOX 3-1 Chemical Structures of Commonly used Local Anesthetics

Ester Anesthetics	Amide Anesthetics
Procaine * Chloroprocaine	Lidocaine Mepivacaine Bupivacaine Etidocaine

* This is no longer a useful local anesthetic in dentistry, because of a high incidence of allergic reactions.[3]

blends into the stylomandibular ligament. The sphenomandibular ligament has a very important influence on the diffusion of anesthetic solution injected into the area. Anteriorly, the pterygomandibular space is bounded by the buccinator muscle.[3]

The contents of the pterygomandibular space include the inferior alveolar and lingual nerves, which separate from each other on the upper surface of the lateral pterygoid muscle and emerge into the space on the lateral surface of the medial pterygoid muscle. The inferior alveolar nerve lies posterior to the lingual nerve and diverges laterally to approach the mandibular foramen where it is situated between the sphenomandibular ligament and the bone. Posterior and lateral to the inferior alveolar nerve are found the inferior alveolar artery and veins, which converge with the nerve to enter the mandibular foramen. The mylohyoid nerve leaves the inferior alveolar nerve at an average of about 14 mm above the mandibular foramen[5] (Fig. 3-1, B). Although the mylohyoid nerve is generally considered to be primarily a motor nerve, there is sufficient evidence to suggest that in some people it does supply sensory innervation to anterior teeth.[5,6]

The buccal nerve (Fig. 3-1, B) travels for a short distance through the upper and anterior part of the space, between the two heads of the lateral pterygoid muscle toward the deep portion of the temporalis. It descends either in the substance of the temporalis muscle or is enveloped in its fascia. The buccal nerve subsequently emerges from beneath the temporobuccinator band to pass forward on the outer aspect of the buccinator muscle.[4]

The Lingula

This ledge of bone is variably developed and guards the mandibular foramen near the center of the ramus. The position of the mandibular foramen is extremely variable. Bremer showed through his research that the position of the lingula relative to the occlusal plane varies considerably[7] (Fig. 3-1, C):

- In 16% of mandibles, the lingula was < 1 mm above the occlusal plane
- 48% were from 1 to 5 mm above the occlusal plane
- 27% from 5 to 9 mm
- 5% from 9 to 11 mm
- 4% from 11 to 19 mm

(In general the "occlusal plane" will correspond to the horizontal plane of the maxillary teeth when the mouth is closed, and will be located 1.5 to 2.0 cm below the maxillary dental plane when the mouth is fully opened. It can often be identified by a line on the mucosa of the cheek.)

Using Bremer's data as a guide, we see that a needle inserted 5 mm above the occlusal plane and parallel to it would lie above the lingula in 64% of mandibles and below it in 36%. A needle placed 11 mm above the occlusal plane would be above the lingula in 96% of mandibles.

In the growing child (ages 10 to 19), the lingula is more posterior and superior on the ramus than in the adult.[8] To perform an inferior alveolar nerve block in the growing mandible, the tip of the needle must reach

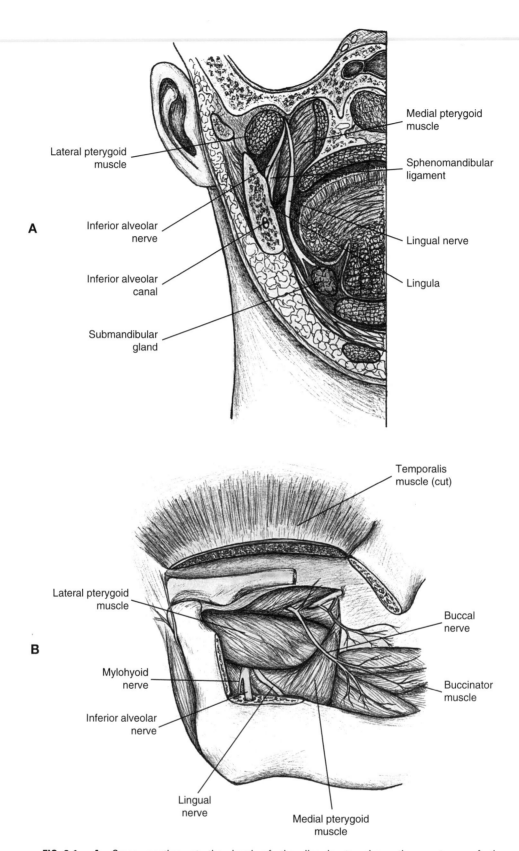

FIG. 3-1 **A,** Cross section at the level of the lingula to show the anatomy of the pterygomandibular space. **B,** Superficial dissection of the pterygomandibular space to show the neural structures.

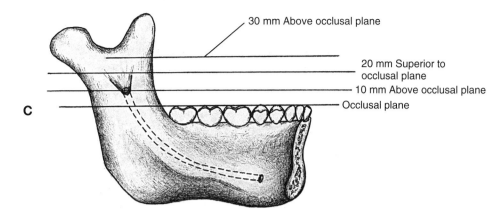

FIG. 3-1—cont'd **C,** Position of the needle for local anesthesia utilizing the occlusal plane as the landmark. Data was taken from 10 mandibles measured in cadavers during surgical anatomy courses.

an area that is high and far back on the ramus. Not accomplishing this goal may result in failure to achieve adequate anesthesia following an attempted nerve block.

TECHNIQUES OF ADMINISTERING LOCAL ANESTHESIA
Maxilla

Infiltration Anesthesia. This is the most common technique for local anesthesia in the maxilla. In this technique, the anesthetic solution is deposited in a supraperiosteal plane in relationship to the buccal and labial periosteum. A subperiosteal injection should be avoided for routine exodontia, soft tissue biopsies, or other minor soft tissue procedures because the detachment of the periosteum from the bone entails the rupture of blood vessels entering the bone, and may cause subperiosteal hematomas and prolonged postoperative pain. The subperiosteal injection will give better local anesthesia when the supraperiosteal method is ineffective. However, Sicher makes the point that if the injected fluid can penetrate the compact bone of the alveolar plate, then the delicate periosteum of the maxilla cannot possibly be a serious barrier.[2] In cases where a mucoperiosteal flap will be raised, the question of subperiosteal injections is moot. The location and level at which the needle is inserted is dependent on what structures the operator is trying to anesthetize (Figs. 3-2 and 3-3).

Maxillary Nerve Blocks. In rare cases when infiltration anesthesia by the supraperiosteal injection fails, or where this technique is contraindicated because of an infection in the area, or when anesthesia of several teeth is required, it may be necessary to block the posterior superior alveolar nerve high on the maxillary tuberosity. The posterior superior alveolar nerve may be

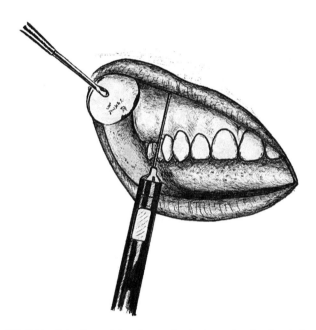

FIG. 3-2 Injection of local anesthesia into the depth of the vestibule to obtain local anesthesia in the maxilla.

blocked before it enters the bony canals located on the zygomatic aspect of the maxilla above the third molar.[9]

Method. The puncture is made high in the mucobuccal fold above the distobuccal root of the second molar. The needle is directed upward and inward to a depth of about 20 mm, keeping the point of the needle close to the periosteum of the tuberosity at all times. This will minimize the chances of entering the pterygoid venous plexus. This block will provide anesthesia on the lateral maxilla from the pterygomaxillary fissure to the distobuccal root of the first molar. The long buccal nerve will also be anesthetized (Fig. 3-4).

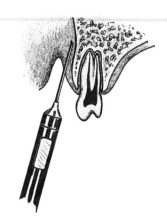

FIG. 3-3 Infiltration anesthesia of the maxillary alveolus. Note the position of the bevel of the needle in relationship to the periosteum. To obtain adequate anesthesia of the tooth, the needle should be above the apex.

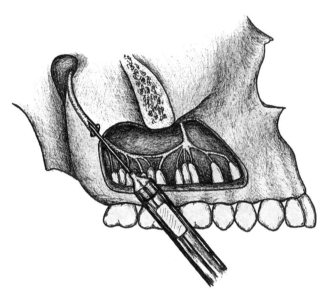

FIG. 3-4 Technique for blocking the posterior superior alveolar nerve close to the pterygomaxillary fissure. The puncture is made high in the mucobuccal fold above the distobuccal root of the second molar.

Infraorbital Injection. This injection is indicated when inflammation or infection contraindicates the use of infiltration anesthesia in the anterior portion of the maxilla, or when an opening into the maxillary sinus is to be performed.

Method. The infraorbital foramen is located by palpation. It is generally found at about 5 mm below the orbital rim on the midpupillary line, but it can sometimes be difficult to palpate the foramen itself. However, a notching of the rim at the zygomaticomaxillary suture line is sometimes easier to identify. The infraorbital foramen will be 3 to 4 mm lateral to this notch,

and 5 mm below the orbital rim. If swelling or pain prevents the palpation of skeletal landmarks the general area should be estimated. Once the area of the infraorbital foramen is identified, the doctor should place a finger on the site. The cheek is then retracted as far laterally as possible, and the needle is introduced about 5 to 7 mm away from the buccal surface of the alveolus. The needle is directed parallel to the long axis of the second premolar, and is advanced until it is below the palpating finger. The distance from the cusp tip of the second premolar to the infraorbital foramen is approximately 40 mm. This can be used as a guide as to how far to advance the needle. (The standard "long" needle used on dental syringes is 30 mm. However, by retracting the cheek laterally the distance from the mucobuccal fold to the foramen is decreased, and the needle will not be completely buried). Once in the area of the foramen the solution of one anesthetic cartridge should be deposited. This block will anesthetize the skin over the lower eyelid, ala of the nose and upper lip, and the lateral maxilla intraorally from the first molar to the central incisor, including the teeth (Fig. 3-5, *A* and *B*.)

Mandible

The majority of surgical procedures performed in the lower jaw will require anesthesia of the inferior alveolar, lingual, and buccal nerves. As previously mentioned, these nerves are accessible in the pterygomandibular space. The most commonly used approach to inferior alveolar nerve anesthesia in the United States is the traditional Halstead method[10] in which the inferior alveolar nerve is approached via an intraoral route just before the nerve enters the mandibular canal (Fig. 3-6, *A* and *B*). A complete block of the inferior alveolar nerve may be produced by placing the anesthetic solution around the nerve before it enters the bony canal of the mandible. This method of blocking the inferior alveolar nerve has a success rate of 71% to 87%,[11] and incomplete anesthesia is not uncommon.

There are two techniques for approaching the inferior alveolar nerve at the point where it enters the mandibular canal. The other two techniques (Akinosi and Gow-Gates) are not done at the point where the nerve enters the mandibular canal but higher up.

Traditional Techniques

Method 1. The thumb of the noninjecting hand is placed in the deepest portion of the concavity of the ramus between the internal and external ridges of the mandible (Fig. 3-7). The other four fingers are placed extraorally on the posterior border of the ramus. The foramen of the mandibular canal will be approximately midway between the internal oblique ridge and the posterior border of the mandible along a line that bisects the thumb. With the barrel of the syringe lying

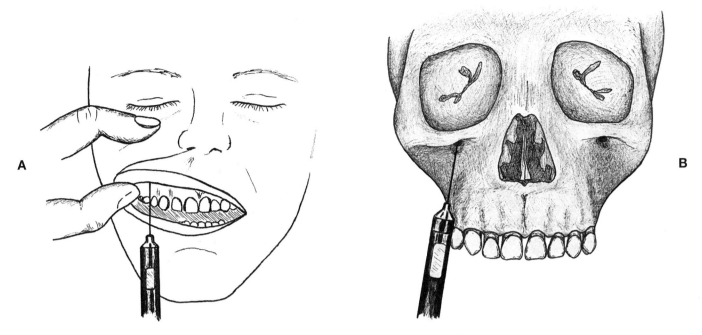

FIG. 3-5 **A,** Infraorbital nerve block. Note the finger over the infraorbital foramen, and the point of entry of the needle at the second premolar tooth. **B,** Infraorbital nerve block. Note the position of the infraorbital foramen in relationship to the orbit, and the maxillary premolar teeth. The needle is superficial to the canal adjacent to where the nerve emerges from the foramen.

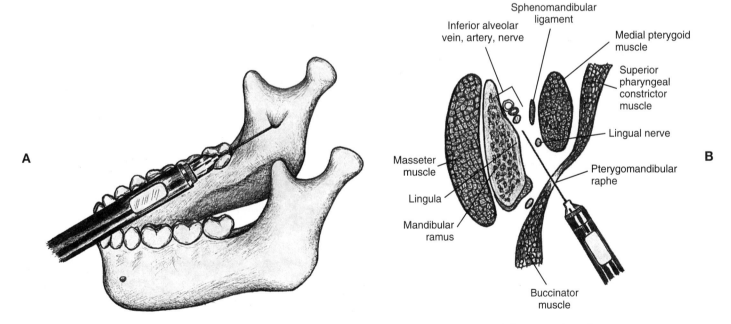

FIG. 3-6 **A,** Inferior alveolar nerve block performed at the entrance of the nerve into the mandibular canal (traditional method). Note that the barrel of the syringe is over the premolar on the contralateral side. **B,** Pterygomandibular space just superior to the lingula. Inferior alveolar nerve block performed at the entrance of the nerve into the mandibular canal. The neurovascular bundle comprises the inferior alveolar vein, artery, and nerve. The needle penetrates the pterygomandibular space through the pterygomandibular raphe. Note the position of the lingual nerve.

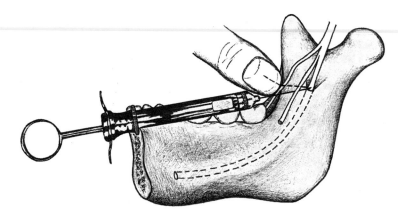

FIG. 3-7 Sagittal view of a hemimandible showing how the thumb is positioned and used as the landmark to perform the traditional block of the inferior alveolar nerve. The position of the inferior alveolar neurovascular bundle, lingual nerve, and buccal nerve is shown. The needle approaches the inferior alveolar neurovascular bundle through the pterygomandibular raphe.

over the premolars of the opposite side (see Fig. 3-6, *A*), the needle is directed parallel to the occlusal plane of the mandibular teeth, bisecting the thumb, and is aimed at the midpoint of the ramus located between the thumb and the extraorally placed fingers. The puncture should be made through the pterygomandibular raphe, and the needle advanced to touch the internal surface of the mandible. Once contact is made with the bone, the needle is then withdrawn approximately 2 mm, aspirated, and the anesthetic solution is deposited. It has been shown that with this technique, 2 mm of anesthetic solution (one cartridge) will be ineffective in 15% of cases.[12]

The lingual nerve can be anesthetized by depositing a small portion from the anesthetic cartridge as the needle is being withdrawn (see Fig. 3-1, *A*). The buccal nerve will not be anesthetized by this technique, and it will be necessary to place a few drops of the anesthetic solution over the external oblique ridge in the vicinity of the third molar and 5 to 7 mm above the occlusal plane (see Figs. 3-1, *A*, 3-6, and 3-7).

Method 2. The patient's mouth is opened to the maximum. The index finger of the noninjecting hand is pressed on the last molar with the nail facing upwards. The barrel of the syringe is placed over the lateral incisor of the same side and the penetration is made right above the nail of the index finger. The needle should first engage the internal oblique ridge, and then advance along the inner aspect of the ramus to a point located in the mid ramus, or about 14 to 15 mm beyond the internal oblique ridge. The mandibular foramen is located halfway between the internal ridge and the posterior border of the mandibular ramus, as well as midway between the condyle and the angle of the mandible. Once this point is determined, the needle should be aimed at it, and the anesthetic solution deposited in the area (Fig. 3-8).

As in Method 1, a separate injection will be required for the buccal nerve. Lingual nerve anesthesia is also achieved in a similar fashion as described in Method 1.

Akinosi Technique.[13] This technique makes use of a more proximal injection level, and anesthetizes the inferior alveolar, lingual, and buccal nerves by a single injection. (See Fig. 3-7 for anatomic rationale.) It is especially useful in patients with limited mandibular opening, particularly in patients with trismus from infection, and in fearful patients who will not open their mouth for administration of traditional block techniques.

The success of this technique (approximately 96%) in producing consistently profound anesthesia is attributable to three factors:

1. Better local anesthesia of the mandibular teeth results when a plexus of nerves, rather than the single inferior alveolar nerve, is blocked.[14] The dental plexus that provides innervation to the mandibular teeth receives major contributions from the inferior alveolar, lingual, mylohyoid, and buccal nerves.[15] With the Akinosi technique all these major nerves will be anesthetized.

2. Superiorly deposited solution results in more effective diffusion of the anesthetic solution throughout the well-defined, closely bound, pterygomandibular space.

3. Larger surfaces of the nerves are exposed to the anesthetic solution. It has been demonstrated that at least 6 mm, and probably more, of inferior alveolar nerve must be exposed to the local anesthetic solution to produce an absolute block.[16] It is more likely that this critical length of nerve will be exposed to the anesthetic solution if the solution is deposited high and allowed to diffuse through the entire pterygomandibular space.[17] Depositing the anesthetic solution 2 to 3 mm above the mandibular foramen may produce an incomplete blockage, because the critical length of nerve was not exposed to the solution.

Method. This injection is given with the mouth closed. The patient is positioned at a 45° angle with the teeth in occlusion. The thumb of the noninjecting hand

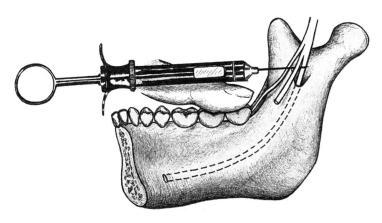

FIG. 3-8 Inferior alveolar block anesthesia performed 12 to 15 mm above the mandibular occlusal plane by placing the index finger on the occlusal surface of the terminal tooth, and entering the pterygomandibular space from the ipsilateral lateral incisor tooth.

is used to reflect the cheek laterally, and to identify the coronoid process. The syringe is placed parallel to the occlusal plane, and is positioned at the level of the mucogingival junction adjacent to the maxillary third molar (Fig. 3-9). The needle is aligned with the mucogingival line of the upper third molar, and penetrates the mucosa just medial to the ramus. It is very important that as the needle advances, it stays close to the bone of the medial aspect of the mandible. A more medial course may place the needle medial to the sphenomandibular ligament, and result in failure (see Fig. 3-1, A). Keeping the syringe parallel to the occlusal plane, direct it posteriorly and slightly laterally until the needle advances approximately 1.5 inches (38 mm). The tip of the needle should now be in the mid-portion of the pterygomandibular space and in close relationship to the main branches of the mandibular nerve. The anesthetic solution is deposited after aspiration and the needle is then withdrawn. Signs of altered sensation should be present after about 2 to 3 minutes, and surgical procedures may be started after 4 to 5 minutes.[14] If the needle is too far medially, anesthesia of the nerve will not occur. It should be noted that with this technique, posterior structures will become anesthetized before anterior structures. The classic sign of tingling of the lower lip will be delayed.

This technique can also be used with the mouth opened, and also gives a very high success rate of obtaining profound local anesthesia. With the mouth wide open the needle is inserted about 15 mm lower than described above, at about the level of the maxillary dental plane, and then advanced as above.

Gow-Gates Technique.[18] This technique uses external landmarks that direct the needle to a higher puncture point, thus ensuring an adequate height for depositing the solution above the lingula (Fig. 3-10). The following two extraoral landmarks are used:

1. The first is a plane that identifies the desired direction for aiming the syringe. This plane extends from the lower border of the tragic notch of the ear through the commissure of the lips (Fig. 3-11).
2. The second is a point, the tragus of the ear, that identifies the landmark toward which the needle is directed.

Method. Because the Gow-Gates technique is more technically difficult to perform it will be outlined in a stepwise fashion below:

1. The head is placed in a horizontal position with the chin raised so that the commissure–tragal line will be almost horizontal. The face is turned slightly toward the dentist in order to allow visual correlation of the puncture point with the external landmarks.
2. The patient is asked to open the mouth as widely as possible so that the condyle will assume a more frontal position and will be in closer relationship to the mandibular nerve. A rubber bite block may also be placed on the contralateral side to keep the mouth opened widely.
3. The anterior border of the ascending ramus is palpated with the forefinger or thumb of the noninjecting hand, and the desired puncture point that would allow the syringe to be positioned as in Fig. 3-11 is visually identified. This puncture point will usually be on the lateral margin of the pterygomandibular depression and just medial to the medial tendon of the temporalis muscle.
4. The syringe and needle are aligned with the plane that extends from the lower border of the tragal notch to the commissure of the lips (see Fig. 3-11). With this alignment the syringe will usually lie over the incisal edge of the cuspid on the opposite side of the mandible, but can vary either anteriorly or posteriorly according to the divergence of the ramus (Fig. 3-12).
5. The oral mucosa is penetrated as close as possible to the anterior border of the ramus, and yet sufficiently medial so as to avoid the medial

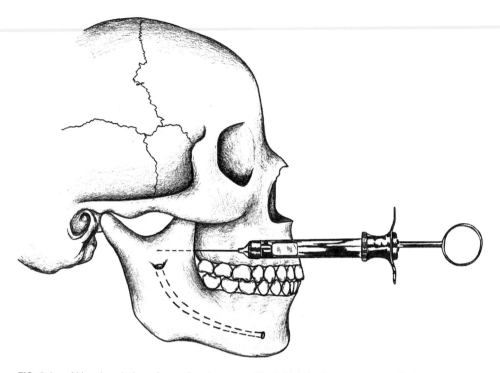

FIG. 3-9   Akinosi technique for performing nerve block high in the pterygomandibular space. The injection is given with the mouth closed. The syringe is placed parallel to the occlusal plane and is positioned at the level of the mucogingival junction adjacent to the maxillary third molar.

FIG. 3-10   The line represents a plane that identifies the desired direction for aiming the syringe when performing the Gow-Gates technique for inferior alveolar nerve block. This plane extends from the lower border of the tragic notch of the ear through the commissure of the lips.

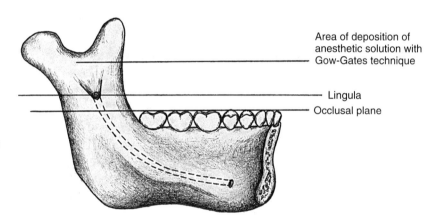

Area of deposition of anesthetic solution with Gow-Gates technique

Lingula
Occlusal plane

tendon of the temporalis muscle and the internal oblique ridge of the mandible. The needle is aimed at the posterior border of the tragus and advanced for about 25 mm. The needle should touch bone at the base of the neck of the condyle. If the needle does not touch bone after it has penetrated a depth of 25 mm, this could indicate that the syringe has been placed too far medially, and that the divergence of the mandibular ramus is significant; or that the needle is too far laterally and too high and has entered the sigmoid notch. (With this approach it is not common that the needle will enter the sigmoid notch, however).

Once bone is identified and the syringe is in the correct location, the needle is withdrawn 1 mm. Aspiration is performed and the anesthetic solution is rapidly deposited in the one position.

6. An alternative method is to have the patient open and close the mouth a few times to permit the operator to identify the head of the condyle. Once identified, the mouth is opened widely, and the operator keeps a finger on this spot. The barrel of the syringe is placed at the occlusal surface of the maxillary first molar on the opposite side, and the needle is aimed for the extraorally placed finger of the operator that is on the condylar head. The

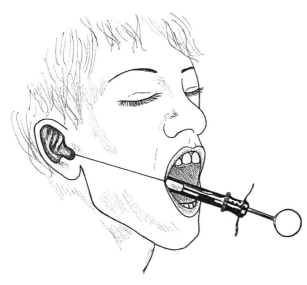

FIG. 3-11 Landmarks for the Gow-Gates technique of mandibular nerve block anesthesia. The extraoral landmarks and the desired plane of injection are shown. This plane extends from the lower border of the tragic notch of the ear to the commissure of the lips.

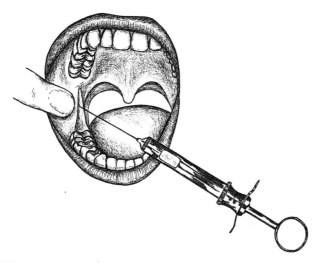

FIG. 3-12 Intraoral site of penetration for the Gow-Gates block of the mandibular nerve. Note the upward slope of the syringe along a plane from the commissure of the lip to the tragic notch, and the position of the syringe from the contralateral canine/premolar teeth.

needle is advanced until it touches the neck of the mandibular condyle. With the mouth wide open, the head of the condyle will assume a more anterior position, making it easier to reach. The operator must make certain that the needle touches the neck of the condyle before depositing the solution. With this alternate technique, it is more common for the needle to enter the sigmoid notch.

7. The mouth is kept opened for another 20 to 30 seconds so that the straightened mandibular nerve will be adequately bathed in the pool of anesthetic solution. The solution will also diffuse better throughout the pterygomandibular space with the mouth opened and will block supplementary innervation in the condylar region, spreading forward under pressure to reach the buccal nerve.

This technique has a reported success rate of 98%,[19] and produces inferior alveolar, lingual, and buccal nerve anesthesia from a single injection.[20]

Complications
- Prolonged postoperative pain at site of injection
- Hematoma formation
- Trismus
- Superficial and deep space infection
- Prolonged paresthesia of the inferior alveolar nerve
- Inadvertent anesthesia of facial nerve or orbital motor nerves
- Psychogenic shock (syncope)
- Broken needle
- Allergic reactions

Allergies. This refers to patients that are allergic to local anesthetics in general. For patients with "caine" allergies diphenhydramine (Benadryl) diluted to 1% may be used. The practitioner should be aware, however, that the manufacturer of Benadryl (Parke-Davis, Morris Plains, NJ) contraindicates the use of this drug as a local anesthetic because of the risk of local tissue necrosis. To use diphenhydramine as a local anesthetic the 5% solution (50 mg/ml) is mixed 1:4 with normal saline to make a 1% solution.[21] (Benadryl is commercially available as a 1% solution, i.e., 10 mg/ml, but the pH is adjusted between 5.0 and 6.0 with either NaOH or HCl. By diluting the 5% solution to 1% the pH becomes more neutralized and may cause less tissue necrosis). I have only used this agent for maxillary infiltration, and never for mandibular blocks. The onset of anesthesia is slower and the anesthesia achieved does not last very long, only about 15 minutes. Tissue necrosis and sloughing of the maxillary gingiva can be a problem if too large a volume is used. I try not to use more than 3 ml and have seen problems with sloughing of the buccal gingiva around a maxillary third molar.

REFERENCES

1. Butterworth JF, Strichartz GR: Molecular mechanisms of local anesthetics: A review, *Anesthesiology* 72:711-734, 1990.
2. Sicher H, DuBrul EL: *Oral anatomy*, ed 6, St. Louis, 1975, Mosby.
3. Wynn RL, Meiller TF, Crossley HL: Procaine hydrochloride, p. 727 and Chloroprocaine, p. 185. In: *Drug information handbook for dentistry*, ed 3, Cleveland, 1997-1998, Lexi-Comp.
4. Barker BCW, Davies PL: The applied anatomy of the Pterygomandibular space, *Br J Oral Surg* 10: 43-55, 1972.

5. Wilson S, Johns P, Fuller PM: The inferior alveolar and mylohyoid nerves: An anatomic study and relationship to local anesthesia of the anterior mandibular teeth, *JADA* 108: 350-352, March 1984.

6. Sillanpaa M, Vuori V, Lehtinen R: The mylohyoid nerve and mandibular anesthesia, *Int J Oral Maxillofac Surg* 17(3): 206-207, 1988.

7. Bremer G: Measurements of special significance in connection with anesthesia of the inferior alveolar nerve, *Oral Surg* 5: 966-988, 1952.

8. Kaban LB: Surgical correction of the facial skeleton in childhood. In Kaban LB, editor: *Pediatric oral and maxillofacial surgery*, Philadelphia, 1990, WB Saunders, p. 425.

9. *Manual of local anesthesia in general dentistry*, New York, Cook-Waite Laboratories, p. 12.

10. Malamed SF. *Handbook of local anesthesia*, ed 4, St. Louis, 1996, Mosby.

11. Kaufman E, Weinstein P, Milgrom P: Difficulties in achieving local anesthesia, *JADA* 108:205-208, 1984.

12. Northrop PM: Practical techniques in administration of local anesthetic agents. Part 11, *JADA* 38:444-448, 1949.

13. Akinosi JO: A new approach to the mandibular nerve block, *Br J Oral Surg* 15:83-87, 1977.

14. Gustains JF, Peterson LJ: An alternative method of mandibular nerve block, *JADA* 103:33-36, 1981.

15. Rood JP: The analgesia and innervation of mandibular teeth, *Br Dent J* 140:237-239, 1976.

16. DeJong RH: Neural blockage by local anesthetics, *JAMA* 238: 1383-1385, 1977.

17. Gow-Gates GA: Mandibular anesthesia, letter to the editor, *Austr Dent* J 23:117, 1978.

18. Gow-Gates GA: Mandibular conduction anesthesia: A new technique using extraoral landmarks, *Oral surg* 36(3):321-330, 1973.

19. Gow-Gates GA, Watson JE: The Gow-Gates mandibular block: Further understanding. *Anesth Prog* 24:183-189, 1977.

20. Watson JE, Gow-Gates GA: A clinical evaluation of the Gow-Gates mandibular block technique, *NZ Dent* J 72:220-223, 1976.

21. Graber MA: General surgery: Wound management. http://www.vh.org./Providers/clinRef/FPHandbook/chapter09/01-9.html. 1998.

4 Oral and Parenteral Sedation

STEVEN R. SCHWARTZ, DDS

HISTORY AND DEFINITIONS

No single medical advance has alleviated more human suffering than the discovery of anesthesia. The contributions of Dr. Horace Wells in utilizing nitrous oxide and Dr. William T.G. Morton using ether anesthesia for surgery in the 1840s, have forever changed the practice of dentistry and medicine.[1] By 1905 with the introduction of procaine local anesthesia, the dental profession had both general and local anesthesia for exodontia. In 1957, Langa and others started promoting the use of nitrous oxide as a "relative analgesic" at low concentrations combined with local anesthesia. This allowed for adequate pain control and light sedation to perform more time-consuming and prolonged restorative procedures. Later work by S.L. Drummond-Jackson in Great Britain and Niels Jorgenson in the United States with IV sedation showed that routine dental procedures could be done more safely with either local or general anesthesia alone. In the wake of these developments numerous routes of administration were tried, including intramuscular (IM), submucosal (SM), intravenous (IV), rectal (PR), and oral (PO). Additionally multiple techniques using various drugs singularly and in combination were promoted.

Defining and understanding the levels of sedation and anesthesia are important for education because the different stages represent different degrees of potential risk (Table 4-1).

Before one can administer sedation/anesthesia to a patient one must understand that the sedative effects of drugs represent a continuum of dose-related responses. These responses vary from light sedation to intense central nervous system (CNS) depression to death (Fig. 4-1).

Additionally, an individual patient's response relies not only on the dose of the drug but on the sensitivity of that patient to the drug. Therefore, a given dose of a particular drug might only result in light sedation in one patient whereas it may produce deep sedation or even general anesthesia in another patient.

PREOPERATIVE PATIENT EVALUATION

Any patient requiring in-office parenteral sedation must be thoroughly and accurately evaluated by the operating surgeon/anesthetist before any procedure commences. This process can be divided into three parts; though listed separately they are all interrelated. These are the history, brief physical examination, and laboratory screening tests, as indicated. The first and foremost is the history. This is the single most important aspect of patient evaluation. In obtaining a medical history many practitioners use a health questionnaire filled out by the patient during the initial visit. This form should cover all pertinent medical information including past and present illnesses, hospitalizations, surgical history, allergies, and current medications. The form should be easily understood by the patient and allow for yes/no answers. The end of the form should always contain an open-ended question such as, "Are there any other medical conditions or treatments past or present that we have not discussed?" This allows the patient to mention any other circumstances that may not be applicable to the yes/no-formatted questions already reviewed. A sample of a health history questionnaire is shown in Fig. 4-2.

The next step is the brief physical evaluation. The emphasis of the physical examination is on the respiratory, cardiac, and neurological systems. The examination includes blood pressure, pulse (rate and rhythm), respiratory rate, and weight. Auscultation of the lungs is necessary in patients with any significant pulmonary disorders to assess current respiratory status. A history of asthma, recent respiratory infection, COPD, or heavy smoking are a few examples. Cardiac auscultation should be performed if there is a question of a heart murmur or valvular abnormality. An overall impression of the patient's body type (that is, well developed versus cachectic versus obese) and general muscle tone can be made by observing the patient walking into the operatory and the ease with which they are able to seat

Normal ⟶ Light conscious ⟶ Deep sedation ⟶ General ⟶ Coma ⟶ Death
activity   sedation   anesthesia

FIG. 4-1 Dose-related responses to sedative drugs.

TABLE 4-1 Definitions of Pain and Anxiety Control Techniques

Category	Definition
Conscious sedation	A minimally depressed level of consciousness that retains the patient's ability to independently and continuously maintain an airway and respond appropriately to physical stimulation and verbal command and that is produced by a pharmacologic or nonpharmacologic method or a combination thereof.
Deep sedation	A controlled state of depressed consciousness, accompanied by a partial loss of protective reflexes, including the inability to continually maintain an airway independently and/or to respond purposefully to verbal commands, and is produced by a pharmacologic or nonpharmacologic method or a combination thereof.
General anesthesia	A controlled state of unconsciousness accompanied by a partial or complete loss of protective reflexes, including inability to independently maintain an airway and respond purposefully to physical stimulation or verbal command, and is produced by a pharmacologic or nonpharmacologic method or a combination thereof.

From the guidelines for teaching the comprehensive control of pain and anxiety in dentistry, ADA, Council on Dental Education, 1992.

TABLE 4-2 American Society of Anesthesiologists Physical Status Classification

Category	Description
ASA I	A normal healthy patient without systemic disease
ASA II	A patient with mild systemic disease (controlled), no functional limitations
ASA III	A patient with severe systemic disease, with functional limitations, not incapacitating
ASA IV	A patient with severe systemic disease, that is incapacitating and a constant threat to life
ASA V	A moribund patient not likely to survive 24 hours with or without an operation

themselves. At this point the patient is assigned a physical status category as per the American Society of Anesthesiologists (ASA) physical status classification system (Table 4-2).

Patients who fall into ASA categories I and II should pose no unusual risks in undergoing properly administered office sedation. Those patients in ASA categories III or IV may require additional evaluation. This may include specific laboratory tests and/or consultation with the patient's physician. Some patients may not be suitable for any office-based sedation technique, or sedation only in a hospital-type setting.

The third component of patient evaluation is the use of laboratory screening tests. This remains the most controversial and least utilized component of patient evaluation. A statistical analysis done by M.F. Roizen found in Miller's text on anesthesia,[2] gives recommended guidelines for screening tests in asymptomatic patients who show up healthy on examination and history. T.A. Nique, in his review,[3]

Have you ever had, or are you presently being treated for any of the following? Please check all that apply.

	Yes	No		Yes	No
Heart disease	___	___	High blood pressure	___	___
Heart murmur	___	___	Low blood pressure	___	___
Rheumatic fever	___	___	Anemia	___	___
Diabetes	___	___	Bleeding disorder	___	___
Asthma	___	___	Thyroid gland disease	___	___
Seizures	___	___	Hepatitis, liver disease	___	___
Artificial heart valve	___	___	Artificial joint(s)	___	___
Stomach ulcer(s)	___	___	Stroke	___	___
Psychiatric care	___	___	Cancer	___	___
Sinus problems	___	___	Venereal disease	___	___
General allergies	___	___	Chemical dependency	___	___
Drug allergies	___	___	Anesthetic allergies	___	___
*AIDS/HIV	___	___	Arthritis	___	___

(*May be illegal to ask in some states)

Please list all medications you are currently taking: _____

_____

Please list all drugs, medications and/or anesthetics you are allergic to: _____

_____

Have you ever responded adversely to medical or dental treatment? Yes ____ No ____

If so how? _____

If patient is a child, what is his or her weight? _____

Women: Do you suspect that you are pregnant? Yes ___ No ___ Are you nursing? Yes ___ No ___

Are there any other medical conditions or treatments past or present that we have not discussed? _____

_____

FIG. 4-2 Sample health history questionnaire.

summarized and tabulated Roizen's work shown in Table 4-3.

As the evaluator, one must remember that patients with systemic disease states (ASA II, III, and IV) should have the appropriate diagnostic tests based on the severity and type of medical problem. As stated previously consultation with the patient's primary physician or appropriate specialist, if applicable, can be helpful. Not only will you get their expert opinion on the patient's status but they may also have results from recent diagnostic tests that you might have ordered.

TABLE 4-3 Recommended Screening Studies for Asymptomatic Patients Who Appear Healthy by History and Physical Examination

Test	Under Age 40	Over Age 40	Over Age 60	On Antihypertensives or Diuretics
Chest x-ray			Yes	Yes
ECG		Yes	Yes	Yes
Hematocrit	Yes (females)	Yes (females)	Yes	
BUN/glucose		Yes	Yes	
Serum Na+/K+				Yes

PATIENT MONITORING

Patients undergoing sedation, whether in a hospital operating room or an outpatient office facility need to be accurately monitored throughout the course of the anesthetic. Monitor by definition can be either an individual who is observing the patient or a machine that is tracking or checking a process. The purpose of patient monitoring is to recognize abnormal changes in physiologic systems (such as respiratory, cardiac, and circulatory) before serious compromise and effect corrections to restore normalcy.

To monitor the respiratory system you need to be able to assess ventilation and oxygenation. Ventilation in the nonintubated, typical office patient can be checked by watching the rise and fall of the chest or movement of the reservoir bag during inhalation and exhalation, or auscultation with a precordial stethoscope placed in the sternal notch. In the intubated patient, a capnograph measuring end-tidal CO_2 is the most accurate breath-to-breath assessment. Previously oxygenation was only monitored visually by observing the color of the blood, oral mucosa, conjunctiva, and the skin. Now with the advent of pulse-oximetry hypoxia can be detected earlier than ever before. Pulse oximeters measure the ratio of oxygenated (saturated) to deoxygenated (desaturated) arterial blood and display a relative saturation value, SaO_2. Values of 90% and above are acceptable. Therefore, alarms should be set at 90% to warn against impending hypoxia.

To monitor the cardiovascular system one must be able to assess circulation, cardiac function, and blood pressure. Heart rate and rhythm were traditionally followed by palpation of a peripheral pulse and/or auscultation with the precordial stethoscope. With the introduction of electrocardiograms (ECG) rate, dysrhythmias, and ischemic changes can be monitored. Lead II is most commonly used in the office setting. Pulse-oximeters monitor heart rate as well as oxygen saturation. Because tachycardia is defined as a heart rate of 120 or greater and bradycardia as a rate of 60 or less, these values are good starting points for

TABLE 4-4 Recommended Monitoring Techniques During Sedation

Monitor	Parenteral Conscious Sedation	Deep Sedation/General Anesthesia
Direct clinical observation	Yes	Yes
Precordial stethoscope		Yes
Pulse oximeter	Yes	Yes
Sphygmomanometer	Yes	Yes
Electrocardiograph	Yes	Yes
Thermometer		Available
Capnograph		Yes (if intubated)

setting internal machine alarms. Blood pressure can be monitored by manual sphygmomanometers or more recently by automated noninvasive blood pressure (NIBP) machines. These devices can be set to automatically take a blood pressure reading at whatever minute interval you elect. Some units will even give you a printed record.

In October 1998, the American Dental Association adopted *Guidelines for the Use of Conscious Sedation, Deep Sedation and General Anesthesia for Dentists.* Section V covers clinical guidelines. Sections V-B, parenteral conscious sedation, and V-C, deep sedation/general anesthesia, are summarized in Table 4-4.

Every sedation should include a record of the anesthesia as well as chart notes for the dental/surgical procedure. Most anesthesia records are abridged versions of the ones used by anesthesiologists in the hospital. This allows you to keep track of the time drugs are given and record the blood pressure, pulse, SaO_2, and ECG in a graphic format. Basic information should include the following: patient's name, age, weight, ASA classification, monitors, medications, vital signs every 5 to 15 minutes, procedure, and surgeon. Many records also have a space for postoperative vital signs and condition at discharge.

The skill and vigilance of a trained, experienced clinician can never be discounted, but the addition of electronic/mechanical monitors should be considered an extra margin of safety to avoid untoward outcomes.

INHALATION ANALGESIA/SEDATION

Nitrous oxide is a colorless nonirritating gas with a mild slightly sweet odor. The gas is stored in a compressed state in cylinders as a liquid at 760 PSI. At 500 PSI only compressed gas remains which will quickly become exhausted.

Nitrous oxide has a blood/gas partition coefficient of 0.47 and is, therefore, poorly soluble in blood. It is excreted unchanged by the lungs. It is nonflammable although it can support combustion in the absence of oxygen. Because of its low solubility in blood nitrous oxide rapidly equilibrates between alveolar and arterial concentration gradients. Hence, both induction and emergence times are very short. The main disadvantage of nitrous oxide is its lack of potency. The highest safe concentration of nitrous oxide is 80%, the remaining 20% being oxygen, the same concentration as found in room air. At this concentration of nitrous oxide and oxygen the deepest plane of anesthesia that can be achieved is Stage I (analgesia). At subanesthetic doses of 30% to 40%, nitrous oxide produces excellent analgesia. Sixty percent is generally the maximum concentration for good analgesia and to allow the patient to maintain verbal contact with the clinician. At 30% nitrous oxide's analgesic effect has been compared to 10 mg of morphine sulfate. It is also useful as a euphoric agent at clinically useful concentrations.

At the conclusion of a nitrous oxide/oxygen sedation, one must remember to administer 100% oxygen for about 3 minutes to avoid diffusion hypoxia. This happens because at the conclusion of a sedation large volumes of nitrous oxide diffuse out quickly into the alveoli of the lung diluting the available oxygen and reducing the alveolar oxygen concentration. Another cause for the hypoxia, is the dilution of alveolar carbon dioxide resulting in the decrease respiratory drive and ventilation.[4]

For the safety of office personnel waste nitrous oxide gas must be kept to the lowest possible levels by using scavenging systems, laminar flow operatory ventilation, and intraoral suction with external exhaust ports.

NARCOTICS

The prototypical narcotic is morphine sulfate, even though it is rarely used for sedation today. Narcotics act primarily in the central nervous system (CNS) on the μ-receptors producing depressed ventilation, euphoria, sedation, and spinal analgesia. By themselves narcotics will not cause loss of consciousness in young healthy patients. Therefore, they are not true sedative or anesthetic agents. Because of their peripheral vasodilating effect a small drop in blood pressure can be expected, but in the semireclining, normovolemic patient it should not be clinically important.

Meperidine (Demerol) has been used successfully for many years in outpatient oral and maxillofacial surgery. At its normal dosage range of 25 to 100 mg its sedative and analgesic effects are useful both intra- and postoperative. The actions of meperidine are similar to morphine except that its onset of action is much quicker (3 to 5 minutes) and its duration of action is shorter. However, it is only 15% as potent. Compared with morphine sulfate, meperidine produces less depression of the cough reflex. It is also metabolized by the liver. Because meperidine can cause significant respiratory depression it should be given slowly over several minutes while being titrated to effect. Because of its ability to cause respiratory depression and release of histamine, meperidine should be avoided in patients with severe asthma. It is also contraindicated in patients taking, or who have taken monoamine oxidase (MAO) inhibitors within the last 14 days. This is because of the possible fatal hypotension and or respiratory depression that can occur. The effects of meperidine can be reversed with naloxone.

Fentanyl (Sublimaze) is a potent narcotic useful in outpatient sedation because of its analgesic and sedative effects. It is approximately 100 times more potent than morphine sulfate and 750 times more potent than meperidine. The approximate equipotent dosages are: fentanyl 0.1 mg, morphine sulfate 10 mg, and meperidine 75 mg. Fentanyl causes decreases in the respiratory rate and alveolar ventilation. These undesirable respiratory effects will outlast its analgesic effects. There is less nausea and practically no release of histamine with fentanyl. The average dosage range is from 0.05 mg to 0.2 mg. Fentanyl's rapid (almost immediate) onset of action and shorter duration of action (about 30 minutes) make it an excellent choice for outpatient sedation. The reported problem of "chest wall rigidity" making it difficult to ventilate the patient seems to be related to a too-rapid injection of the drug. Because of its negative respiratory effects it should be used with great care in patients with pulmonary compromise. Fentanyl's effects can also be reversed with naloxone. However, one must remember that the respiratory depressant effects of fentanyl will outlast the reversal effects of naloxone.

BENZODIAZEPINES

Since benzodiazepines were introduced into outpatient sedation in the mid 1960s, they have dominated the field as both single agents and as part of multiple agent techniques. The two most popular benzodiazepines are diazepam (Valium) and midazolam (Versed), introduced in the 1980s.

Benzodiazepines act upon the limbic system (an area of the brain associated with emotion and behavior), thalamus, and hypothalamus. It also interacts with gamma aminobutyric acid (GABA) receptors. These sites of action account for benzodiazepines' calming and antiemetic effect, euphoria, amnesia, and muscle relaxation. However, benzodiazepines have no inherent analgesic properties.

The cardiac effects of the benzodiazepines are negligible. They can cause a minimal decrease in cardiac output as a result of a mild negative inotropic effect and venodilation. Typically a compensatory positive chronotropic response maintains the cardiac output. As the aforementioned effects are so minimal, benzodiazepines are often used in cardiac patients as premedication and as part of the induction sequence for general anesthesia.

The respiratory consequences of the benzodiazepines are their most serious side effect when being administered as part of a conscious sedation. Usually the tidal volume decreases while the respiratory rate increases. The net effects of these changes essentially cancel each other and the patient maintains an adequate minute ventilation. Benzodiazepines, particularly midazolam, depress the ventilatory response to increasing levels of $PaCO_2$ to a clinically significant effect. This undesirable effect is more marked in patients with pre-existing respiratory disease (such as COPD). Because the degrees of respiratory depression and sedation do not necessarily coincide, monitoring of the patient's oxygen saturation (SaO_2) is important.

Benzodiazepines are contraindicated in patients with acute narrow angle glaucoma, and open-angle glaucoma unless they are receiving appropriate treatment.

Diazepam is lipophilic (insoluble in water) and compounded with propylene glycol and ethyl alcohol to make it suitable for intravenous use. The same compounds that enable diazepam's parenteral use are attributed to its vascular irritating effect which can lead to pain and/or local phlebitis. Therefore, it should not be used in small veins, such as the wrist or the dorsum of the hand. Diazepam should not be mixed or diluted with other drugs. It should be injected slowly, no more than 5 mg (1 ml) per minute. Extreme care should be taken to avoid inadvertent intraarterial injection or extravasation into the subcutaneous tissues. Diazepam's lipophilic property accounts for its rapid absorption and onset (peak, 3 to 5 minutes). In addition, diazepam's lipophilic properties cause it to be accumulated in body fat and then slowly re-released into the circulatory system and ultimately metabolized. This in addition to its active metabolites (desmethyldiazepam and

oxazepam) account for diazepam's prolonged half-life of 20 to 50 hours. When diazepam is used in a sedative technique including narcotics, the calculated narcotic dose should be reduced by one third and administered in small increments.

Diazepam has a long and proven track record in outpatient sedation in oral and maxillofacial surgery. It is readily available, relatively inexpensive, and has a proven safety record.

Midazolam is a short acting benzodiazepine that unlike diazepam is soluble in water making it less irritating to veins and surrounding tissues. It is approximately two to three times as potent as diazepam. The onset of action is dependent on concomitant narcotic premedication and the total dose of midazolam administered. In sedative doses, with healthy patients under 60 years old, midazolam should be given slowly, no more than 2.5 mg per 2 minutes, to allow time to fully evaluate the sedative effect. With patients over 60, chronically ill, or debilitated, the rate of administration should be decreased to 1.5 mg per 2 minutes. The onset of action of midazolam alone for sedation is 3 to 5 minutes. At induction doses for general anesthesia it decreases to 2 to 2.5 minutes. With narcotic premedication, onset times further decrease to 1.5 minutes. If other CNS depressants are used concomitantly the midazolam dose should be reduced by about 30%. Even though midazolam's half-life is only 2 to 4 hours, much shorter than diazepam's, clinical recovery from sedation is much the same.

In pediatric sedation several routes of administration are available depending on the child's age and degree of cooperation. Techniques include intranasal and oral. An intranasal dose of 2 to 3 mg will usually provide sedation in 5 to 10 minutes, depending on the child's size. Oral midazolam at 0.5 mg/kg mixed with fruit juice produces sedation in 5 to 10 minutes with the peak effect at about 15 minutes.

KETAMINE

Ketamine (Ketalar) was introduced into human clinical practice as an anesthetic in 1965. In 1970 it was introduced into the United States. Ketamine was a new type of anesthetic classified as "dissociative anesthesia." Ketamine is a derivative of phencyclidine (PCP/"angel dust"). Undesirable side effects elucidated in early trials adversely affected ketamine's use. Later, newer techniques including dosage adjustments and combining it with other sedative drugs have decreased the incidence of its unpleasant side effects.

Ketamine is a slightly acidic sterile solution (pH 3.5 to 5.5) that is water-soluble. It can be administered either IV or IM and is nonirritating. It is highly lipid-soluble and therefore readily crosses the blood–brain barrier. Administered intravenously at doses of 2 mg/kg the onset of dissociative anesthesia is 30 to 60 seconds, the duration of anesthesia being about 5 to 10 minutes. Given intramuscularly, at doses ranging from 9 to 13 mg/kg, the onset of surgical anesthesia is about 3 minutes, lasting 12 to 25 minutes. When used intravenously ketamine should be administered slowly, over 60 seconds, to decrease the incidence of respiratory depression and/or a hypertensive response. The elimination half-life of ketamine varies from 1 to 2 hours in children to 2 to 3 hours in adults.

The central nervous system effects of ketamine are profound. The state described as "dissociative anesthesia" is characterized by intense analgesia, amnesia, and catalepsy. Patients appear to be in a cataleptic state in which their eyes remain open with slow nystagmus and intact corneal reflexes. The dissociation component refers to a disruption of the pathways between the thalamoneocortical and limbic systems. This prevents the higher cortical centers from receiving painful stimuli as well as visual and auditory signals. Generally the patient is noncommunicative, though he appears to be awake. Varying degrees of muscle hypertonus may be seen, including twitching and random limb movements. These should not be mistaken for seizure activity as EEGs have not shown seizure-like activity associated with ketamine administration. Ketamine may even possess anticonvulsant properties. Ketamine is a potent dilator of the cerebral vasculature. This in turn, along with increases in blood pressure, is responsible for increased intracranial pressure.

Emergence phenomena have been the most often reported unfavorable side effects of ketamine. The reactions have been described as a feeling of floating, vivid dreams (pleasant and unpleasant), hallucinations, and delirium. This occurs more commonly in female patients between the ages of 16 and 65. Patients younger than 16 or older than 65 seem to have a much lower incidence. Emergence phenomena may be reduced by intramuscular administration. Allowing the patient to recover in a quiet area with subdued lighting and minimal physical contact can also help lessen the severity of emergence reactions. The most effective way of reducing unpleasant emergence reactions is the prior administration of certain sedative drugs. The benzodiazepines are the most effective agents thus far.

The effects of ketamine are multifocal. The cardiovascular system is stimulated following ketamine administration. The heart rate, systemic vascular resistance, and systolic blood pressure all increase. This causes an increase in myocardial oxygen consumption. In the healthy patient this is accommodated by increased coronary artery blood flow. This is one reason why ketamine must be used with caution in patients with coronary artery disease. They may not be able to satisfy the extra myocardial oxygen demands. These cardiovascular changes are not dose-specific. They may occur with low to dissociative (0.5 to 1.5 mg/kg) doses. Oddly enough, a second dose of ketamine can produce cardiovascular effects exactly opposite to those of the first dose.

One special feature of ketamine is its minimal negative respiratory effects even at full anesthetic doses, as long as it is given slowly. The patient will be able to maintain her own airway. Both protective airway reflexes as well as spontaneous respirations remain intact. Ketamine can significantly stimulate tracheobronchial secretions and salivation, which can make a patient prone to laryngospasm. Premedication with either atropine or glycopyrrolate is beneficial, however scopolamine is best avoided because of its possible side effects including hallucinations and confusion. Ketamine's beneficial respiratory effects include decreased airway resistance and increased lung compliance. Bronchodilation induced by ketamine via sympathetic stimulation and direct smooth muscle relaxation protects the patient from the development of bronchospasm. Because ketamine can also reduce symptoms of acute asthma present at the time of induction it would therefore appear to be indicated in the asthmatic patient.

BARBITURATES

Since 1960 methohexital (Brevital) has been used for the induction of general anesthesia as well as an anesthetic maintenance agent for brief surgical procedures. Methohexital is an ultra–short-acting barbiturate and is the most commonly used barbiturate by oral and maxillofacial surgeons for office-based outpatient sedation. Compared with its predecessors, thiamylal (Surital) and thiopental (Pentothal), methohexital is twice as potent with one half the duration of action. Though not fully understood, the CNS effects of barbiturates seem to depress ascending neuronal activity through the reticular activating system (RAS). The degree of this depressive effect is dose-dependent, progressing from sedation to hypnosis to anesthesia, through coma, and ultimately death. Barbiturates have no inherent analgesic properties; in fact they may actually be antianalgesic and enhance painful stimuli. There are no specific reversal agents for the barbiturates.

Methohexital comes as a freeze-dried, sterile powder that is reconstituted with either sterile water or 0.9% sodium chloride (normal saline). The instructions for dilution/preparation must be followed exactly. When used in adults for intravenous injection methohexital is usually prepared as a 1% (10 mg/ml) solution. The average adult general anesthesia induction dose of methohexital is 1.0 mg/kg to 1.5 mg/kg given at a rate of 1 ml/5 seconds. The usual duration of anesthesia is 5 to 7 minutes. Maintenance doses of 20 mg to 40 mg every 4 to 7 minutes or a continuous drip of a 0.2% solution at about 3 ml/minute should be adequate. When used in pediatric anesthesia either intramuscularly or rectally it is diluted to either a 5% solution or 1% solution, respectively. When reconstituted methohexital has a basic pH of 10 to 11. Therefore, it should not be mixed or given simultaneously with acidic drugs (such as atropine, succinylcholine, and scopolamine) because a precipitate of free barbituric acid may form. Additionally, because of its high pH, methohexital is caustic and can lead to superficial tissue sloughing and necrosis if extravasated subcutaneously during injection. If inadvertently injected intraarterially the results can range from thrombosis to distal necrosis to gangrene, which may require amputation. Previously, for years, reconstituted methohexital that was refrigerated was usable for up to 6 weeks. Although the chemical formulation has not been changed, the current manufacturers' recommendation is that reconstituted solution should be used within 24 hours. Methohexital should not be used on patients with known barbiturate allergy or with porphyria.

Methohexital is lipid-soluble at physiologic pH and rapidly diffuses into the vessel-rich group (that is, the brain) within 30 seconds of intravenous injection. This accounts for its rapid onset of action. The short duration of action is attributable to its speedy redistribution into skeletal muscle, fat, and other vessel-poor groups. Secondly, since methohexital does not appear to concentrate in fat as much as the other barbiturates do, cumulative effects are less and recovery is faster. Methohexital is eliminated through the liver by demethylation and oxidation and excreted via the kidneys.

In addition to the previously mentioned CNS effects barbiturates exert other effects. They decrease intracranial pressure by reducing cerebral blood flow. There is also decreased cortical brain activity as seen on an EEG. Methohexital, however often increases EEG activity which is why it is the anesthetic of choice of some psychiatrists for electroconvulsive therapy (ECT). Yet this is a relative contraindication for methohexital's use in patients with a history of seizures. In some patients methohexital will cause an idiosyncratic reaction eliciting excitement rather than depression and the patient may appear inebriated. If this occurs, discontinue the methohexital and either modify your sedation plan or finish the case under local anesthesia.

Methohexital is a direct myocardial and medullary vasomotor center depressant. This causes a temporary drop in blood pressure of anywhere from 10% to 25% because of the decreased stroke volume and peripheral vasodilation. A mild compensatory tachycardia develops as a result of the decrease in peripheral vascular resistance. The resulting cardiac output is only mildly decreased from the baseline in healthy individuals.

Barbiturates including methohexital produce a dose-related depression of the medullary and pontine areas of respiratory control. They also decrease the brain's sensitivity to changes in blood pH and CO_2 levels ("CO_2 drive") and depress the sensitivity of the chemoreceptors in the carotid and aortic bodies to O_2 concentration (hypoxic drive). This respiratory depression is characterized by a reduced rate and tidal volume, which can significantly diminish minute ventilation. At the point where all three of the above mechanisms are abated respiration ceases altogether.

Previously it was thought that barbiturates themselves caused laryngospasm and bronchospasm. This is not true at sedative/hypnotic doses. However, if a patient passes into the plane of deep sedation or general anesthesia, and is not be able to protect his airway, direct laryngeal stimulation from saliva, blood, irrigation, or instrumentation will trigger a laryngospasm or bronchospasm.

REVERSAL AGENTS

At this point in time specific reversal agents only exist for the opioid and benzodiazepine classes of drugs commonly used for office-based sedation in oral and maxillofacial surgery.

Naloxone (Narcan) is the only pure opioid antagonist available for parenteral use. It reverses all of the effects of opioids including respiratory depression, sedation, analgesia, and hypotension. Naloxone accomplishes this by competitively binding to all of the various narcotic receptor sites in the CNS. By replacing the agonists at the receptor sites the prenarcotized state is rapidly restored.

Naloxone can be administered intravenously, intramuscularly, and subcutaneously. The onset of action is about 2 minutes after intravenous injection. It is only slightly slower when administered intramuscularly or subcutaneously. The duration of action of naloxone varies from 31 to 81 minutes (mean time 64 minutes) and is dose and route of administration dependent. Intramuscular dosing results in a prolonged release and therefore prolonged duration of action compared with intravenous administration. Even so, the respiratory and sedation reversal effects of naloxone are shorter than many narcotic agonists and patients must be carefully monitored for possible renarcotization. Although large doses of naloxone can be and are used in life-threatening situations it is more advisable to use it in smaller doses titrated to effect if the situation permits. Incremental doses of 0.1 mg to 0.2 mg intravenously every 2 to 3 minutes allows for partial reversal of the respiratory depression and sedation without significant reversal of the analgesic effects. Large rapid doses may completely reverse the analgesia and have been shown to cause hypertension, tachycardia, nausea, and vomiting. A total dose of 10 mg is considered a maximal reversal dose and no additional benefit is expected after that. Doses approaching this are usually only seen in cases of illicit narcotic overdose.

Flumazenil (Romazicon) is a recently available benzodiazepine-specific reversal agent. Other nonspecific agents previously used, including physostigmine and aminophylline, will not be discussed as they have been replaced by flumazenil.

Flumazenil is an imidazobenzodiazepine that is a pure benzodiazepine antagonist in humans. It reverses the effects of benzodiazepines on the CNS by competitively binding with the benzodiazepine receptors in the GABA complex. It does not inhibit other depressant drugs that bind to other sites in the GABA complex such as barbiturates, ethanol, and general anesthetics. Neither will it antagonize narcotic effects.

Intravenous flumazenil will reverse sedation, amnesia, psychomotor impairment, and respiratory depression. The degree and duration of the antagonistic effects are dependent upon dose and plasma concentration over time. The reversal effects are apparent within 1 to 3 minutes, with the peak effect attained at 6 to 10 minutes. With a terminal half-life of approximately 60 minutes flumazenil's effect is shorter than that of diazepam or midazolam. Therefore, resedation is possible when large doses of agonists are used. However, the doses usually employed in office sedation should avoid this problem.

Flumazenil is recommended for intravenous use only. It is packaged in multidose vials containing 0.1 mg/ml. It is a mildly acidic solution (pH 4) and should be given through a free flowing intravenous line into a large vein. The initial dose to counteract the benzodiazepine effect is 0.2 mg (2 ml) given over 15 seconds. If the desired endpoint is not reached after waiting another 45 seconds, additional doses of 0.2 mg (2 ml) may be administered up to a total dose of 1.0 mg (10 ml).

ADMINISTRATION TECHNIQUES

Numerous routes of administration are available for sedation techniques including, inhalation (IH), oral (PO), submucosal (SM), intramuscular (IM), intravenous (IV), and rectal (PR).

For the purposes of conscious sedation, inhalation techniques of sedation are limited to N_2O/O_2. Its ease of use, rapid onset, and rapid recovery are its advantages. The disadvantages are its relative impotence and how nasal hoods can interfere with the surgical procedure.

Oral is probably the easiest and most convenient route while at the same time being the least predictable. Between the effects of gastric enzymes, contents, and rate of emptying, gastric absorption is unpredictable. Add to that emesis following ingestion or expectoration because of bad taste, and you have no idea of the dose actually received.

The number of drugs that can be given subcutaneously for conscious sedation is few. Most of the medications are too irritating and would cause sloughing. Two useful medications that can be administered SC in the oral cavity are atropine and succinylcholine.

Intramuscular is the second most rapid rate of absorption of a parenterally administered medication. Only intravenously injected drugs act faster. The ability to administer IM injections even to uncooperative patients make this technique particularly suited for pediatric and uncooperative mentally disabled adults. Three main anatomic areas are suitable for IM injection. The most commonly considered site is the buttock, specifically the gluteus medius muscle. This area is well suited for adults. In children the gluteus medius muscle is small and composed mostly of fat. To give this injection in the proper area and avoid the sciatic nerve and superior gluteal artery, draw an imaginary diagonal line from the posterior superior iliac crest down to the greater trochanter of the femur. Insert a 22-gauge 1-1/2 inch needle above the imaginary line perpendicular to the skin deep into the muscle layer (Fig. 4-3), and aspirate to ensure the needle is not within a blood vessel; if so withdraw the needle and select another site. If the aspiration is negative, inject slowly and smoothly emptying the syringe completely. The vastus lateralis muscle of the lateral aspect of the anterior thigh is another recommended site, particularly for children. To administer the injection aim for the lateral aspect of the anterior thigh, pointed from anterior to posterior about 1 inch deep (Fig. 4-4). Finally, the deltoid muscle of the upper arm is an often-used site because it is the most easily accessed. However, it is generally the smallest muscle mass of the three and the number of injections and volume of the injection should be limited (Fig. 4-5).

Intravenous administration allows introduction of the medications directly into the bloodstream and therefore has the most rapid effect. Medications administered IV bypass the problems of variable absorption and the most predictable and consistent blood levels are obtained. Sedative agents can be given as multiple small doses allowing the patient to be "titrated to effect," to achieve the desired level of sedation. Because the technical aspects of IV cannulation are more demanding, practice is required. Additionally, a relatively cooperative patient is required.

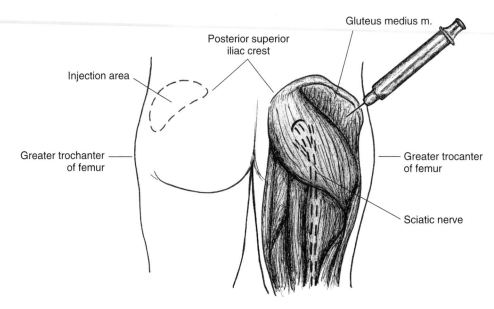

FIG. 4-3   The dorsogluteal site for an intramuscular injection.

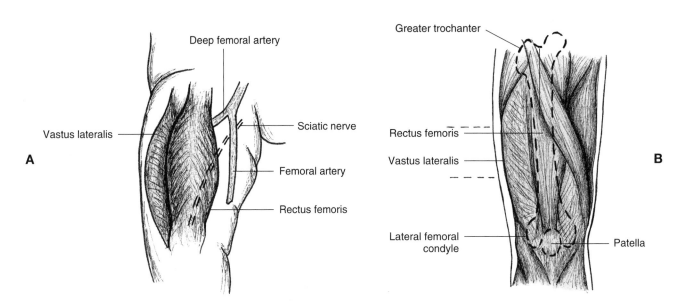

FIG. 4-4   **A,** The vastus lateralis muscle of the upper thigh, used for intramuscular injections on children. **B,** The vastus lateralis site for intramuscular injections on adults.

Therefore, not all patients, such as very young children, are good candidates.

Three basic types of cannulas are generally used for short outpatient office-based sedation cases. They are the traditional hollow "straight" needle, a winged or "butterfly needle," and an indwelling plastic catheter over the needle units. The basic technique of venipuncture is the same for all three. Except with the plastic catheter units, once the vein is entered, the catheter is advanced over the needle into the vein and the needle is withdrawn. As important as technique is proper venipuncture site selection. Although most superficial veins are suitable for use, the veins of the antecubital fossa are most commonly utilized. The median basilic (ulnar side) and median cephalic (radial side) veins of the arm are usually large caliber and easily accessible. The basilic and cephalic veins immediately above the antecubital fossa and of the forearm below are also commonly selected sites for venipuncture (Fig. 4-6). Usually an 18 or 20 gauge needle/catheter is sufficient for conscious sedation. However, small veins will necessitate using smaller needles/catheters.

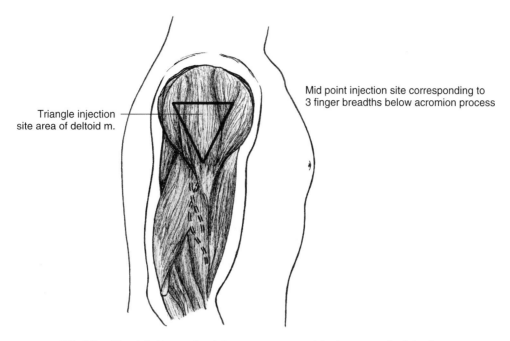

Triangle injection
site area of deltoid m.

Mid point injection site corresponding to
3 finger breadths below acromion process

FIG. 4-5   The deltoid muscle of the upper arm, used for intramuscular injections.

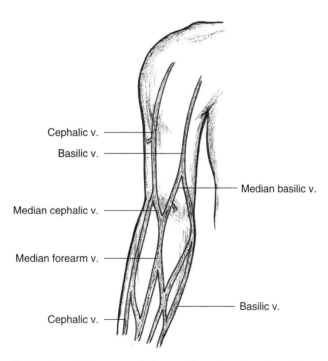

Cephalic v.

Basilic v.

Median basilic v.

Median cephalic v.

Median forearm v.

Basilic v.

Cephalic v.

FIG. 4-6   Superficial veins of the upper limb, anterior view. Note the difference in arrangement in front of the elbow; the median basilic and median cephalic veins are variants of the vena mediana cubiti.

SEDATION TECHNIQUES
Adult

Patients presenting for conscious sedation should have refrained from eating (NPO) solids for 8 hours. Clear noncarbonated liquids can be imbibed up to 3 hours preoperatively. The patient is placed in the chair and all necessary monitors for the type of anesthesia planned are attached. Presedation vital signs are obtained and recorded. Based on the patient medical evaluation, psychological state, and type and length of procedure to be performed suitable agents are selected. Nitrous oxide/oxygen inhalation is started via nasal hood, gradually being increased to the desired level. Intravenous access is obtained and continuous infusion started. Usually the sedative/anxiolytic agent (benzodiazepine) is administered first. After waiting a sufficient length of time to gauge its effect an analgesic agent (narcotic or ketamine) may be added. Finally, as needed on an individual basis, an amnesic agent (barbiturate) can be added. Specifically diazepam starting with a test dose of 2.5 mg or midazolam at 0.5 to 1.0 mg may be given. This is followed by either meperidine at 25 to 100 mg or fentanyl at 25 to 100 µg. Lastly, methohexital can be given at a 20 mg test dose, followed by incremental doses of 20 to 60 mg to achieve the desired level of sedation or anesthesia. A second technique including a benzodiazepine and substituting ketamine at 0.5 to 1.0 mg/kg for the narcotic and eliminating methohexital is also an option to be considered.

Pediatric

Those who routinely treat children are well aware that the surgery is the easy part; it is the anesthetic management that presents the greatest difficulty. Children (ages 2 to 8) often are not suitable candidates for venipuncture and, therefore, require alternate routes of administering sedation. The most commonly used by dentists are oral (PO) and intramuscular (IM). Table 4-5 lists commonly used single- and multiple-agent techniques by route of administration.

MEDICAL EMERGENCIES DURING OUTPATIENT SEDATION
Recognition and Management

When taking on the responsibility of administering outpatient sedation one must also be prepared to handle the associated complications that can arise. These can be secondary to either the sedation and/or the surgical procedure. Box 4-1 includes some of the more commonly discussed emergencies. Remember, in all cases terminate the procedure, pack the surgical site to control bleeding, and monitor the patient's vital signs.

TABLE 4-5 Commonly Used Single- and Multiple-Agent Techniques by Route of Administration for Pediatric Sedation

Drug	Dose	Onset of Action	Duration of Action
ORAL REGIMENS			
Single Drug			
Diazepam	0.3-0.7 mg/kg	30-45 min.	1-2 hr.
Midazolam	0.5 mg/kg (mixed with sweetened juice)	5-10 min.	30 min.
Ketamine	5-6 mg/kg	20-25 min.	30-45 min.
Combined Oral			
Midazolam	0.4 mg/kg	20 min.	30-45 min.
Ketamine	4.0 mg/kg	20 min.	30-45 min.
INTRAMUSCULAR			
Single Drug			
Midazolam	0.1-0.2 mg/kg	5-15 min.	30 min.
Ketamine	1.0-4.0 mg/kg	5-15 min.	15-30 min.
Combined Intramuscular			
Midazolam	0.03 mg/kg	5-15 min.	30 min.
Ketamine	3.0 mg/kg	5-15 min.	30 min.

BOX
4-1 Common Medical Emergencies During Outpatient Sedation

SYNCOPE / PSYCHOGENIC SHOCK

Signs and Symptoms
Pallor
Diaphoresis
Nausea
Lightheadedness
Hypotension
Tachycardia progressing to bradycardia

Treatment
Trendelenburg position
100% oxygen
Ammonia inhalants
0.5 mg Atropine for persistent bradycardia

LARYNGOSPASM

Signs and Symptoms
High pitched "crowing" on inspiration with partial obstruction
Absence of breath sounds with total obstruction
Suprasternal retraction on inspiration

Treatment
Pull tongue forward
Suction oral cavity and pharynx
Push on chest to break spasm
If not successful give 10 mg succinylcholine IV

BRONCHOSPASM

Signs and Symptoms
Impaired respiratory exchange
Inspiratory and expiratory wheezing
Decreased lung compliance
Cyanosis

Treatment
100% positive pressure oxygen
Intubation
Epinephrine 0.3-0.5 mg SC or 0.3-0.5 mg of 1:10,000 IV Aminophylline up to 50 mg/min

ASPIRATION

Signs and Symptoms
Patient seen aspirating
Wheezing, rales and rhonchi
Tachypnea, tachycardia, cyanosis
Progressive hypotension

Treatment
If patient coughing allow to do so
If not, Trendelenburg on right side
Suction/clear oral cavity, pharynx
100% oxygen
Consider intubation
Activate EMS

ANGINA PECTORIS

Signs and Symptoms
Intense substernal chest pain
Pain lasts only a few minutes
Related to increased emotional stress

Treatment
Sublingual nitroglycerin tablets every 5 minutes, up to 3 times
100% oxygen
IV narcotics for pain relief
If no improvement after nitro X3 consider myocardial infarction

MYOCARDIAL INFARCTION

Signs and Symptoms
Severe "crushing" substernal chest pain radiating to left arm
Pain not relieved by nitroglycerin
Pallor
Diaphoresis
Anxiety
Hypotension

Treatment
Sublingual nitroglycerin tablets every 5 minutes, up to 3 times
100% oxygen
Activate EMS
IV Morphine 2-10 mg for pain relief and preload reduction
Monitor ECG and treat arrhythmias

REFERENCES

1. Ring ME: *Dentistry: An illustrated history*, St. Louis, 1986, Mosby.
2. Roizen MF: Preoperative evaluation: laboratory tests in asymptomatic populations. In Miller, RD: *Anesthesia*, 3e, New York, 1990, Churchill-Livingstone.
3. Nique TA: Preanesthetic evaluation of the ambulatory oral surgery patient, *Oral Maxillofac Surg Clin North Am* (4):743-751, 1992.
4. Rackow H, Salamitre E, Frumin MH: Dilution of alveolar gases during nitrous oxide excretion in man, *J Appl Physiol* 16:723, 1961.

5 Perioperative Hemorrhage

ORRETT E. OGLE, DDS

Successful management of perioperative hemorrhage in the patient undergoing a minor oral surgical procedure will entail three aspects:

1. Preoperative identification of patients with a possible bleeding diathesis
2. Minimization of blood loss during the surgical procedure
3. Identification and elimination or correction of the causes of postsurgical bleeding and reestablishment of adequate hemostasis

PREOPERATIVE IDENTIFICATION OF PATIENTS WITH A POSSIBLE BLEEDING DIATHESIS

Because of the potentially high morbidity associated with hemostatic failure in the surgical patient, each patient should be carefully assessed before surgery for risk of bleeding. Several studies have shown that the most valuable preoperative screen to predict bleeding complications is a comprehensive clinical history. In a review by Peterson and colleagues only 2 of 17 patients (12%) who experienced excessive bleeding at surgery were prospectively classified as "high risk" based on the results of bleeding time tests.[1] Because the history is so important the dental surgeon should try to elicit information from the patient about known hemostatic disorders, any history of bleeding from previous surgery, and a history of current medication usage, including both prescription and nonprescription drugs (Box 5-1). Drug usage is the most common undocumented cause of bleeding in the oral surgical patient. A special emphasis should be placed on nonsteroidal antiinflammatory drugs (NSAIDs), because they are currently the most widely used drugs that may cause bleeding. Anticoagulants and antibiotics are another important group of drugs that should be investigated.

Bleeding disorders may either be intrinsic or acquired. Intrinsic disorders are inherited and bleeding results from congenitally deficient or dysfunctional components of the hemostatic system. Acquired disorders result because of an underlying condition or disease (Box 5-2).

Based on the history, the patient may be placed into a risk category as outlined in Box 5-3. From this classification the procedures listed in Table 5-1 should be followed.

Management of Specific Problems Affecting Hemostasis

Aspirin and NSAIDs. NSAIDs are a widely used group of drugs. Prescribed or purchased over the counter, they are taken for pain or chronic inflammatory conditions. Aspirin in low dosage is used as an anticoagulant in patients following bypass surgery.

Both aspirin (ASA) and NSAIDs inhibit thromboxane A_2 synthesis, causing a decrease in ADP release and ultimately a decrease in platelet aggregation. In these patients bleeding time will be prolonged. It should be noted that ASA can inhibit platelet function even after as low a dose as 300 mg, and that its effect may last for several days until sufficient new platelets have been produced to correct the defect.

For patients on low-dose aspirin therapy the drug should be stopped 7 to 10 days before the dental procedure because aspirin affects platelet function for up to 7 to 10 days after its use has been stopped. However, the treating physician must be consulted before the aspirin is stopped. If the risk of discontinuing the aspirin is high, and the surgical procedure is minor, the problem of bleeding may be managed by local methods. Gelfoam or Gelfoam soaked with topical thrombin may be placed in the extraction site and the gingival margins tightly secured with sutures. The purpose of sutures here is to maintain pressure on the wound for initial hemostasis. At other surgical sites where the use of Gelfoam may be impractical, then a layer of topical collagen may be used.

The effects of NSAIDs on platelets is quantitatively less and of shorter duration than aspirin. NSAIDs should be stopped 2 to 3 days before surgery.

Warfarin (Coumadin). Anticoagulation with warfarin is often used as a preventive measure for embolic phenomena related to several conditions. Some of the most common ones are atrial fibrillation, dilated car-

BOX 5-1 History to Assess Surgical Risk for Bleeding

Major Risk Factors	Minor Risk Factors

1. Bleeding with prior surgical procedures:
  • Extraction of teeth or periodontal surgery
  • Excess bleeding following any minor surgical procedure.
2. Obstetric Bleeding:
  • Heavy menstrual flow
3. Liver Disease:
  • Hepatitis B and C
  • Cirrhosis
  • Chronic alcohol abuse
4. Renal Disease
5. Known hereditary diseases:
  • Hemophilia
  • Von Willebrand's disease
  • Other inherited coagulopathies
6. History of abnormal blood count:
  • Leukemia
  • Thrombocytopenia
7. Medication:
  • NSAIDs
  • Aspirin
  • Anticoagulants
  • Antibiotics
  • Chemotherapeutic agents
	1. History of unusual bleeding
	2. Frequent episodes of epistaxis
	3. Unusual mucosal bleeding
	4. Abuse of illicit drugs

BOX 5-2 Bleeding Disorders

Intrinsic Bleeding Disorders	Acquired Bleeding Disorders

Hemophilia A
Hemophilia B
Von Willebrand's disease
	Thrombocytopenia:
	  • Decreased production of platelets
	  • Increased destruction of platelets
	The medicated patient:
	  • Heparin
	  • Warfarin
	  • Aspirin
	  • NSAIDs
	Liver disease
	Systemic diseases

diomyopathy, systolic congestive heart failure with poor ejection fraction, valvular heart disease, metallic cardiac valve replacement, and deep vein thrombosis/pulmonary embolism prevention.[2] The drug inhibits the production of vitamin K-dependent factors II, VII, IX, and X. It should be stressed that the use of vitamin K to correct an acute bleed in this patient population should be discouraged. Vitamin K will require 12 to 36 hours before its coagulating action can be seen. More important, however, is the fact that vitamin K administration will make renewed oral anticoagulation very difficult for a number of days. Reestablishing therapeutic INR (International Normalization Ratio) levels will be prolonged, thus exposing the patient to the risk of embolism.*

Dental Procedures. The intensity of anticoagulation is measured by the prothrombin time (PT). Patients with PT less than 1.5 times control (e.g., 18 sec with a control of 12 sec), or an INR no greater than 2.8 can safely undergo minor oral surgical procedures without alteration of medication. Patients with PT of 1.5 to 2 times control may also be managed without stopping the anticoagulant if the procedure is minor, such as a simple extraction of a tooth. In this case, the use of a local antifibrinolytic agent should be adequate. Tranexamic acid (10 ml of a 5% aqueous solution† used to irrigate the socket before suturing the operative field, followed by a mouthwash of the same solution for 2 minutes, 4 times a day for 1 week) has proven successful in preventing excessive bleeding following dental extraction and periapical surgery in patients on warfarin without withdrawing this drug either before or after the procedure.[3,4] Sutures should also be placed over the extraction site. This method of management will eliminate the risk of potential thromboembolism related to the lack of warfarin anticoagulant action during the pre - and postoperative period.

Patients should also be instructed to apply direct local pressure at the extraction site (biting on a piece of gauze for 20 minutes) to control bleeding. A full liquid diet is recommended for the first 24 to 48 hours; followed by a soft diet for another 5 days. They should also avoid drinking hot liquids as increased temperature promotes clot lysis.

It is important that the patient not be given ASA or NSAIDs for postoperative pain. Acetaminophen when

---

*The INR that is used to monitor warfarin therapy allows comparison of PT assays performed in laboratories using different thromboplastin reagents. It is calculated by the formula: $(PT_{patient}/PT_{control})^{ISI}$. ISI (International Sensitivity Index) is a measure of thromboplastin sensitivity.

†Preparation of solution: tranexamic sterile solution for intravenous injection contains 100 mg/ml of the acid. To prepare a 5% solution, take a 10 ml ampule and dilute with 10 ml of saline.

5-3 Categorizing Patients into Risk Groups for Possible Surgical Hemorrhage

Low-Risk Patients*	Moderate-Risk Patients**	High-Risk Patients**
• No history of bleeding from previous surgery • No family history of coagulopathies • No history of excessive bleeding • No history of liver disease • No history of heavy alcohol usage • Not taking any medication known to cause bleeding	• History of abnormal bleeding following tooth extraction or other minor surgery • A family history for bleeding • Abnormal bruising without trauma • Menorrhagia • History of liver disease • Alcoholic • Use of NSAIDs or ASA • History of malabsorption • Long term antibiotic usage	• Patient is known to have a coagulopathy • Documented family history of bleeding • Patient taking warfarin or heparin (within 4 hours)

*All factors must be present.
**Any one factor is significant.

TABLE 5-1 Procedures to Follow Based on Patient's Risk Category for Surgical Hemorrhage

Risk Category	Action Required
Low-risk patient	• Proceed with surgery. No further investigation or laboratory testing is required.
Moderate-risk patient	• A more detailed history should be obtained and the potential risk assessed. • Laboratory testing: PT, bleeding time, and platelet count. Consult with physician if necessary. • Optimize patient preoperative: the treatment to optimize the patient will depend on the results of the findings that contribute to the risk factors.
High-risk patient	• Consult with a hematologist. • Laboratory testing: PTT, PT, bleeding time, and platelet count. • Management of bleeding problems before surgery. • Postoperative management.

PT, Prothrombin time; *PTT,* partial thromboplastin time.

used in patients on warfarin has been reported to increase the risk of intracranial bleed ten fold.[5] Codeine or oxycodone (Roxicodone®: Roxane Lab, Columbus, OH) may be used to manage pain.

In more extensive oral surgical procedures where the risk of bleeding is much higher than with simple dental extraction the warfarin should be stopped 5 to 7 days before surgery. In order to keep a protective anticoagulation level, subcutaneous low molecular weight heparin should be substituted to keep a partial thromboplastin time (PTT) ranging from 1.25 to 2:1 compared with the PTT control. Subcutaneous heparin is stopped 2 to 4 hours before the procedure, and in this way the procedure can be safely performed without risk of excessive bleeding. Warfarin can be restarted in the postoperative period. Clinical judgement and individualization of each case are the factors that will determine the appropriate postoperative day when warfarin should be restarted. Warfarin is started at the same dose that the patient had been using. It must be remembered that warfarin's anticoagulation effect does not start before the third day. Heparin dosages can be adjusted to maintain anticoagulation during this transition phase.

Heparin is used for acute and short-term anticoagulation. One commonly seen clinical scenario is the dialyzed patient. Surgical procedures can safely be performed 4 hours after the heparin is terminated.

Antibiotics. Long-term antibiotic usage can cause defects in the coagulation system because of their effect on vitamin K production and absorption. A PT should be done. If the PT is elevated, these patients will benefit from administration of vitamin K_1 (Phytonadione). An initial dose of 15 to 20 mg IV will return the PT to normal within 6 to 12 hours. Usually a smaller dose of 10 mg IV or subcutaneous is used in controlling hemorrhagic episodes. The initial dose should be followed by one-third the dose every 8 to 12 hours. When given IV, vitamin K_1 must be given slowly (<5 mg/min) to avoid the precipitation of a hypotensive episode.

Platelets. Platelets play a key role in surgical hemostasis, and an adequate quantity and satisfactory functioning of platelets are required for successful hemostasis.

Platelet Count. This is usually obtained as a part of the CBC. Normal platelet numbers are 190,000 to

400,000/µl. Thrombocytopenia in the range of 50,000 to 100,000 will elevate the bleeding time; however, minor surgical procedures like extraction of teeth and biopsies are usually tolerated without need for platelet transfusion. In the case of tooth extraction, placing Gelfoam or microfibrillar collagen (Avitene) in the socket is useful because these substances accelerate formation of the platelet plug; Avitene also stabilizes the plug.[6] Elective oral surgical procedures should not be performed on patients with platelets less than 50,000/µl.

Hemophilia A/B and von Willebrand Disease. These congenital coagulation disorders should be managed in conjunction with a hematologist. The details of their management are beyond the scope of this Atlas. (The reader can refer to Ogle and Hernandez[2] for a detailed discussion on the management of these patients.)

MINIMIZATION OF BLOOD LOSS DURING THE SURGICAL PROCEDURE

The surgeon should attempt to perform the planned surgical procedure with the smallest amount of blood loss possible. The less blood that the operator has to contend with, the better will be the visibility and the surgical outcome. It is very difficult to perform competent surgery in a bloody field. Bleeding should be controlled during surgery not solely for the purpose of improved visibility, but also to prevent postoperative clots inside the wound. Clots will separate the periosteum from the bone, interfere with blood flow to the area, act as a foreign body, and provide an excellent culture medium with an increase in the infection rate.

Preincision. In minor oral surgery, control of bleeding should start with the injection of a vasoconstrictor. This may be achieved simultaneously when infiltration anesthesia is administered. In the case of a nerve block, which is done away from the immediate surgical area, local infiltration of the vasoconstrictor into the surgical field will be necessary to achieve vasoconstriction. Epinephrine is the most commonly used vasoconstrictor. The recommended maximum amount is 0.04 mg (2 cartridges of epinephrine 1/100,000 or 4 cartridges of epinephrine 1/200,000) in the patient with significant cardiovascular disease and 0.2 mg (11 cartridges of epinephrine 1/100,000 when used with 2% lidocaine) in a nonimpaired person. Simultaneous injection with lidocaine, with its antiarrhythmic effect, may explain why greater than 0.2 mg rarely precipitates arrhythmias in the dental setting.[6]

Lidocaine is commercially available with epinephrine in concentrations from 1/50,000 to 1/200,000. Following the injection of the local anesthesia with epinephrine, the decrease in gingival blood flow will be readily apparent in 5 minutes.[7] It is advisable, however, to wait for about 6 to 7 minutes for maximum vasoconstriction before making the incision. Increasing the concentration of epinephrine will give longer periods of decreased gingival blood flow.

Incision and Intraoperative Considerations. The incision must be planned with care so that adequate exposure of the surgical field will be obtained. However, it should be kept in mind that the longer the incision, the greater will be the blood loss. The incision should be designed so that the wound may be closed on bony support, even if bone removal will be extensive. This will permit the application of pressure directly to the incision site for control of bleeding. It should also be planned so as to avoid injury to the following vascular structures: the mental vessels, the greater palatine artery, the lingual artery and vein, and the vessels on the ventral surface of the tongue.

In dentoalveolar surgery, a full thickness mucoperiosteal flap is the most common surgical access. Making sure that the periosteum is sharply incised and reflected will minimize bleeding and also inadvertent tearing of mucosal tissue. Once the mucoperiosteal flap is fully reflected, the oozing from the incision will stop. The mucoperiosteal flap should be elevated with a periosteal elevator in an atraumatic manner. The periosteal elevator must be placed in direct contact with the bone. If the Cambian layer of periosteum (seen as a thin veil of tissue over the bone) is not being reflected, then the incision should be repeated. To avoid tearing, the elevation should be started at the gingival margin or in the attached gingiva. The attached gingiva should be reflected and loosened along the entire length of the incision before progressing to more extensive mucoperiosteal dissection. If the attachment of the attached gingiva to the bone is tenacious, or if the mucosa is adherent to underlying pathology, then sharp dissection is indicated.

In oral surgery the majority of incisions will be made over bone. This means that it will always be possible to control bleeding by applying pressure to compress the wound against the underlying bony surface. In the case of a bleed, the application of pressure should always be the first method used to attempt control of the bleeding. The patient may be asked to bite on a gauze or exodontia sponge. For a gingival bleed, the pressure should be maintained for about 3 to 5 minutes. If gauze is used to apply pressure to the bleeding site, then it should be removed slowly, as the interlaced fresh clot may be pulled away with the gauze, and the bleeding may begin anew. Usually, however, the saliva will prevent this from happening by keeping the gauze wet.

In the case of injury to the inferior alveolar artery pressure will be required for a longer period of time. In this circumstance, a moistened 2×2 gauze may be packed into the extraction socket for 7 to 10 minutes. After this time, the packing should be slowly removed so as not to dislodge the clot. At the moment that the pack is being removed the operator should be ready to replace the packing in case the bleeding is not controlled. After initial control of the bleeding by pressure, Gelfoam or other hemostatic agents may be placed into the socket, and sutures used to further apply pressure to the soft tissue. Biting on a wad of gauze for 20 minutes will further aid hemostasis. Keeping hot liquids and cigarette smoke out of the mouth for the first 24 hours is also helpful.

When injury has occurred to the vascular structure within the inferior alveolar neurovascular bundle, direct pressure should still be placed to control bleeding. The pressure may cause injury to the nerve, but the immediate control of the bleeding is more significant, and must be the primary objective.

The greater palatine artery and the vessels in the floor of the mouth may not be easily controlled by pressure, and packing is difficult. Bleeding at these sites may have to be controlled by ligatures, sutures, or electrocoagulation. The ligation of the divided vessel may be done with a nonabsorbable material such as silk or nylon, or an absorbable material such as catgut (natural collagen) or synthetic collagen (Dexon or Vicryl). In the oral cavity, silk is the ideal material. It has the best handling qualities and knot-setting accuracy of all surgical sutures, plus it is flexible and soft so that it does not irritate the patient. Its multi-strandedness and wicking effect keep it moist and soft during the healing phase. Nylon tends to be firm and not very comfortable to the patient when used intraorally. Catgut and Dexon/Vicryl are acceptable alternatives.

In intraoral surgery, ligation of vessels will most often involve the techniques of instrument ties around a clamp, or suture of a buried bleeder. Hand ties will be difficult because of access.

Instrument Tie Around a Clamp. This technique may be applicable in the floor of the mouth. Pressure should first be applied to slow the bleeding. After gauze is packed into the floor of the mouth, bidigital compression should be used to apply pressure to the bleeding area (Fig. 5-1). After about 2 to 4 minutes the pressure may be slowly released and an attempt made to identify the bleeding vessel. High evacuation suction should be available. When the end of the lacerated vessel is identified, it should be clamped with a hemostat. Only the vessel should be clasped with the hemostat. Grasping large bites of tissue in the floor of the mouth may cause irreversible damage to the lingual nerve or to the submandibular duct.

Once the bleeding vessel is clamped, a slender needle

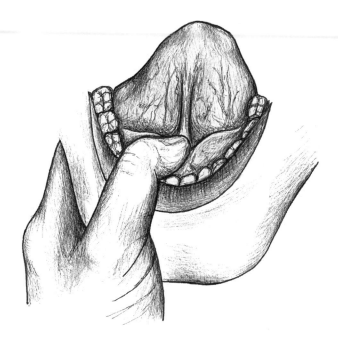

FIG. 5-1 Pressure being applied by bidigital pressure to control bleeding from the floor of the mouth.

holder or a Kelly clamp should be used to pass the tie around the vessel. The short end is then placed toward the incisors so that it is in view and is readily accessible. Outside of the mouth a loop in the long end of the suture is thrown in a clockwise direction around the tip of the needle holder (Fig. 5-2, *A*). The tip with the loop is then directed into the floor of the mouth to secure the short end of the suture (Fig. 5-2, *B* and *C*). Once the short end is grasped the loop is tightened around the vessel by applying tension to both ends of the tie suture (Fig. 5-2, *D*). After this first throw is tightened, the surgeon returns the short end to a visible location and throws a second loop in a counterclockwise direction and then snugs down this second throw (Fig. 5-2, *E* and *F*). If the surgeon has difficulty securing the knot, then a hemostat may be placed on the short end and used to counterpull the short end in a direction 180° to the long end (Fig. 5-2, *G*). Three or four throws will be required to secure the vessel. A commonly used technique is to make two throws clockwise in the first loop and then one counterclockwise in the second throw. The suture is cut approximately 3 to 5 mm away from the knot.

Suture of a Buried Bleeder. This technique may be applicable in the hard palate. The greater palatine artery, if sectioned, may not be readily clamped. In such a case, a suture may be placed around the vessel to produce local constriction. A large non-cutting (tapered) needle is passed below the vessel along the bony

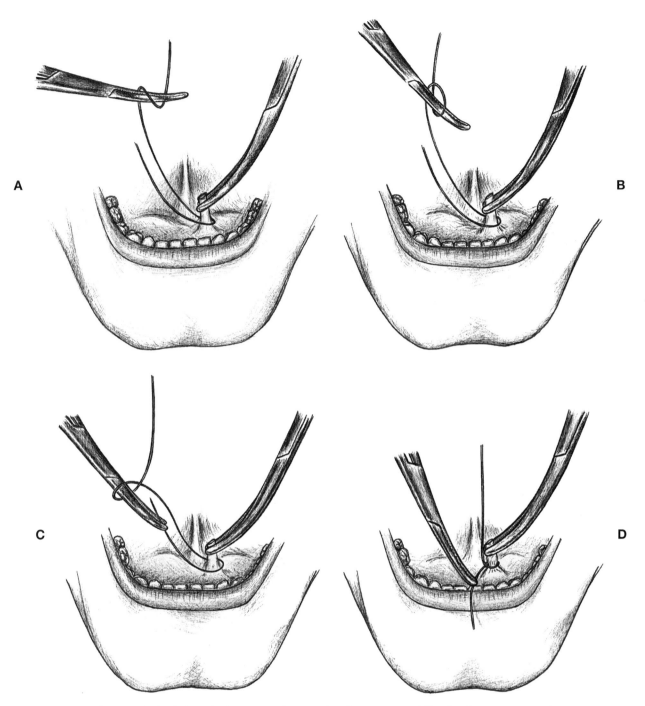

FIG. 5-2 **A,** Technique for instrument tie around a clamp to control bleeding from a transected vessel. The bleeding vessel is identified, isolated, and the lumen closed by securing it with the tips of a small hemostat. The vessel is raised and the tie placed around the vessel. The knot is started by making a loop in a clockwise direction around the needle holder. **B,** The short end of the tie is placed in a position where it can easily be reached by the needle holder. **C,** The tip of the needle holder with the loop is used to secure the short end of the suture. **D,** The short end is securely grasped and the loop is pulled down around the vessel by applying tension to both ends of the tie suture. The knot is pulled tightly to close the lumen of the vessel and to be sure that it will not slide away from the vessel. *Continued*

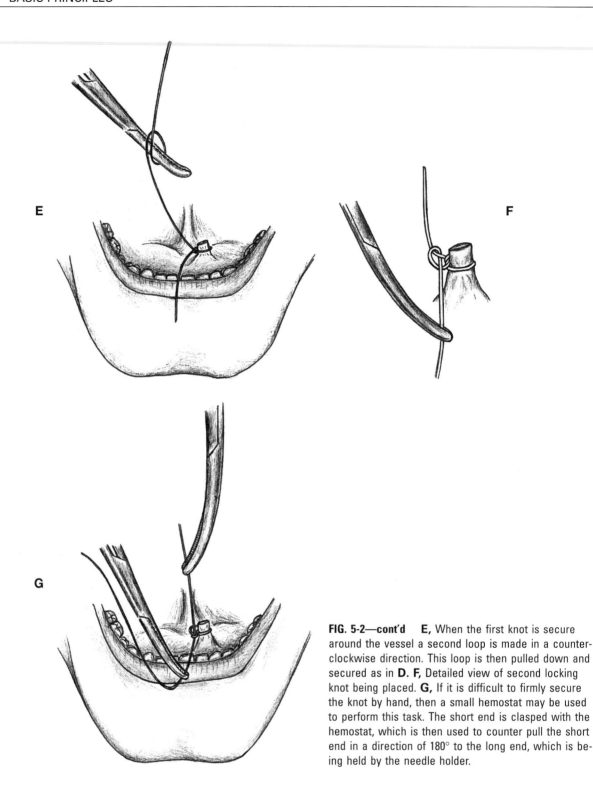

FIG. 5-2—cont'd **E,** When the first knot is secure around the vessel a second loop is made in a counter-clockwise direction. This loop is then pulled down and secured as in **D. F,** Detailed view of second locking knot being placed. **G,** If it is difficult to firmly secure the knot by hand, then a small hemostat may be used to perform this task. The short end is clasped with the hemostat, which is then used to counter pull the short end in a direction of 180° to the long end, which is being held by the needle holder.

palate and is tied on the palatal mucosa (Fig. 5-3). (This may only be practical in the posterior part of the hard palate, however, as often the palatine artery will be in a bony groove anteriorly, and difficult to get below. In this case pressure or electrocautery may be the best options.)

Electrocautery. Electrocoagulation is achieved by the passage of a small quantity of electrical current through a bleeding vessel. The electrical frequency generates heat, which coagulates protein and controls bleeding by thrombosis of vessels. Electrocautery in minor intraoral surgery is indicated when the bleeding is not controlla-

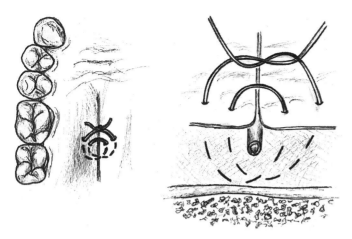

FIG. 5-3 Technique for ligating a buried bleeder. Using a tapered needle, the suture is passed blindly beneath the vessel. The first pass should be approximately 6 mm from the vessel and aimed to exit about 2 mm from the vessel. A second pass is now made starting it at approximately 2 mm from the vessel. This second pass should be aimed to exit at about 6 mm from the vessel. Tension is then applied to the free ends to put pressure on the source of bleeding. The knot is made by making loops around the needle holder and throwing them around the short end as shown on the right.

ble by pressure, and the surgeon is further unable to control the bleeding with sutures. Coagulation will be achieved by applying the tip of the cautery directly to the bleeding mucosa. Every attempt should be made to minimize the amount of tissue that is damaged. Electrocautery will cause tissue damage from 3 to 7 mm. beyond what is clinically observed, depending on the energy applied to the tissue.

When using electrocautery on oral mucosa, the power should be set to the lowest level that will rapidly produce localized vessel thrombosis without charring the tissues. The coagulation button should be depressed to the "on" position before the current is applied to the tissue. If the current is applied after the tip is in direct or indirect (via a clamp) contact with the bleeder, the surgeon will find that it is much more difficult to control the amount of current with sufficient accuracy. If, however, the current is "on" at the moment of contact, the surgeon may instantly break the circuit by withdrawing the tip of the cautery immediately on seeing the first darkening of tissue as the coagulation begins about the vessel.[8]

If the electrocautery is applied directly to a very small bleeding vessel in the gingiva or the oral mucosa, it should be done rapidly and with a light touch. Excessive heat will cause necrosis and subsequent sloughing of the tissue. This will increase postoperative pain and cause delayed healing.

To avoid injury to the lip, tongue, or other soft tissue the tip of the cautery should be covered with a rubber catheter. Only about 5 mm of tip should be exposed. The tips available with the small electrosurgical units used in dental offices will often meet this criterion and need not be further protected.

Hemostasis in Bleeding Bone. While reflecting a full thickness mucoperiosteal flap, at times small vessels may be seen emerging from the cortical plate of the maxilla or the mandible. As the dentist develops the flap, these vessels will rupture and bleed. Bleeding from

these vessels can be controlled by burnishing the entrance of the bony canal with the sharp end of the periosteal elevator (Fig. 5-4) or with a small hemostat. The tip of an electrocautery unit also works very effectively.

Bleeding within an extraction site can be controlled by packing the socket with a 2×2 gauze for 3 to 5 minutes, then slowly removing it. After initial control by pressure, Gelfoam, Avitene, or topical Thrombin may be placed into the socket to maintain hemostasis. The patient should be instructed to further maintain pressure by biting firmly on a wad of gauze for 20 minutes, and to avoid spitting or the application of heat to the clot. Because heat is known to cause lysis of the clot, smoking should be avoided for at least 6 to 8 hours postoperatively.

Bone wax is possibly the most effective way to plug blood vessels in bleeding bone. A small piece of the wax is warmed to the desired consistency by manipulation with the fingers. With gloves this may take a few minutes as the body temperature will be poorly transmitted through the gloves. After softening, the wax is forced into the bleeding channels to mechanically plug them (Fig. 5-5). Excess bone wax should be removed.

Suction. Suction plays a valuable role in the control of bleeding during surgery. Its function is to remove the blood and saliva from the surgical field, giving the operator optimal visibility to perform the surgery. In surgery, high-speed evacuation should always be used.

During the surgery the tip of the suction cannula should always be near to the instrument that the surgeon is using, and it should be confined to the surgical field. The assistant must keep in mind at all times that during the procedure the suction will be needed at the location where the surgeon is working and not at another portion of the oral cavity. If excess fluid must be removed from the floor of the mouth, the surgeon should stop and allow the assistant to suction remote parts of the mouth. Care must be taken not to

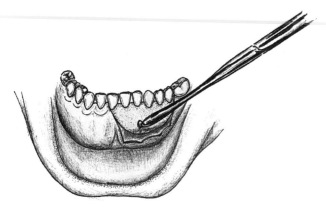

FIG. 5-4 Burnishing of buccal cortical bone in the anterior mandible to control bleeding from a small foramen in the cortical plate.

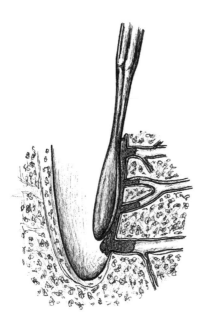

FIG. 5-5 Technique for placing bone wax into an extraction site to control bleeding from cancellous bone. The bone wax is forced into the bleeding channels to mechanically tamponade the vascular flow. A periosteal elevator or curette may be used to perform this function.

traumatize the oral mucosa with the suction cannula. The dental assistant who is suctioning for the dentist must also make certain that neither her hand nor the suction tip blocks the surgeon's vision.

Topical Hemostatic Agents

Absorbable Collagen Hemostatic Sponge or Plugs (Helistat, CollaPlug, CollaCote, CollaTape). This material is fabricated from collagen obtained from bovine deep flexor (Achilles) tendon. This tendon is known to be one of the purest sources of collagen that can readily

be obtained and processed in commercial amounts. These sponges are soft, pliable, and nonfriable. Because of the nonfriable, coherent structure of these sponges, application to a bleeding site is easily achieved. On contact with blood, collagen is known to cause aggregation of platelets. Platelets will deposit in large numbers on the collagen sponge or plug, degranulate, and release coagulation factors that, together with plasma factors, enable the fabrication of fibrin. Bleeding will be controlled within 2 to 5 minutes. The material is completely absorbed within 14 to 56 days. The sponge or tape may be laid against a bleeding surface or packed into an extraction site.

Microfibrillar Collagen (Avitene, Helitene, Instat, Collastat). This is bovine collagen that is shredded into fibrils. Physically, microfibrillar collagen yields a larger surface area than do sponges and plugs. Chemically, Avitene is collagen with hydrochloric acid noncovalently bound to some of the available amino groups in the collagen molecules. The properties and function are identical to the sponges. Avitene is very light, and when used in the fibrous (flour) form can sometimes be difficult to use intraorally. When the mouth is open, patients may tend to mouth breathe, and on exhalation will blow away the material. In such a case, the dentist should ask the patient to take a deep breath and hold it until the material has been placed. The use of microfibrillar collagen in dental extraction sockets has been reported to increase the incidence of alveolalgia.[9] Also, transient laryngospasm caused by aspiration of the dry, powdery material has been reported following the use of microfibrillar collagen in tonsillectomy.[9]

Absorbable Gelatin (Gelfoam*). This material is a sponge prepared from specially treated and purified gelatin solution that is beaten to a desired porosity and then dried, sterilized, and packaged. It is capable of absorbing and holding within its mesh many times its weight in whole blood. When placed in an extraction site it aids in hemostasis by absorbing blood and expanding within the socket. It also provides a matrix on which the clot may be organized. Gelfoam is completely absorbed within 4 to 6 weeks, without inducing excessive fibrosis. To use Gelfoam, a piece is cut to the desired size and rolled between the fingers to lightly compress it to the size that will fill the bony cavity or extraction socket. Following insertion of the rolled pack, light finger pressure should be applied for 1 to 2 minutes.

Gelfoam should not be used in the presence of frank infection, as it will absorb infected fluids and serve as a nidus for abscess formation. If signs of infection or abscess develop in an area where Gelfoam has been

*Manufactured by Upjohn, Kalamazoo, MI 49001, USA.

placed, the area should be reoperated and the infected material removed.

Bone Wax. This is a mixture of beeswax and isopropyl palmitate, a wax-softening agent. It achieves local hemostasis of bone by acting to tamponade (a mechanical barrier) bleeding channels within bone. It is minimally resorbable, and as such should not be used where rapid osseous regeneration is desired, because it may inhibit osteogenesis and act as a physical barrier to the reparative process. It should be used to stop bleeding from small channels on the cortical plate, or in lower third molar sites. Its usage in the anterior portion of the jaws at sites into which implants may be placed should be discouraged. When used, it should be used sparingly, and all excess should be removed. Bone wax should not be used in an area that is infected, or in which periapical pathology is present, because studies have suggested that it impairs the ability of cancellous bone to clear bacteria.[10]

Oxidized Regenerated Absorbable Cellulose (Surgicel Absorbable Hemostat). This is an absorbable knitted fabric prepared from the oxidation of regenerated cellulose. It accelerates clotting by serving as a matrix for the formation of a clot. After it has been saturated with blood, it swells into a brown/black gelatinous mass that aids in clot formation. When used in minimal amounts, it is absorbed from the site of implantation with little or no tissue reaction. Absorption, however, depends on several factors, including the amount used, degree of saturation with blood, and the tissue bed. When used in bony cavities, it is not advisable to leave the material in the bone because of possible interference with osteogenesis, and a risk of cyst formation. It is best to remove the material once hemostasis has been achieved. It should not be used in an infected area.

Oxidized cellulose should be used dry. It should never be impregnated with antibiotic solutions or with thrombin. The hemostatic effect of oxidized cellulose is not enhanced by thrombin, because the activity of thrombin is destroyed by the low pH of the product.

Oxidized Cellulose (Oxycel, Surgicel). A knitted fabric prepared by the controlled oxidation of cellulose, this material is not resorbable, and should be removed once hemostasis is achieved. The information provided for Surgicel Absorbable is also applicable to Oxycel and Surgicel.

Thrombin (Thrombostat, Thrombinar, Thrombogen). This is of bovine origin and catalyzes the conversion of fibrinogen to fibrin. It is applied directly to the bleeding site, either in solution or in the powder form. A dose of 100 units/ml is customary to control bleeding from mucosa.

Tranexamic Acid (Cyklokapron Injectable). This derivative of the amino acid lysine is an analog of epsilon-aminocaproic acid (Amicar) and is 6 to 10 times as potent as Amicar. It forms a reversible complex that displaces plasminogen from fibrin, resulting in inhibition of fibrinolysis. It also inhibits the proteolytic activity of plasmin and the conversion of plasminogen to plasmin by plasminogen activators.[11]

Fibrin-Sealants (Tisseel). This is a synthetic fibrin-type glue. It is a new product, and not much information is available about its usage in oral surgery or orthopedics. It has been used very successfully to control bleeding in cardiovascular surgery.

IDENTIFICATION AND ELIMINATION OR CORRECTION OF THE CAUSES OF POSTSURGICAL BLEEDING AND REESTABLISHMENT OF ADEQUATE HEMOSTASIS
Postoperative Hemorrhage

This will be the most common bleeding emergency that the dentist will encounter. It is usually the result of the patient's failure to apply constant pressure to the surgical site, or is the result of prolonged hemostasis. When applying pressure, the patient should be advised not to chew on the gauze or remove it from the mouth too frequently. Spitting should be discouraged, as well as smoking and excessive rinsing within the first 12 hours.

When postoperative bleeding occurs first aid measures should be the first methods used to try to control the bleeding. The following are a series of sequential steps that should be used to control postoperative bleeding:

1. Ask the patient to rinse with warm saline to remove clotted blood. Then have him/her bite firmly on a clean gauze sponge for 20 minutes. Educate the patient that constant pressure is required. Do not change the gauze or chew on it. After 20 minutes, slowly remove the gauze and observe the area. The patient should avoid putting the tongue or fingers into the site, and avoid spitting or further rinsing for 24 hours.

2. If the bleeding does not stop, then repeat the above, except that a tea bag should now be used and the patient asked to bite on it for another 10 minutes. Most tea bags are strong enough for the patient to bite on without risk of the bag rupturing, and will give faster and better results than if it is wrapped in gauze. Because the taste from a moistened tea bag is slightly bitter and may cause nausea, I do not ask the patient to keep it in the mouth for longer than 10 minutes. The patient should be advised that the fresh tea bag is bitter, and asked to cooperate in this respect. The tannic acid in the tea bag often accelerates clotting. Most

good brand-name tea bags are strong and do not rupture easily by pressure alone, but if the bag ruptures and tea leaves are escaping, the patient should change the tea bag at once and clean the area lightly with a moistened gauze. If this fails to arrest the bleeding, or if the bleeding is brisk, this patient must be seen by the dentist either in the office or in the emergency room.

3. If the patient has to be seen, then the first step should be to obtain vital signs: blood pressure and pulse. A history of bleeding abnormalities should also be reassessed. Next, the surgical site should be examined to identify the cause of the prolonged bleeding. This exploration of the surgical site should be done with good lighting, high speed suction, and irrigation. If a large blood clot is present over the extraction or other surgical site, it should be removed grossly with a hemostat, college pliers, or a moistened gauze wrapped around the operator's index finger. Once the clot is grossly removed, the area may be irrigated with saline. High-speed suction should be available to rapidly remove the irrigant. As long as the large blood clot is present, hemostasis will not occur.

4. The surgeon should now try to determine if the bleeding is from bone (the extraction socket) or from the soft tissue associated with the surgery.
   - If the bleeding is from soft tissue, this may be controlled by sutures, or in rare cases with cautery. In periodontal surgery, a periodontal pack may be used to provide stable, constant pressure to support the gingival flaps. If the bleeding is from a denuded area, as for example, the donor site of a palatal graft, a topical hemostatic agent such as a collagen sponge

(Helistat) should be used to cover the area. Avitene or thrombin may also be used. When the blood is oozing from the surrounding soft tissue, then a figure-8 suture should be placed to apply pressure on the area (Fig. 5-6 *A* and *B*).
   - If the bleeding is coming from the bone, the surgeon should try to determine if the source is a nutrient vessel, excess granulation tissue in an extraction socket, diffused bleeding from cancellous bone, or from a fracture of the alveolus. If the bleeding is from a nutrient canal, burnishing the bone over the bleeding point should compress bone over the bleeding canal resulting in control of the hemorrhage. Granulation tissue should be curetted from the extraction site or debrided from periodontal lesions. Granulation tissue is rich in small capillaries, the walls of which will not constrict, and profuse bleeding will continue. Diffuse bleeding from cancellous bone can be managed by packing the area with Gelfoam, or Gelfoam impregnated with topical thrombin in the case of an extraction site or other bony cavities. If this is for an extraction site, a figure-8 suture should also be placed (see Fig. 5-6). If the bleeding removes the Gelfoam, use a larger amount of the material or use bone wax. A fracture of the alveolus can be stabilized by tension sutures over the socket. This suture should be left in place for 10 days. Collagen may also be placed, followed by pressure from gauze.

5. Following any of the above interventions, pressure should again be applied by biting on a wad of gauze for 20 minutes. This will further apply pressure to the area, plus prevent the patient from

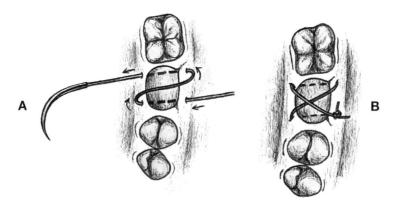

FIG. 5-6   **A, B** Technique for placing a figure-8 suture to apply pressure to the soft tissues at an extraction site. The first pass is from the buccal to the lingual/palatal mucosa at the anterior of the extraction site. The suture is next passed diagonally over the extraction site to the buccal gingiva at the posterior portion of the extraction site. It is again passed from buccal to lingual/palatal. To complete the figure 8, the suture is again passed diagonally across the extraction site and tied where the first pass was made on the buccal.

playing with the area before the clot is fully organized.

6. Local anesthesia will be necessary to adequately manage the patient. A local anesthesia without a vasoconstrictor must be used, because the operator will never be sure if the control of the bleeding is a result of the therapy administered, or only a temporary arrest of the hemorrhage secondary to local vasoconstriction. The use of a vasoconstrictor will cause the vessels responsible for the bleeding to constrict, and the hemorrhage may reappear once the chemical is metabolized.

Lasers and Bleeding

When used for surgical procedures such as gingivectomy or the ablation of intraoral lesions, the laser light is absorbed by the soft tissue. The absorption of the radiation causes local tissue destruction. The electromagnetic energy that is absorbed by the tissue is transformed instantaneously into heat energy. This heat energy causes a sudden temperature rise in a small tissue volume. This process is called photocoagulation.[12] As the laser vaporizes tissue, the exposed blood vessels are simultaneously coagulated.

Management of Uncontrollable Bleeding in the Dental Office

When bleeding cannot be controlled by local means in the dental office the patient should be transported to a local hospital. In this situation epinephrine 1/50,000 may be injected into the bleeding area to provide vasoconstriction. The bleeding site should be packed as tightly as possible with gauze, and the patient asked to apply pressure by biting firmly on the pressure gauze placed on the bleeding site. If the blood loss is significant (>500 ml) then an IV line should be started with normal saline or lactated Ringers solution, and the patient transported to the hospital.

REFERENCES

1. Peterson P, Hayes TE, Arkin CF, et.al: The preoperative bleeding time test lacks clinical benefit, *Arch Surg* 133:134, 1998.
2. Ogle OE, Hernandez AR: Management of patients with hemophilia, anticoagulation and sickle cell disease, *Oral Maxillofac Surg Clin North Am* 10(3):401-416, 1998.
3. Sindet-Pedersen S, Ramstrom G, Bernville S, et. al: Hemostatic effect of tranexamic acid mouthwash in anticoagulant-treated patients undergoing oral surgery, *New Engl J Med* 320:840-843, 1989.
4. Ramstrom G, Sinedet-Pedersen S, Hall D, et al: Prevention of postsurgical bleeding in oral surgery using Tranexamic acid without dose modification of oral anticoagulants, *J Oral Maxillofac Surg* 51(11):1211-1216, 1993.
5. Hylek EM, Heiman H, Skates SJ, Sheehan MA, Singer DE: Acetaminophen and other risk factors for excessive warfarin anticoagulation, *JAMA* 279(9):657-662, March 4, 1998.
6. Bavitz JB: Perioperative hematologic management, *Oral Maxillofac Surg Clin North Am* 4(3):629-637, 1992.
7. Dodson TB, Bays RA, Paul RE, Neunschwander MC: The effect of local anesthesia with vasoconstrictor on gingival blood flow during Lefort 1 osteotomy, *J Oral Maxillofac Surg* 54(7):810-814, 1996.
8. Edgerton, MT: Hemostasis and removal of blood from the surgical field. In: *The art of surgical technique*, Baltimore, Williams and Wilkins, pp. 71-106; 1988.
9. Avitene Product Information, Davol, Inc. 1996. http://www.medchemproducts.com/avinsrt.htm
10. Johnson P, Fromm D: Effects of bone wax on bacterial clearance, *Surgery* 89(2):206-209, 1981.
11. Levy, AF: Antifibrinolytics: epsilon-aminocaproic acid, tranexamic acid and aprotinin, *The Internet Journal of Anesthesiology* Vol 1 N2. 1997. http://www.ispub.com/journals/ISA/Vol 1 N2/antifibr.htm.
12. Golman L: *The biomedical laser: Technology and clinical applications*, New York, 1981, Springer-Verlag.

EXODONTIA

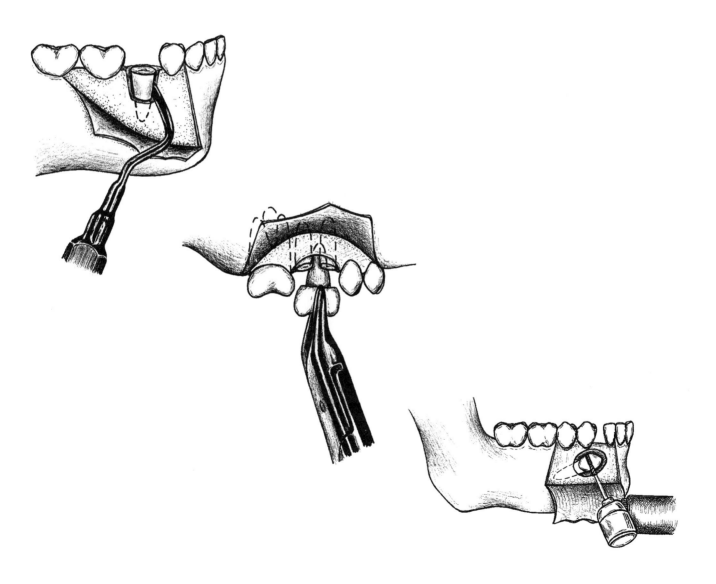

6 Simple and Surgical Exodontia

HARRY DYM, DDS

BASIC PRINCIPLES

This chapter will outline the basic principles involved in the extraction of teeth, with detailed description of the appropriate techniques for specific situations. Exodontia is not merely an exertion of brute force, but is based on biological science and sound fundamental concepts common to all surgical procedures. Prior to any planned exodontia an appropriate medical/dental history must be completed and diagnostic x-rays taken and reviewed (Box 6-1). The radiograph must clearly show the entire tooth structure (crown and roots) and be available for review during the planned procedure. In addition to providing clinical information regarding contiguous vital structures (inferior alveolar canal, mental foramen, maxillary sinus position) quality radiographs will allow you to evaluate the root configuration and assess the relative degree of difficulty related to the particular extraction. Additionally, apical pathologic cystic lesions are often associated with extracted teeth and should be removed along with the offending tooth. A film with good contrast that is well fixed will provide the surgeon with the necessary information.

Before any surgical procedure an assessment of the type of anesthetic required must be made. Most patients can be managed with local anesthesia; however, in some cases the patient's level of anxiety will require additional therapeutic modalities. Oral or intravenous sedation should be used when needed; otherwise a simple procedure can quickly transition into an unmanageable situation.

Principles of Exodontia

Extraction of teeth is perhaps the oldest historical surgical procedure performed by mankind, and will undoubtedly continue to be practiced well into the next millennium (Box 6-2).

As with all surgical procedures, the practitioner should be armed with all the necessary biological information as well as surgical techniques and principles so that he/she can perform this procedure with a minimal amount of complications.

Basic Techniques

Many factors are involved in obtaining the best visibility and access for extractions. Proper lighting and retraction must be available and the Minnesota retractor is an excellent instrument that can help provide atraumatic retraction (Box 6-3).

High-speed surgical suction along with a variety of different-sized suction tips must also be available. The patient must be positioned appropriately in the dental chair to allow for maximum doctor comfort and leverage. The patient's head should be at the level of the operator's elbow for maximum comfort and control during surgery. For maxillary extractions, the upper arch should be perpendicular to the floor with the operator positioned in front of the patient, whereas surgery in the mandible is best performed with the lower arch parallel to the floor.

During difficult mandibular extractions, significant forces are transmitted to the patient's temporomandibular joint, which can be most painful. A bite block is most helpful in stabilizing the arch and reducing temporomandibular joint pain and should be routinely used.

Instrumentation

In order to properly incorporate and perform exodontia in one's dental practice, the dentist must have adequate instrumentation as well as the knowledge and ability to use them.

Dental Forceps. A large variety of forceps designed for the extraction of each tooth is currently available. The correct forceps is the one that fits comfortably in the dentist's hand, adapts well to the contours of the tooth needing extraction, and applies the forces along the long axis of the tooth.

Extraction Forceps for Maxillary Teeth. The upper universal forceps #150 is designed for the removal of all maxillary teeth. The #1 forceps is a straight forceps used for the extraction of maxillary anterior teeth, whereas the #286 is a bayonet forceps designed for the removal of maxillary bicuspids and single roots. The #65 forceps

BOX 6-1 Documentation

The doctor performing any surgical procedure should make certain to enter a complete note in the patient's record. The important elements of a note include the following:
1. Date
2. Review of significant medical history and allergies
3. Significant clinical findings
4. Operative note
5. Anesthesia used
6. Medication prescribed
7. Return follow up appointment
8. Signature

BOX 6-2 Indications for Extraction of Teeth

1. Extensive dental decay
2. Serious infection
3. Preirradiation
4. Advanced periodontal disease
5. Teeth that interfere with placement of prosthesis
6. Orthodontic reasons
7. Malposition
8. Teeth in line of fracture
9. Teeth associated with pathology
10. Economics

BOX 6-3 Fundamental Elements in Exodontia

1. Properly position the patient and chair so that the treating doctor can keep his arms close to his body.
2. For maxillary extractions the chair should be tipped back so that the maxillary occlusal plane is 60 to 90° to the floor.
3. For mandibular extractions the occlusal plane is parallel to the floor.
4. Always be prepared with necessary instrumentation and rotary instruments in case a simple planned extraction converts suddenly into a complex surgical procedure.
5. Reflect cervical gingiva to expose crestal bone.
6. All teeth should be luxated in their socket prior to forceps extraction.
7. Always avoid excessive forces and use controlled force.
8. Use a mouth prop to aid the patient in opening the mouth as this will help to alleviate facial muscle pain and temporomandibular joint discomfort.
9. If no tooth mobility is seen after various attempts at forceps extraction, stop and plan on surgical extraction.
10. The degree of postoperative pain, swelling, and discomfort correlate to the amount of trauma received during the extraction procedure.

is a narrower version of this instrument and is used for root tip removal.

The #53R and #53L forceps are bayonet forceps designed specifically for maxillary molars. They engage the buccal bifurcation with a projection from the buccal beak and adapt smoothly to the palatal root for maximum contact by a broad-based concave-shaped beak.

Extraction Forceps for Mandibular Teeth. The lower universal forceps #151 are very similar in design and function to the maxillary universal forceps. They are designed for removal of all the lower teeth. The #23 (cowhorn) forceps is designed for only the mandibular molars. This forceps functions quite differently than the other extraction forceps. The beaks of the cowhorn forceps are not designed to grip the tooth but rather to elevate the molar tooth from its socket. The sharp beaks are firmly seated in the mandibular molar bifurcation and apical pressure is applied along with a pumping action. This motion, when properly applied, will lift the tooth from the alveolus.

Dental Elevators. Dental elevators are available in a wide variety of designs and configurations and their use depends on their function and the experience and preference of the treating dentist (Table 6-1).

The dental elevator is not designed to extract but to loosen teeth. They are placed between the alveolus and root surface and gently rotated apically to luxate the teeth. The #301 and #34S are the standard instruments found in all basic extraction kits. In addition to luxating teeth, the dental elevator is able to generate significant "lever" forces, using the alveolar crest as the fulcrum, to gently lift a tooth or root from its bony crypt (Fig. 6-1). These forces must be applied in a slow, deliberate, and controlled fashion to avoid any unwanted trauma to both the adjacent soft and hard tissues.

Forceps Techniques and Principles

Regardless of the tooth to be extracted, some common principles are applicable to all dental extractions. Before engaging the tooth with the appropriate dental forceps, a periosteal elevator should be used in an atraumatic fashion to gently release the gingival cuff and interdental papillae to allow placement of the forceps' beaks in an apical direction. When the forceps has been positioned beneath the soft tissue cuff, a strong apical seating force is applied which helps to significantly increase the mechanical advantage. When the forceps are seated, the handles are squeezed to engage the tooth and the operator's free hand is positioned to stabilize the alveolus with the tooth. This allows the practitioner to feel if the alveolus is moving along and to then alter his technique, perhaps by doing a surgical extraction, before causing any serious problems.

The force generated during forceps extraction is applied in both an apical and buccal-lingual direction. The apical force will act to break the periodontal ligament attachment while the lateral forces will cause the alveolus to expand. The technique should be modified somewhat in the posterior maxilla where more buccal than palatal forces should be used during posterior maxillary extractions, as it is easier to surgically retrieve a fractured buccal maxillary molar root than a fractured palatal root.

Additionally, one should be more careful and deliberate when extracting maxillary first bicuspids for orthodontic reasons, as removing buccal plate during attempted root retrieval can detrimentally affect future planned orthodontic movements.

In all cases, however, all forces used during extractions should be applied in a slow and deliberate fashion to allow for expansion of the alveolus. Rapid, jerky movements of either elevators or forceps are more likely to lead to fracture of teeth (Fig. 6-2) and associated bony alveolar fractures. Rotational forces can be applied during the removal of teeth with single conical roots such as maxillary cuspids and incisors and lower mandibular canines.

When it becomes clearly obvious that the routine exodontia cannot be accomplished or if the crown has snapped off during the attempted extraction, a surgical technique must be then employed.

Surgical exodontia involves reflection of a full thickness mucoperiosteal flap and exposure of the underlying bone with possible bone removal (Figs. 6-3 through 6-6). The design of the flap is varied but all are based on a common surgical principle.

Flap Designs

1. Incisions should be made over bone not planned for removal.
2. Flaps should be the full thickness of the underlying mucoperiosteum.
3. Flaps should allow clear and adequate hard tissue visualization to avoid tearing the soft tissue and increase ease of bone removal.
4. Avoid placing incisions over vital structures (such as the mental nerve/foramen and lingual nerve).

The actual soft tissue flap configuration can be of two basic designs.

The first design is the envelope flap, made by using a #15 blade on a #3 scalpel handle and sharply incising

TABLE 6-1   Types of Dental Elevators

Type	Description
Straight	The blade of the straight elevator has a concave surface on one side and is used to luxate erupted teeth prior to seating of forceps.
Triangular (East-West or Cryer)	These elevators are paired instruments and have a pointed triangle shape. They are best used for removing broken roots from sockets, especially multi-rooted sockets.
Crane pick	This elevator possesses a sharp and thick point used for removing roots. It is best used by inserting it into a small hole drilled into the remaining root and elevating fragment out.
Root Tip Elevators	Delicate instruments that are used to gently tease small root tips from their sockets.

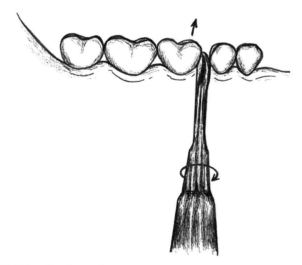

FIG. 6-1 Small, straight elevator inserted perpendicular to tooth after reflection of interdental papilla. Use the adjacent bone as a fulcrum to luxate the tooth.

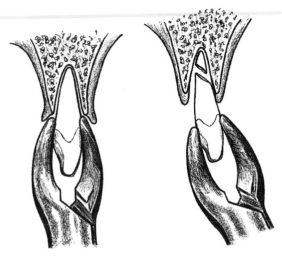

FIG. 6-2 Extraction forceps should be seated as far apically as possible. Lack of apical seating will increase incidence of root fracture.

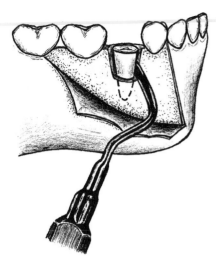

FIG. 6-5 Root is removed with elevator wedged between root and alveolar bone. Controlled luxation is performed to avoid root displacement and soft tissue injury.

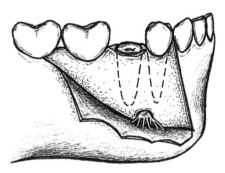

FIG. 6-3 In the area of the mental foramen, note how a vertical releasing incision is placed anteriorly and away from any possible damage to the mental nerve. When extracting lower bicuspid root tips, one should always be cognizant of the mental nerve and foramen.

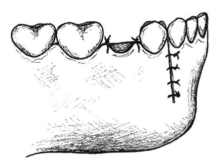

FIG. 6-6 Replace buccal flap and suture vertical flap first to better establish presurgical anatomic flap relationship.

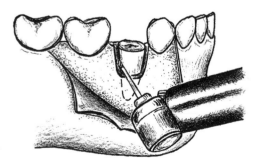

FIG. 6-4 Teeth often fracture during extraction leaving root fragments in alveolar bone. Adequate access must first be established by either an envelope or three-cornered triangle flap. Buccal plate is removed with a bur to expose root fragment. Space should be made to allow introduction of narrow elevator.

the fibers around the involved tooth and one tooth on either side in a circumdental fashion. A sharp periosteal elevator then firmly lifts all the involved dental papillae and gently reflects a full thickness mucoperiosteal flap. Care must be taken not to place undue pressure on the flap, causing it to tear. If more access and visualization are needed a vertical incision can be incorporated into the flap, converting it into a three-cornered flap, which is the other most common basic design.

Occasionally two vertical incisions are used to create a four-cornered flap. Once an adequate flap has been reflected, the surgeon can now make a better determination as to his next move. The dentist may, if enough tooth structure remains, attempt to reseat the extraction forceps and remove the tooth with no bone removal at all. If this is not possible he may grasp a bit of buccal bone to obtain a better mechanical advantage and grasp the tooth root.

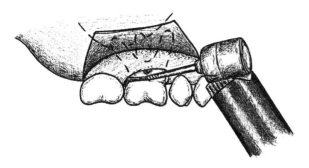

FIG. 6-7 When intact maxillary molar proves too difficult for routine extraction, it should be extracted surgically. A mucoperiosteal flap is raised and a small amount of crest bone is removed. Buccal roots are then sectioned with a surgical bur from the crown of the tooth.

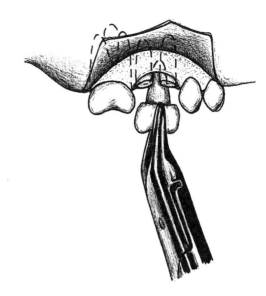

FIG. 6-9 Upper molar forceps are then used to remove the crown portion of the tooth along with its palatal root.

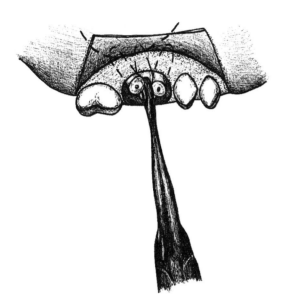

FIG. 6-8 If crown of the upper molar has been lost to caries or fracture, a flap is raised and the roots are sectioned into three independent roots and delivered with a straight elevator.

If the surgeon feels that buccal bone needs to be removed at this time, a surgical handpiece with a bur can be used to carefully remove bone to about one half of the root length and then use either a straight elevator or forceps to remove the tooth. In multi-rooted teeth, the roots should be sectioned and divided and each root then removed separately (Figs.6-7 through 6-13).

The surgical site is irrigated with copious water and bone edges are smoothed with a bone file before reapproximation of the mucoperiosteal flap and closure. Interrupted 3-0 or 4-0 black silk suture should be used to reapproximate the interdental papillae (Boxes 6-4, 6-5, and 6-6).

Removal of Root Tips

Despite good technique and procedure, teeth will fracture during routine exodontia leaving small roots in their socket. If this should occur, good lighting and small diameter suction are critically important to allow for good visualization. With the use of very fine apical root tip elevators (and if the tooth had significant mobility prior to fracturing) the root tip can most often be carefully elevated out of its bony crypt. If repeated attempts prove fruitless one should then immediately convert this to a surgical open procedure.

A full thickness mucoperiosteal flap is reflected and the buccal plate is removed with the root delivered buccally with a straight elevator (see Figs. 6-4 and 6-5).

In some cases, a modification of the open surgical procedure should be performed in order to preserve the buccal cortical crestal bone. In cases where an endosseous implant is planned or in bicuspid extractions for planned orthodontia a "window" technique is employed. In this procedure a small window is drilled and opened in the buccal plate adjacent to the root fragment and a fine instrument is then inserted into the window and the root pushed out through the socket (Figs. 6-14 and 6-15).

Leaving Root Fragments In Bone

At times during planned surgical extractions a decision will have to be made whether retrieving a fractured root is in the patient's best interest. Clearly, various reasons exist to abort an extraction when the risk of removal, in the treating doctor's opinion, outweighs the benefits.

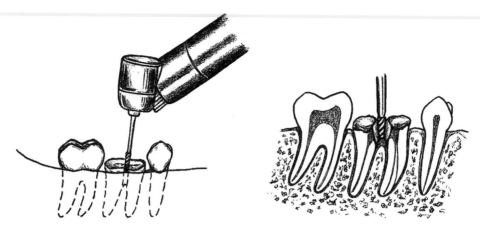

FIG. 6-10 If lower molar tooth proves difficult to extract, it is sectioned through the furcation area, resulting in two single-rooted teeth.

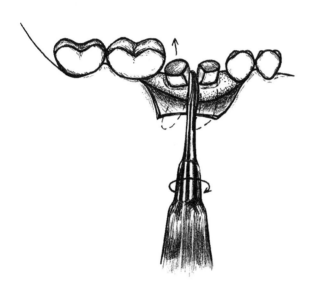

FIG. 6-11 After the lower molar has been surgically sectioned, a straight elevator is used to mobilize and deliver roots.

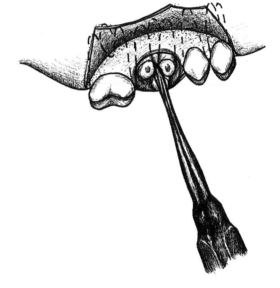

FIG. 6-12 Buccal roots are then separated and delivered with a straight elevator.

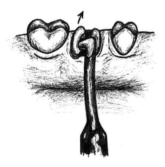

FIG. 6-13 After one root of molar roots has been removed, the Cryer elevator (East-West) is placed into empty mesial socket and turned with sharp point engaging interseptal bone and root to elevate remaining distal root.

BOX 6-4 Post Operative Surgical Management

1. Always remember to irrigate the extraction socket to remove all bone dust and tooth particles that may be present.
2. Always be certain to irrigate under the soft tissue flap before closure.
3. Compress buccal and lingual plates before closure (avoid in orthodontic extraction and implant sites).
4. Replace soft tissue flaps and close wound with 3-0 black silk.
5. Check for hemostasis prior to discharge.
6. Appropriate prescription for analgesic medication should be given.
7. Postoperative instruction should be given personally and patient informed of common postextraction sequelae such as swelling, facial bruising, etc.
8. Advise against spitting and rinsing for the first 24 hours.

Instructions Following Extractions

1. Avoid vigorous exercise
2. No smoking for 3 days
3. No rinsing or spitting for 24 hours
4. No drinking with straws
5. No alcoholic beverages while on narcotic medications
6. Rest for remainder of day
7. Elevate head for 24 hours
8. Take medications as instructed
9. Soft foods and liquids for 24 hours
10. Keep gauze in place for 2 hours upon leaving office
11. Ice packs to face 20 minutes on and 20 minutes off for 1 day
12. Call emergency number if any problems occur

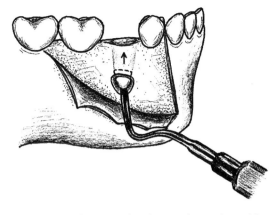

FIG. 6-15 An angled root tip elevator is used to drive root apically through window in bone, helping to preserve buccal plate.

Suture Material

- Two basic types of suture material exist: resorbable (material is broken down by the body) and nonresorbable, and both can be used in the oral cavity.
- The three types of resorbable sutures commonly used in the oral cavity are gut, polyglycolic, and polygalactic acids.
- Plain gut sutures retain their strength for approximately 5 to 7 days whereas the chromic-treated catgut will last for a slightly longer period of about 9 to 14 days.
- Polygalactic and polyglycolic acid sutures may take up to 4 weeks to resorb.
- Silk, nylon, polyester and polypropylene are types of nonresorbable sutures, with silk (4-0 or 3-0) being the most commonly used in the oral cavity. Whether resorbable or nonresorbable sutures are used, they should be removed in a week, when the patient returns for a follow-up visit.

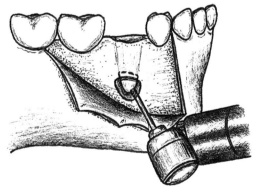

FIG. 6-14 In an attempt to maintain buccal plate and alveolar bone, a bony window can be opened at the apical root area with a bur.

The following are indications for leaving root fragments behind:

1. If root fragment is tiny (4 mm or less) and its removal will result in significant trauma to the patient.
2. There is no infection or apical pathology associated with the root fragment.
3. Root fragment is in close proximity to mental or inferior alveolar nerve.
4. Uncontrolled hemorrhage exists.
5. Patient is feeling ill.
6. Root is in close proximity to maxillary sinus.

If the surgeon elects to leave a root fragment behind, she should inform the patient and document reasons in the patient's chart. An immediate follow-up x-ray should be taken and the patient followed up during the course of the year to determine the fate of the remaining root.

The patient is also instructed to notify the office if any problems with the retained root develop.

Surgical Handpiece

The type of handpiece used for surgical sectioning of teeth is of vital importance. The ideal handpiece must be autoclavable, possess high torque, and not force air into the surgical field. Air forced directly under a periosteal flap can cause the development of air emphysema that can possibly lead to life-threatening airway problems. Copious irrigation must always accompany the use of a surgical handpiece to prevent overheating and necrosis of bone that will lead to postoperative pain and infection.

A backup spare handpiece should always be readily available in case of machine breakdown.

Swelling and Trismus

Postoperative swelling following surgical extractions is a usual and expected complication and should be considered surgical edema until proven otherwise. This edema may continue to increase for 2 to 3 days. Ice packs applied externally immediately following surgery for the first 24 hours is helpful in reducing this swelling. Postoperative infection is usually not a factor until 4 days following surgery and is associated with pain, overlying erythema, lymphadenopathy, fever, trismus, and fluctuance.

EXTRACTION TECHNIQUES
Maxillary Incisors and Canines

Gently reflect labial and palatal gingival cuff with periosteal elevator, then use straight elevator to develop some mobility of tooth. A straight upper forceps (#1) is placed on the crown and controlled force is used to seat the beaks at the neck of the tooth. Careful labial and palatal pressure is then applied along with mild rotation (Fig. 6-16).

Maxillary Premolars

Upper universal forceps (#150) is used and seated along the long axis of the tooth after some mobility is obtained with a straight elevator. Sustained apical pulling force is maintained after gentle buccal and palatal movement. Because the first premolar often has two fine roots it is important to attempt to avoid palatal

root fracture as this will be the harder of the two roots to recover and so a buccal delivery of the tooth is best performed (Fig. 6-17).

Maxillary Molars

The upper universal forceps (#150) is used for most maxillary molars whereas more difficult molar teeth may be removed with the upper molar cowhorn forceps (#88-R or 88-L). After attempting to achieve some mobility with the straight elevator the forceps is seated and buccal and palatal forces are applied; however the predominant direction of force should be buccal. If limited mobility is obtained the tooth should be surgically removed by sectioning the buccal roots from the palatal root, splitting the tooth with a straight elevator, and then delivering each root segment separately.

Mandibular Anterior Teeth

The mandibular incisors and canines are similar in shape but the incisors are shorter and thinner and more likely to fracture during extraction. Lower universal forceps (#151 type) are generally used for their extraction and are firmly seated followed by short labial and lingual luxating movements performed with teeth delivered in a labial direction.

A vertical hinge-type forceps known as the Ashe Forceps (also known as the English or European style) can also be used for the extraction of lower single-rooted teeth including incisors, canines, and bicuspids.

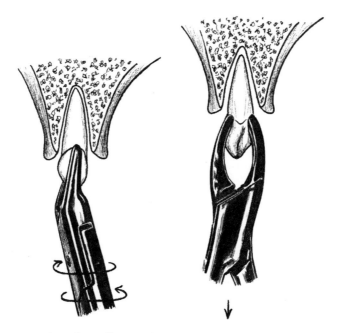

FIG. 6-16 For extraction of maxillary canine teeth, forceps are seated as far apically as possible. The tooth is extracted using pendulum movements along with careful rotation.

However, more caution is required as great forces can be generated with these forceps resulting in a higher incidence of root fracture(Fig. 6-18).[3]

Mandibular Premolars

The mandibular premolars tend to be conical root shaped and are extracted with #151 universal lower forceps using buccal and lingual movements.

Mandibular Molars

Mandibular molars are two-rooted teeth often with divergent roots. The lower universal forceps (#151) can and is often used but the lower molar cowhorn forceps is more helpful in extracting difficult molars(#23). The cowhorn forceps has sharp buccal and lingual beaks that seat between the mesial and distal roots. As the forceps is firmly seated between the roots an apical force is applied with a gentle pumping action which forces the tooth superiorly out of the tooth socket (Fig. 6-19).

Multiple Extractions

With the extraction of multiple teeth one should follow the following guidelines:

1. Maxillary teeth should be extracted first as the onset of local anesthesia is usually quicker in the upper jaw.

2. Begin with extraction of posterior teeth.
3. Following multiple extractions replace overlying mucosa and palpate bony ridge for obvious sharp bony ridges or severe undercuts. If any exist perform osteoplasty with bone rongeur and smooth with bone files. Irrigate copiously before closure.
4. Maintain as much of the alveolar bone and ridge as possible to allow for better bone contour and possible later implant placement.
5. Replace mucosal tissue and close with papillary sutures.

Extraction of Primary Teeth

Extraction of primary teeth includes all of the basic principles involved with adult permanent exodontia. Other than the forceps being smaller because of the smaller size of the teeth involved, separation of the gingival cuff followed by gentle elevation and forceps extraction is the standard technique of primary tooth extraction.

However, because of the significant divergence of the roots found in nonresorbed primary molar teeth, early consideration should be directed toward sectioning the teeth and performing individual root retrievals. One should always be aware of the close proximity of the primary tooth to the succedaneous permanent tooth and be most careful to avoid damaging them.

If root fracture should occur an attempt should be made to surgically retrieve any residual root if, in the

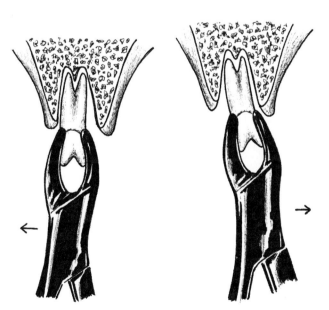

FIG. 6-17 The first maxillary premolar most often has bifid roots with slender root tips. It should be handled with caution using pendulum movements only and no rotational movements. Deliver the tooth buccally.

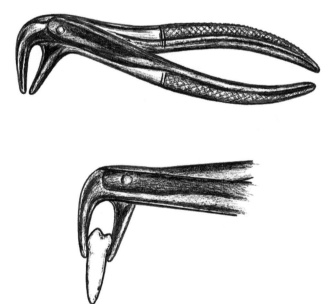

FIG. 6-18 Ashe (English or European style) forceps have hinge in vertical direction and are held in a vertical direction. These forceps are used for extraction of single rooted lower teeth.

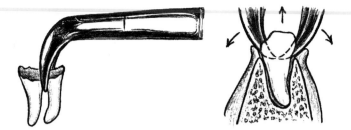

FIG. 6-19 Cowhorn forceps beaks are pressed into the lower molar bifurcations during extraction. As the handles of the forceps are squeezed, upward extraction forces are generated.

opinion of the treating doctor, such an attempt will not result in any permanent injury to the permanent tooth. If residual roots are allowed to remain in the bone, most often no adverse sequelae will result but the patient's guardian or parent should be informed.

EXTRACTIONS IN THE SPECIAL HIGH-RISK PATIENT
Patients Undergoing Radiotherapy

Clinical Findings. It is very likely that the average dental practitioner will in her lifetime be asked to examine and treat patients who have either undergone radiotherapy for the treatment of head and neck cancer or who are scheduled for such treatment. It is imperative that the treating doctor be aware of the special precautions necessary before initiating any therapy.

Radiotherapy when delivered in cancerocidal doses to the oral cavity results in the destruction of neoplastic cells as well as affecting both normal epithelial and endothelial cells also found in the oral cavity. Clinically this results in the patient possibly developing various clinical hard and soft tissue complications.

1. *Mucositis:* severe painful erythematous mucosal reaction with or without ulceration
2. *Xerostomia or dry mouth:* secondary to radiation damage to the salivary glands
3. *"Radiation caries":* severe cervical decay secondary to the decreased salivary flow
4. *Osteoradionecrosis:* a noninfective bone destruction with resultant nonvital dead bone or sequestra formation as a result of the destruction of the mandibular vasculature.

Extraction Protocol

Patients who are scheduled for radiotherapy should be sent routinely to a dentist for screening and treatment. All teeth with a questionable or poor prognosis should be extracted and only those teeth with a healthy periodontium should be retained. If extractions are to be performed, they should be done at least 3 weeks before starting the radiotherapy to ensure soft tissue healing[1]

The extractions should be performed atraumatically with careful attention to the overlying soft tissue. Primary soft tissue closure should be achieved even if it means removing some extra bone. All sharp bony margins should be carefully smoothed out and well irrigated before closure. A custom tray should be fabricated for the remaining teeth and topical self-administered fluoride applications should be started.

The postirradiated patient who requires extraction poses a difficult clinical dilemma. The incidence of developing postextraction osteoradionecrosis in this patient population is high because of the decreased blood supply in the involved jawbones.

If extractions must be performed these patients are probably best managed by oral and maxillofacial surgeons. It is recommended that these patients be placed on systemic antibiotics prior to and following extractions and Marx advises they be given hyperbaric oxygen therapy both before and following surgery.[2]

Dental Extraction in Chemotherapy Patients

Chemotherapy like radiotherapy has a cancerocidal effect based on its ability to destroy rapidly dividing cells. Unfortunately, normal cells are also affected in patients receiving chemotherapeutic drugs, especially the epithelium cells of the oral cavity and the bone marrow. The bone marrow suppression seen in patients on chemotherapy leads to a decreased number of circulating white blood cells and red blood cells and platelets.

Obviously surgical extraction in patients currently being treated with chemotherapy can result in severe hemorrhage and infection. However, cell recovery from myelosuppression after cessation of chemotherapy is usually complete in 3 weeks and patients with nonhematologic neoplasms can than be treated.

It is good practice to consult with the patient's private physician to determine the patient's exact blood profile before surgical intervention especially if the patient has received chemotherapy within 3 weeks of any planned surgical procedure.

The patient's white blood cell count should be at least 2000/mm^2 with a platelet count of 50,000/mm^2 before undergoing routine surgery.

REFERENCES

1. Ellis E: Management of the radiotherapy or chemotherapy patient. In Peterson LJ: *Contemporary oral and maxillofacial surgery*, St. Louis, 1988, Mosby.
2. Marx RE: A new concept in the treatment of osteoradionecrosis, *J Oral Maxillofac Surg* 41:351, 1983.
3. Peterson LJ et al: Armamentarium for basic oral surgery. In Peterson LJ: *Contemporary oral and maxillofacial surgery*, ed 3, St. Louis, 1998, Mosby.

Management of Impacted Third Molar Teeth

HARRY DYM, DDS

One of the most common surgical procedures performed in the United States is the surgical removal of impacted third molars or "wisdom teeth." The impacted third molar fails to erupt into the dental arch because of some interference including:

1. Dense overlying bone
2. Thick overlying fibrous tissue
3. The tooth's angulation
4. Adjacent teeth

The NIH Consensus Development Conference for the Removal of Third Molars, held in 1979,[1] developed a series of guidelines and statements that provide important information to practitioners involved in the treatment of patients with impacted third molars.

INDICATIONS FOR REMOVAL OF IMPACTED THIRD MOLARS[2]

1. Infection
2. Nonrestorable dental caries
3. Compromise of periodontal status of adjacent teeth
4. Cyst formation
5. Interference with orthodontic treatment
6. Presence of impacted tooth in the line of jaw fracture
7. Persistent pain of unknown origin
8. Preirradiation
9. Resorption of adjacent teeth
10. Preceding fabrication of adjacent restorative crowns and dentures

Additional comments from the consensus study include:

1. The least morbidity associated with third molar removal occurs when they are removed between the ages of 15 and 25 or when the roots are only two-thirds formed. This opinion is formed based on many reasons associated with the anatomic development of wisdom teeth in patients at this stage including:

a. Roots are generally straight and not curved
b. Bone is softer and more pliant
c. Inferior alveolar nerve is more distant from the root apices
d. Healing is more rapid

2. Overwhelming clinical evidence clearly shows that patients with impacted teeth who wait until symptoms occur before seeking removal have greater morbidity associated with their surgery. Clearly, early intervention in the surgical removal of impacted third molars will benefit most patients.

CONTRAINDICATIONS TO REMOVAL OF IMPACTED TEETH

Elective removal of third molar teeth, like all surgical procedures, should not be performed if the potential damage outweighs the benefits to be obtained. Clearly, patients with significantly compromised medical conditions are not candidates for elective third molar removal. It is also the consensus of most surgeons that symptomatic third molars in the mature (over 50) adult population should not routinely be removed.

Indications For Removal of Impacted Teeth—Pericoronitis

A common finding in patients presenting with lower third molar pain is a clinical condition referred to as pericoronitis. Pericoronitis is an infection of the soft tissue surrounding a partially erupted third molar and can be caused by multiple factors.

1. Food debris is often trapped under the soft tissue flap overlying the impacted wisdom tooth and cannot be effectively cleansed. As a result, bacteria (streptococci and a variety of anaerobic organisms) invade the site and initiate the infectious process.

2. The opposing maxillary third molar will often cause constant occlusal trauma to the overlying soft tissue of the lower third molar, which will result in a highly swollen and inflamed tissue mass. This clinical condition is referred to as operculitis.
3. Pericoronitis can present as a mild infection or as a severe fulminating infection requiring hospitalization and aggressive surgical and medical treatment.

Mild to moderate acute pericoronitis can be best managed by the removal of the impinging maxillary third molar, followed by irrigation of the pericoronal tissues with saline, hydrogen peroxide, or chlorhexidine solution, along with a prescription for antibiotics, such as penicillin or clindamycin.

In some patients, pericoronitis can lead to serious systemic illness that will require hospitalization and intravenous antibiotic therapy. These patients will usually present with fever (greater than 101° F) malaise, trismus (inability to open greater than 20 mm), and severe facial swelling.

Though removal of the overlying soft tissue (operculectomy) has been advocated by some rarely is it successful and only delays the inevitable surgical extraction.

Odontogenic Cysts and Tumors

Impacted third molar teeth are often associated with cysts and tumors and screening panoramic x-rays are most helpful in early diagnosis and detection. As the impacted teeth develop, the surrounding follicular sac in most patients maintains its original size but in some cases may undergo cystic degeneration and develop into a dentigerous cyst or keratocyst. As a general guideline, if the follicular space around the crown of the tooth is greater than 5 mm, a diagnosis of dentigerous cyst can be made.

Similarly, odontogenic tumors can arise from the epithelial cell lining within the dental follicle and screening panoramic x-rays are important in the thorough dental and medical evaluation of the patient.

CLASSIFICATION OF IMPACTED THIRD MOLARS

Impacted third molar teeth can be classified by a variety of descriptive terms. The one classification system most commonly used refers to the tooth's angulation as compared with the long axis of the adjacent second molar. The mesioangular impaction, tilted toward the second molar, is the most commonly seen variety of impacted third molars.

The vertical impaction is the second most commonly occurring type of third molar impaction and has its long axis parallel to the second molar. In the distoangular impaction, the crown faces distally or posteriorly and is the most difficult of all to remove.

INSTRUMENTATION

Appropriate instrumentation is as critical to the successful removal of impacted third molars as is good surgical technique. Before attempting any surgical third molar removal one should have the following instruments available (Table 7-1):

1. #15 blade
2. Periosteal elevator
3. Seldin retractor
4. Minnesota retractor
5. Elevators (thin and wide)
6. Bone files
7. Needle holder
8. Suture scissors

Rotary instruments for cutting both tooth and bone are essential, whether they be air/nitrogen driven or electrical; they must be autoclavable and not exhaust air into the surgical field. Burs used are either round or fissured and irrigation during bone/tooth cutting must be available (sterile or tap water).

SURGICAL TECHNIQUE (Box 7-1)
Step 1—Access (Figs. 7-1 through 7-3)

Adequate visibility at the surgical site is essential to good surgical technique, and the surgical extraction of impacted third molar teeth is no different. The #15 blade is the instrument of choice for use in incising the soft tissues necessary for wisdom teeth extraction.

Incision design for third molar surgery falls basically into two broad categories:

1. Envelope design
2. Triangular flap, an envelope design with a vertical releasing incision

Obviously, the degree of soft tissue reflection is dependent on the type of impaction being removed and the quantity of bone removal required. The ability to limit the flap design will help decrease postoperative swelling and pain but should never be done at the expense of compromising technique or tearing of the flap because of decreased visibility.

The soft tissue incision is intrasulcular beginning from the distal of the lower first molar and extending directly behind the second molar, making certain to be over bone. The incision is always made lateral to the

TABLE 7-1 Basic Instruments for Third Molar Surgery

Technique	Instruments
Cheek retraction and visualization of the surgical area	Mouth mirror, wide retractor (Seldin #23, Minnesota)
Incisions	Scalpel handle with #15 blade
Flap development and reflection	#9 periosteal elevator, Woodson, Molt
Flap retraction	Wide retractor (Seldin #23, Minnesota)
Bone Removal	Handpieces: high-speed surgical handpiece (no air blown into the surgical field), two-speed straight handpiece (using the higher speed), surgical straight handpiece (used by many oral surgeons)
	Burs: crosscut tapered fissure (702, 558), nontapered crosscut fissure, round (high speed burs should be surgical length)
Luxation and sectioning	Straight elevators, such as the 301, and 34 or 34S and Cryer (East-West) elevators
Tooth removal	Forceps, such as 150 and 151
Suture cutting, distal wedge excision, severing fibrotic tissue	Surgical scissors, such as Dean
Tying sutures, traction on follicle removing loose pieces of tooth	Needle holder, such as Mayo-Hegar 6"
Suturing material	4-0 or 3-0 silk or chromic gut suture with 3/8 circle reverse cutting needle
Curetting follicle or infection	Surgical spoon curette
Suctioning	Surgical suction tip, preferably tapered, plastic or metal
Irrigation	Device: (1) through the handpiece or (2) with three-way syringe (irrigation medium from a reservoir); (3) 15-30 ml irrigation syringe with a blunt irrigation needle; (4) bulb syringe; or (5) plastic molded irrigation syringe
	Medium: sterile saline or sterile water

BOX 7-1 General Principles for Surgical Technique of Impaction Removal

1. Reflect mucoperiosteal flap to obtain good visual access.
2. Remove labial bone with high speed surgical drill using round or cross cut bur.
3. Expose crown of impaction up to CEJ and make room to allow for elevator placement.
4. Attempt to gently evaluate for mobility with elevator (straight or angled).
5. Section crown (either horizontally or vertically depending on angulation of impaction) with high-speed surgical handpiece. Be careful of lingual soft tissue and depth of surgical cut.
6. Straight elevator should be used to separate crown from tooth.
7. Deliver roots with root tip elevators or crane pick. Be prepared to remove additional superior and labial bone and section roots if no mobility present.
8. Inspect bony crypt for loose debris and any bleeding problems and smooth bone margins with bone file.
9. Carefully remove follicular soft tissue and tease it out from surrounding mucosa.
10. Copious irrigation of socket and beneath soft tissue flap prior to closure.
11. Reapproximate soft tissue flap and close with 3-0 or 4-0 chromic or black silk sutures.
12. Consider intraoral injection of steroids if extensive bone surgery performed. 4mg of dexamethasone (Decadron) can be injected into masseter muscle on each side.
13. Evaluate for post surgical bleeding prior to discharge.

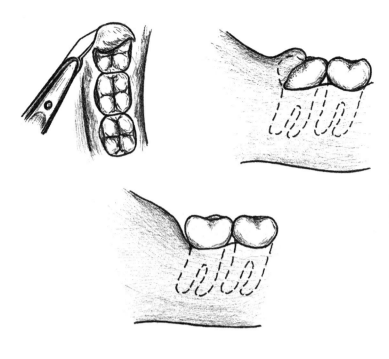

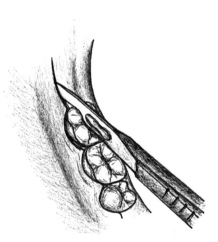

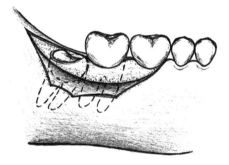

FIG. 7-1 The soft tissue impaction can sometimes be treated by surgically removing the overlying (operculum) distal soft tissue flap. This can be done with either a scalpel blade or electrocautery. This procedure is often referred to as an operculectomy.

FIG. 7-2 The surgical incision begins posterior or distal to the impacted third molar along the external oblique ridge. Be certain to stay to the buccal and cut along the bone. The incision is then extended anteriorly and intrasulcularly to the first molar.

FIG. 7-3 An envelope flap is developed with a periosteal elevator. In some circumstances, when dealing with deeply impacted teeth it may be necessary to incorporate a vertical anterior release and create a triangular flap.

midcrestal bone to assure that the lingual nerve is not damaged. If greater visibility is required a vertical incision can be generated by incising the papilla and extending it through the attached gingivae at the mesial aspect of the second molar. When using a vertical releasing incision, it is always important to make certain that the incision can be closed over bone and not a bony defect.

The full thickness mucoperiosteal flap is then reflected, starting anteriorly with a periosteal elevator. The

flap can be retracted during surgery with either a Selden or Minnesota retractor.

Removal of Surrounding Bone
(Figs. 7-4 through 7-21)

After adequate flap retraction, bone removal is then performed. A high torque handpiece with a special surgical attachment that will not blow air into the surgical field must be used. A variety of

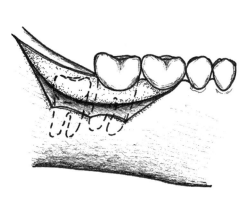

FIG. 7-4 Remove adequate amount of bone to fully expose the crown of the vertical impaction. This will require bone removal on the occlusal, buccal, and distal aspects of the crown. Be certain to expose the crown to the cervical line.

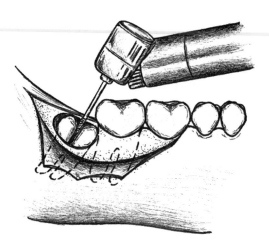

FIG. 7-6 Buccal bone is removed to reveal the crown of the impacted tooth. Distal bone is also removed to fully expose the crown. In this mesioangular wisdom tooth, a surgical bur will attempt to section the roots through its bifurcation. Be careful not to cut completely through to the lingual side to avoid possible damage to the lingual nerve.

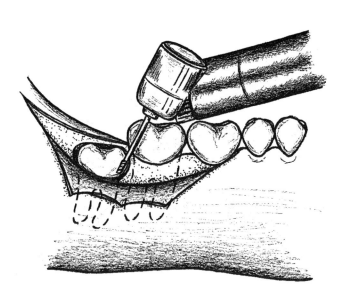

FIG. 7-5 Reflected mucoperiosteal envelope flap and outline of vertically impacted third molar tooth.

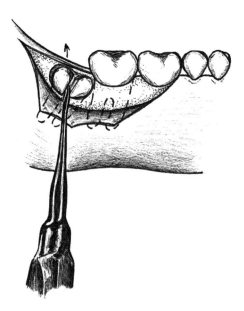

FIG. 7-7 A straight elevator is then inserted into the cut section of the tooth and turned sideways. This will cause the tooth to fracture into two. The distal half is then elevated upward.

45°-angled surgical handpieces are currently available and are quite useful. Of course, all equipment used must be capable of undergoing frequent sterilization procedures.

The type of drill used is operator-dependent but large round burs (#6 and #8) or crosscut fissured burs are most often used.

A trough should be cut between the crown and the lateral buccal alveolar bone exposing the entire crown to the cementoenamel junction. A con-

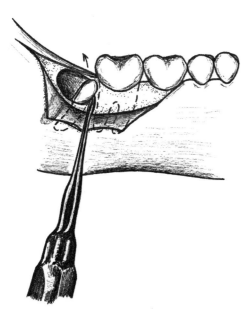

FIG. 7-8 With the distal half of the tooth removed, the mesial half can now be elevated out to the distal.

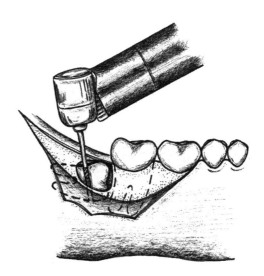

FIG. 7-10 Crown is sectioned with surgical bur and removed with narrow elevator. When sectioning crown, leave lip of root structure to help in its removal.

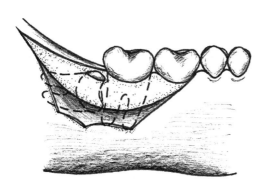

FIG. 7-9 Outline of reflected envelope flap before removal of full bony horizontal impaction.

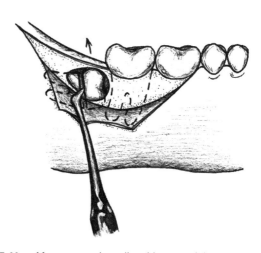

FIG. 7-11 After crown is split with a straight elevator, it is rolled out with an East-West or Cryer elevator.

stant stream of water irrigation must accompany the drilling to avoid overheating the bone as well as improving visibility by removing the cut bone and tooth debris.

After the crown is exposed on both its occlusal and buccal aspect, the crosscut fissure bur should be placed on the mesial aspect of the tooth to create a space between the tooth and bone in a vertical right angle fashion. This squaring of the bone will allow a small narrow straight elevator to be introduced to attempt to

luxate or move the tooth even before actual sectioning of the tooth.

At this stage in the procedure, the crown should be sectioned and delivered in segments. When sectioning teeth, always be careful not to completely drill through the entire crown to the lingual, or this will significantly increase the chance of causing actual lingual nerve damage. Always cut through three fourths of the way and split the remaining tooth with a straight elevator.

It is also good technique to gently place a throat

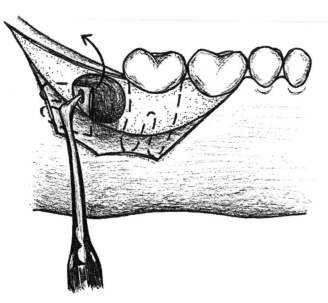

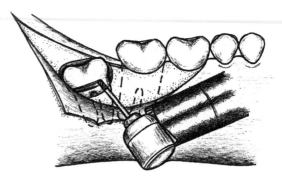

FIG. 7-15   Crown of tooth is sectioned off with bur and split with straight elevator.

FIG. 7-12   The remaining roots are then elevated out with an angled elevator after a purchase point has been drilled into roots with a bur.

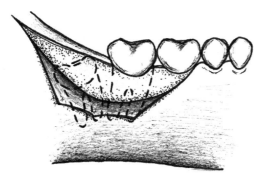

FIG. 7-13   Outline of soft tissue flap prior to extraction of disto-angular impaction.

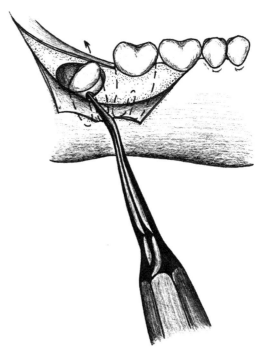

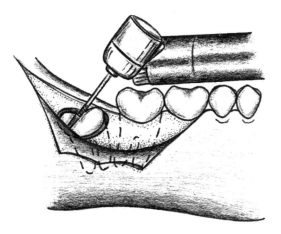

FIG. 7-14   Occlusal, buccal, and distal bone is removed in the distoangular impaction. It is important to remember that more distal bone will need to be removed in this type of impaction.

FIG. 7-16   Sometimes only distal portion of the crown needs to be removed to allow for tooth to be elevated out distally.

curtain in the mouth (4×4 sponge) before luxation and actual tooth removal. Be prepared to section the crown in multiple segments, as it is sometimes difficult to remove the entire crown after only one split. After the crown has been sectioned and removed the roots should be luxated out with straight and offset elevators. If no or limited movement follows, continue to carefully trough the bone and prepare to section the roots. Narrow root tip elevators are very helpful in loosening and prying the roots free.

Once the tooth is completely extracted, pay close attention to the debridement and closure of the surgical site. Inadequate debridement is a primary cause of postoperative pain and infection. A gentle

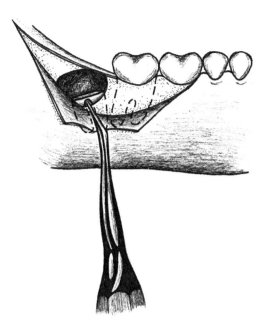

FIG. 7-17 Purchase point is placed into remaining root structure and delivered by east-west or angled elevator.

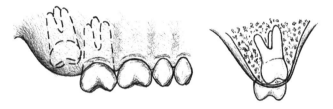

FIG. 7-18 Maxillary third molars most often present as vertical type of impaction (63% of the time).

stream of water should be directed at both the bony crypt and beneath the soft tissue flap only after a bone file has been used to smooth out the cut bone. In addition, the attached third molar follicular sac should be gently detached from the surrounding soft tissue and socket (making very certain not to cut any lingual attached mucosa) and removed with a curved hemostat.

Wound Closure (Fig. 7-22)

The mucoperiosteal flap is gently repositioned under firm pressure for closure. The suture material often used is 3-0 or 4-0 black silk but many doctors prefer resorbable materials. The author prefers silk sutures as they are easy to remove and allow for the patient to be seen for a postoperative visit. The flap should not be closed

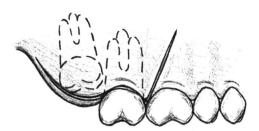

FIG. 7-19 A vertical incision is extended mesial to the maxillary second molar and then follows posteriorly around the sulcus. The incision then extends backwards over the maxillary tuberosity to allow for better access. The triangular flap is difficult, but an envelope flap can also be used for less complex third molar impaction removals.

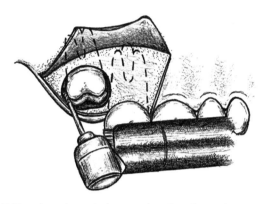

FIG. 7-20 A periosteal elevator sharply reflects the mucoperiosteal flap and a surgical handpiece is then used to carefully expose the crown of the impacted maxillary third molar.

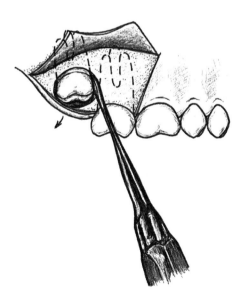

FIG. 7-21 Using a straight or contraangled elevator from the mesial side, the tooth is then elevated out of its bony crypt in a distobuccal direction.

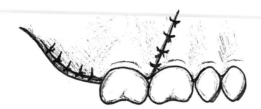

FIG. 7-22 Replace flap in its proper presurgical position. It is important to secure the corner of the flap first to help achieve correct anatomic flap closure.

watertight with multiple sutures but rather closed with two or three sutures to allow for some limited opening and drainage.

PREOPERATIVE MANAGEMENT OF THE IMPACTED THIRD MOLAR PATIENT

All patients scheduled for removal of impacted wisdom teeth should first be seen for a separate extensive consultation visit. It is at this time that diagnostic x-rays are taken, medical history reviewed, and clinical exam performed. Clinical teaching aids should be used to review and discuss the nature of the planned surgery and review possible intraoperative complications; it is also at this visit that a decision should be made as to the type of anesthetic technique to be used during the actual surgical encounter (Box 7-2).

Though local anesthesia used appropriately can provide a complete pain-free environment many patients will require some form of additional IV sedation to allow them to calmly endure the surgical removal of multiple impactions. The technique used is the surgeon's preference, but whichever method is chosen, intraoperative amnesia should be a desired end result.

Because the neurovascular canal carrying the inferior alveolar nerve bundle is in close proximity to the apices of the lower third molar teeth, a discussion of lower lip and chin numbness or paraesthesia should take place. Though the incident of permanent paraesthesia (greater than 12 months duration) is only 1%, the patients should be made aware of this as well as other more commonly occurring postoperative sequelae.

POSTOPERATIVE INSTRUCTIONS
(Box 7-3)

Before patient discharge following third molar removal, close inspection of the surgical site should be performed to check for hemostasis. The patient should be given both verbal as well as written postoperative instruction with a contact number to access the treating doctor in case of emergency. Additional gauze

pads should also be given along with appropriate prescriptions.

MANAGEMENT OF INTRAOPERATIVE COMPLICATIONS
Bleeding

Intraoperative hemorrhaging can sometimes occur during lower third molar surgery and can be rather disconcerting. Frequently, this bleeding is secondary to the patient's underlying medical history or caused by medication the patient is currently taking.

A review of the patient's surgical history, with emphasis on past bleeding episodes is essential and can alert the dentist/oral surgeon to potential bleeding complications. Aspirin therapy and anticoagulation medication, often used to manage cardiac patients, interfere with the blood clotting mechanisms and should be, in consultation with the patient's physician, stopped before extensive surgical extractions.

However, if intraoperative bleeding does occur, careful suction should be used first to accurately determine the source of bleeding. Sometimes, the bleeding can be seen coming from a soft tissue injury: tongue, floor of mouth, and lingual or buccal mucosa. These injuries will respond well to firm direct pressure with a 2×2 sponge followed by direct suturing if possible.

Most often the oozing stems directly from the open bony extraction socket. First, direct pressure with a 2×2 sponge applied to the site and maintained for 10 minutes should be attempted. If after this time it appears that the bleeding seems unabated, Gelfoam

BOX 7-3 Sample Postoperative Instructions

1. Bite down on gauze pad for 1 hour after leaving the clinic.
2. *Do not* spit. Swallow your saliva continuously to keep your mouth dry.
3. On arrival home, place ice bag on face for 20 minutes, take off for 20 minutes, but do not freeze the skin. If too cold, place a thin towel on skin and apply ice bag on towel.
4. Upon removal, gauze pad may be stained pink. This does not mean there is bleeding-bite down on another clean gauze pad for 1 hour and repeat if necessary, but *do not* rinse.
5. For bleeding, bite down on another clean gauze pad for 1 hour and repeat if necessary, but *do not* rinse.
6. Some swelling or discoloration may follow oral surgery and would cause no concern.
7. *Do not* rinse today. Tomorrow, rinse after meals, using 1/4 teaspoon salt in a large glass of warm water.
8. *Do not* smoke for 24 hours.
9. Diet: any soft food that you can mash with a fork (cold or warm, but not hot).
10. Brush all teeth carefully and gently, especially the teeth around the area of operation. Use a soft toothbrush.
11. If you were given any prescriptions, take the medicine as directed.
12. *Do not take aspirin* if you have pain, take Tylenol or Advil.
13. If constipated, take a mild laxative tonight.
14. In case of emergency the Doctor's access number is_____.

TABLE 7-2 Commonly Prescribed Analgesics

Drug Name	Dosage	Frequency
Tylenol No. 3	codeine 30 mg and 300 mg acetaminophen	q4h-q6h
Percodan	oxycodone 5 mg and 325 mg aspirin	q6h
Percocet	oxycodone 5 mg and 325 mg acetaminophen	q6h
Vicodin	hydrocodone 5 mg and 500 mg acetaminophen	q6h
Vicodin ES	hydrocodone 7.5 mg and 500 mg acetaminophen	q6h
Vicoprofen	hydrocodone 7.5 mg and 200 mg ibuprofen	q6h
Lortab (Liquid)	hydrocodone and acetaminophen elixir 7.5 mg/500 mg per 15 ml	q6h
Motrin	600 mg ibuprofen	q6h

(bioabsorbable gelatin sponge) should be packed directly into the surgical extraction socket. If this maneuver proves unsuccessful, the author prefers packing collagen pads (they work better than the soft collagen-powder/fibers currently available) directly under pressure into the socket and then applying pressure with 2×2 sponge over the filled socket, after firmly closing the socket with multiple sutures for 20 minutes.

Patients over the age of 60 who undergo surgical tooth extractions should be cautioned about the possibility of developing perioral facial ecchymosis 2 to 4 days following the extraction. This black and blue appearance is the result of bleeding into the subcutaneous soft tissues and other than practicing as atraumatic a surgical procedure as possible, little can be done to prevent and treat it, once it occurs.

Teeth Displacement

Maxillary and mandibular third molars can quite accidentally because of their presenting anatomic position be inadvertently displaced into various anatomic extra-oral positions. The upper third molar can most often be displaced into the maxillary sinus or the infratemporal fossa with the lower third molar sometimes pushed through the lingual plate into the parapharyngeal and submandibular spaces.

This misadventure, though sometimes unavoidable, can best be prevented by

1. good access.
2. good visibility and suction.
3. good retraction.
4. appropriate and well directed mechanical forces.

If displacement does occur retrieval (if the tooth can be directly visualized) should be tried with a long tissue forceps or rongeur instrument. If the displaced tooth can be palpated, it may be directed back into the socket for retrieval. No blind attempts should be made at this time and often the best procedure is to close the wound and refer the patient to an oral and maxillofacial surgeon for treatment.

MANAGEMENT OF POSTOPERATIVE COMPLICATION PAIN (Table 7-2)

Once patients are reassured that they will not experience any intraoperative surgical pain they are still very much concerned about postoperative pain and their ability to tolerate such discomfort. Patients should be advised at the presurgical consultation meeting of the dentist's/surgeon's concern for their postsurgical well-being and a prescription for appropriate analgesic should be given and filled before the actual surgery.

This allows the patient to begin immediate pain therapy while he is still anesthetized, and not have to wait hours for potential drugstore deliveries.

It is well documented that patients who take analgesic medication before the onset of pain, while the local anesthesia is still in effect, will experience a milder and less intense postsurgical pain that will be more easily managed with the usually prescribed analgesic medications. Two basic types of analgesic medication are currently available: those that act peripherally by interfering with prostaglandin synthesis (aspirin, acetaminophen, and the nonsteroidal antiinflammatory agents) and the narcotic medications, centrally acting analgesics (most commonly codeine or its congeners such as oxycodone and hydrocodone).

The narcotic medications are formulated either with aspirin, acetaminophen, or nonsteroidal antiinflammatory medication. Many surgeons prefer not using any aspirin-based compounds, which cause a decrease in platelet aggregation, and tend to limit analgesics to acetaminophen compounds. The first 2 days following third molar surgery are probably the most painful with the pain diminishing in intensity from that point onward.

Nerve Dysfunction (Figs. 7-23 and 7-24)

The postoperative complication most distressing to both patient and surgeon alike is damage to either the lingual or inferior alveolar nerve resulting in an altered sensation (paresthesia) or total anesthesia of the lip and tongue. Obviously this is one complication, though according to the literature quite uncommon with a permanent paraesthesia of the lower lip reported to be about 1% and that of the tongue occurring in about one in 1000 extractions, that should be explained thoroughly to any patient undergoing third molar removal.

The literature states that over 96% of patients who experienced inferior alveolar injuries and 87% of those with lingual nerve injuries recovered spontaneously.[3] Most spontaneous recovery occurs within 9 months and after 2 years there is little likelihood of further spontaneous recovery but the possibility of further recovery several years after injury cannot be dismissed.[4,5]

If nerve damage does occur, its extent should be documented in the chart, and the patient followed every 2 weeks for 2 months then every 6 weeks for 6 months followed by every 6 months for 2 years.

Opinions differ as to the best timing for surgical intervention with a microsurgical nerve repair, with advocates from 3 months to 1 year following surgery. This is one complication that should be thoroughly discussed with all patients before any third molar surgery and documented in the chart.

Postoperative Hemorrhage

If bleeding occurs after the patient has left the office, the patient should be instructed to avoid constant expectoration and to replace the gauze sponge directly over the socket for 20 minutes. If bleeding is persistent and continues, the patient should be advised to place a dry tea bag over the site and apply pressure.

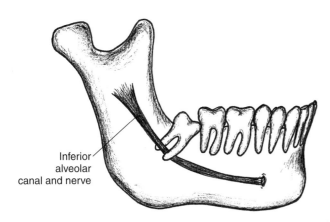

FIG. 7-23 Prior to lower third molar surgery, a quality panoramic radiograph should be available so that the proximity of the anterior alveolar canal to the tooth can be visualized. This will give both the patient and treating doctor a better indication of the possibility of post extraction nerve dysfunction. It is generally believed, however, that differences in surgical techniques have little influence on the overall incidence of inferior alveolar nerve damage.

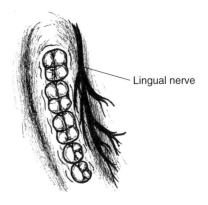

FIG. 7-24 The clinician should always be aware of the close proximity of lingual nerve to the medial aspect of the third molar tooth and should be extremely careful when sectioning the crown near the lingual side of the tooth. Overly aggressive curettage and follicle removal should also be avoided on the lingual aspect of the socket.

If bleeding still continues the patient should be seen on an emergency basis for evaluation and treatment.

Treatment Steps

1. Give local anesthesia with epinephrine to allow for complete and adequate inspection.
2. Remove any existing clot from the socket and explore the site and surrounding tissues.
3. Apply direct pressure with gauze sponge for 10 minutes.
4. If bleeding still persists and is emanating from the bony socket, place a hemostatic agent such as Gelfoam, Surgicel, or Avitene (collagen pads or in fiber form) into the socket; suture over the site and apply digital pressure with a gauze sponge for 10 minutes.
5. The patient should only be discharged after complete hemostasis is achieved.

A more in-depth discussion on this topic appears in Chapter 5.

Maxillary Tuberosity Fracture

A complication associated with extraction of upper third molar teeth is fracture of the posterior maxillary tuberosity. If a large segment of tuberosity is removed along with the third molar, a significant sinus opening can occur which will be difficult to close.

Early recognition that a tuberosity fracture may occur is essential to avoiding this problem. Lone longstanding maxillary third molars in close proximity to the maxillary sinus should be approached with great caution and surgical extraction should be considered early on if the tooth exhibits no mobility during luxation.

During maxillary third molar extraction the surgeon should visualize the tooth and surrounding soft tissues at all times and palpate the area as pressure is applied.

When tuberosity fracture does occur, the clinician should immediately stop the extraction and leave the segment in place. If little mobility exists, place the patient on appropriate pain medications, wait 6 weeks and plan for surgical extraction at that time.

If significant mobility exists it will be necessary to splint the tooth with either brackets or wire for 6 weeks, to allow for bone healing to occur.

Maxillary Sinus Involvement

Because of the intimate relationship between the maxillary sinus and the roots of the upper molar teeth, especially third molar teeth, a real risk of developing an oral antral communication exists following third molar removal. This risk should therefore be discussed before the procedure and is routinely part of the informed consent process. Evaluation and treatment of sinus exposure is discussed in detail in Chapter 12.

Alveolar Osteitis (Dry Socket)
(Box 7-4)

Perhaps the most common complication, seen following 3%[6] of all third molar extractions, is the "dry socket" or alveolar osteitis. Rarely seen in the maxilla, the dry socket is thought to arise secondary to either a subclinical infection or bone inflammation, resulting in early lysis of the socket blood clot. This empty socket results in denuded bone that is very sensitive and painful. The patient who has a dry socket will classically complain of lessening pain that begins to increase in severity 3 or 4 days following surgery. Upon examination no clinical signs of infection are seen (swelling, purulence, lymphadenopathy) except for an exquisitely painful socket that appears empty.

Treatment is principally directed toward decreasing the patient's pain while the socket gradually fills in with soft tissue coverage. Under local anesthesia (although not always necessary), the socket is irrigated copiously with sterile saline or water and suctioned dry. Then a commercially prepared "dry socket" paste (eugenol is the primary compound) is then applied to 0.25-inch plain or iodoform gauze or to Gelfoam (an absorbable gelatin sponge) and placed directly into the socket. Patients normally have significant decrease in pain immediately thereafter. The socket should be irrigated every 24 to 48 hours and the dressing replaced, depending on the patient's pain response. This pain usually lasts for 4 to 8 days and resolves with no need for follow-up. Antibiotics are rarely necessary unless there are systemic symptoms.

BOX 7-4 Dry-Socket Treatment Regimen

1. Confirm Diagnosis
   a. Continued presence of pain that begins to worsen on third or fourth post operative day.
   b. Fetid odor.
   c. Socket extremely painful upon light palpation.
   d. Socket devoid of any clot or tissue upon close inspection.
2. Use irrigation syringe to flush loose debris from socket.
3. Place socket dressing with dry-socket paste on 1/4-inch gauze strip and pack to top of socket.
4. See patient in two days for evaluation and if pain persists remove packing irrigate and replace packing.
5. Continue patient on appropriate pain medication while under treatment for dry socket.
6. Patient may benefit from additional week's course of antibiotic therapy if there are any systemic symptoms.

Predisposing factors for dry socket development may include:

1. Patients with smoking history
2. Patients on birth control medication
3. Preexisting infection
4. Extensive bone removed during extraction.

Possible means of preventing dry socket include:[7]

1. Constant irrigation of bone including during cutting phase of extraction.
2. Careful irrigation and debridement following procedure and prior to suturing.
3. Limiting trauma and bone removal.
4. Some practitioners feel that placing either an antibiotic-saturated dressing (like clindamycin or tetracycline saturated Gelfoam) or steroid paste directly into the socket will decrease the incidence of dry sockets.
5. Pre- and postoperative rinsing with 0.12% chlorhexidine solution.
6. Prescribing systemic prophylactic antibiotics.

Trismus

The inability to open one's mouth maximally following any extraction, but especially after lower third molar surgery, is not an unusual finding. This trismus is most often the result of inflammation of the muscles of mastication secondary to the surgical procedure but may also be the result of multiple injections of local anesthetics used in achieving local anesthesia with an inferior alveolar block; with the medial pterygoid being the most likely muscle involved. The treatment includes reassurance, soft diet, hot and cold compresses to the face, nonsteroidal antiinflammatory medication, and possibly antibiotics. Prolonged or worsening trismus should be referred to an oral surgeon for evaluation because a deep space infection of the pharyngeal space is possible.

Edema

Postoperative soft tissue swelling or edema following multiple impaction surgery is a common finding, and patients should be made aware of this fact prior to surgery to avoid any undue alarm.

Peak swelling will usually occur 48 to 72 hours after surgical insult. Immediate application of ice packs (not directly applied to the skin) following the completion of surgery for the first 24 hours will help to decrease swelling. Ice packs should be applied in 20-minute increments. Intravenous or intramuscular administration of glucocorticoids is helpful in decreasing postoperative edema. In very extensive surgery an additional prescription for oral steroid medication can be given to help decrease postoperative edema.

DIET AND ORAL HYGIENE

In the immediate postsurgical period (12 to 24 hours) the patient should be advised to maintain a diet of soft foods and avoid anything too hot. Patients should be told to avoid brushing the teeth in the surgical site in the immediate postoperative period and not perform any oral rinsing and spitting for 24 hours to prevent bleeding.

REFERENCES

1. Al-Khateeb TL, el-Marsafi AI, Butler NP: The relationship between the indications for the surgical removal of impacted third molars and the incidence of alveolar osteitis, *J Oral Maxillofac Surg* 49:141-145; discussion 145-146, 1991.
2. American Association of Oral and Maxillofacial Surgeons: Position paper on impacted teeth, Chicago AAOMS, 1983; January, 1989.
3. Alling CC: Dysesthesia of the lingual and inferior alveolar nerves following third molar surgery, *J Oral Maxillofac Surg* 44:154, 1986.
4. Girard KR: Consideration in the management of damage to the mandibular nerve. *JADA* 98:65, 1979.
5. Mozsary PG: Editorial comment, *J Oral Maxillofac Surg* 45:204, 286, 1987.
6. Heasman PA, Jacobs DJ: A clinical investigation into the incidence of dry socket, *Br J Oral Maxillofac Surg* 22:115, 1984.
7. Kaban LB, Pogrel MA, Perrott DH: *Complications in oral and maxillofacial surgery*, Philadelphia, 1997, WB Saunders.

CHAPTER 8

The Impacted Canine

HARRY DYM, DDS

After the mandibular and maxillary third molars, the next most commonly impacted tooth is the maxillary canine.[1] Because of the esthetic and functional significance of the canine teeth, an orthodontic consultation should be sought as soon as the diagnosis of delayed canine eruption and impaction is confirmed and surgical plans for its exposure should be made. It is far more difficult to orthodontically move an impacted canine in the older child/adult patient than in the younger child and consequently early intervention is advised.

POSITION

The impacted maxillary canine is most commonly situated on the palatal side and less often on the buccal or lateral aspect. Though panoramic (Fig. 8-1) and occlusal (Fig. 8-2) x-rays are helpful in both diagnosing and evaluating impacted teeth, they are not able to precisely aid the practitioner in determining the exact position of the impacted maxillary canine. To locate the exact position, dual periapical x-rays must be taken in the same position while shifting the central x-ray beam in a mesial or distal direction, utilizing the buccal object rule[2] (Figs. 8-3 and 8-4). The literature offers many techniques for the uncovering of impacted maxillary cuspids and suggests various attachments to aid in their traction. These include uncovering the teeth and packing them open with iodoform gauze or paste, using friction pins, wrapping ligature wire around the crown, or using cemented crowns. Although all these methods are used and often successful, a far easier, predictable, and ultimately less traumatic method is the use of a bonded bracket or the gold-chain bonded bracket as the sole means for assisting in the orthodontic movement of the impacted canine.

SURGICAL PROCEDURE

Local anesthesia is obtained with 2% lidocaine with 1:100,000 epinephrine infiltrated into the palatal mucosa near the palatal incisal foramen and in the area of the impacted canine. Additional anesthesia is infiltrated in the depth of the buccal vestibule in the anterior maxilla near the infraorbital foramen. Care should be taken to aspirate before injecting anesthesia in the area of the palatal foramen. The surgical approach for exposure of a palatal impacted canine is through an intrasulcular incision around the palatal aspects of the bicuspid teeth on the involved side and extending over to the opposite central incisor. If bilateral cuspid exposure is to be performed, the entire palate can be elevated from bicuspid to bicuspid.

It is critical to remember that the incision is a full thickness one and a subperiosteal elevation should be done carefully to avoid perforating the mucosal flap and possibly injuring the greater palatine artery that runs along the palate.

One should not hesitate to transect the neurovascular bundle that emanates from the incisal foramen, as it will allow for more ease in flap retraction (Fig. 8-5).

Traction sutures can then be placed through the elevated palatal flap to allow for easier retraction. A slow-speed handpiece with a #6 or #8 round bur under constant irrigation is then used to expose the impacted crown without damaging the tooth itself.

After the crown is exposed a periodontal currette should be used to remove the associated follicular cyst that contributes to bleeding which will make bonding of any orthodontic bracket difficult (Fig. 8-6). Placing cotton pledgets soaked with hydrogen peroxide adjacent to the exposed crown is helpful in achieving hemostasis as is applying pressure and infiltration of local anesthesia. Once the entire crown is exposed and hemostasis achieved the tooth is then acid-etched in the usual manner and the orthodontic bracket bonded (Figs. 8-7 through 8-10).

Maxillary labially impacted cuspids can be approached via a trapezoid-shaped incision, making certain to maintain the attached gingiva. This flap can then be repositioned in an apical direction and sutured in its new position (Fig. 8-11). Alternatively, another surgical approach is to make an intrasulcular incision around the maxillary central and lateral incisor with a distally placed vertical releasing incision. The tooth is then

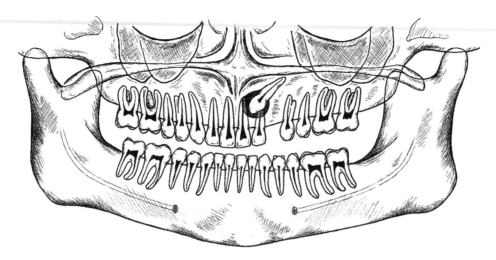

FIG. 8-1 Impacted cuspid teeth are often only discovered after routine panoramic x-ray screening. Periapical x-rays will still be required to establish exact anatomical position before exposure.

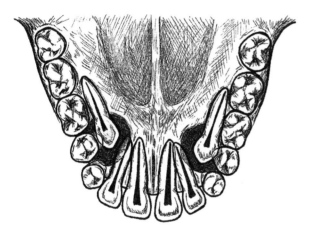

FIG. 8-2 Occlusal x-ray offers an excellent radiographic view of impacted cuspids and any associated cystic pathology and their anatomic relationship to surrounding teeth and vital structures.

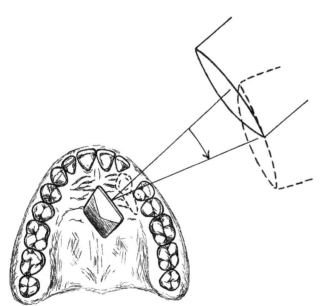

FIG. 8-3 The buccal object rule is used to help determine the exact anatomic position of the impacted canine. A periapical film is positioned and the initial film is taken. A second x-ray is then taken, making certain to place the x-ray packet in the exact position, with the x-ray head positioned and shifted to a posterior and distal direction. If the impacted tooth appears to shift with the x-ray beam, it is in the palatal or lingual position. This is often referred to as the rule of S.L.O.B. (same lingual opposite buccal).

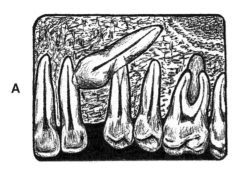
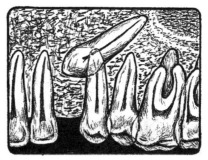

FIG. 8-4 Comparison of two periapical x-rays taken and knowledge of the buccal object rule, allows one to determine the exact position of the impacted canine. **B** shows the impacted canine in a more distal or posterior position as compared to **A.** As the x-ray head has been shifted back (posteriorly), when **B** was taken, it is clear that the tooth has shifted in tandem with the x-ray beam and is, therefore, in the palatal position.

FIG. 8-5 Palatal flap reflected and nasopalatine duct exposed. Impacted canine is now ready for exposure. Note, envelope flap used with no vertical releasing incision, though one can be used if treating doctor is so inclined. The neurovascular bundle is cut as this may be done with no complications. The flap can be sutured to posterior teeth to aid in retraction.

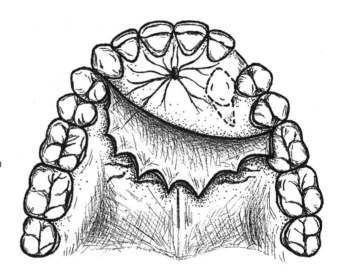

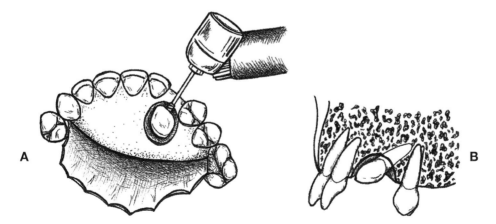

FIG. 8-6 It is critical that one go slowly in exposing impacted palatal cuspids, as it is possible to inadvertently drill into enamel tooth structure. After crown is exposed a periodontal curette should be used to remove follicular tissue that surrounds the tooth which will contribute to bleeding into site and make it difficult to establish a dry operating field. **A,** Exposing canine; **B,** Side view after exposed.

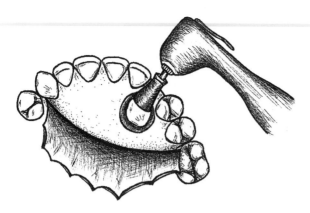

FIG. 8-7 Shows entire crown exposed and rubber cup on slow speed handpiece used to pumice and clean exposed cuspid crown.

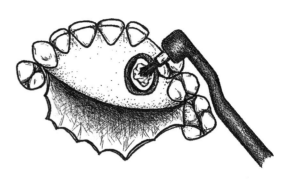

FIG. 8-8 Once impacted cuspid is fully exposed and hemostasis established, the tooth is prepared for bracket placement. Tooth is acid etched using standard techniques after crown is pumiced and dried. Echant used can be either liquid or paste type.

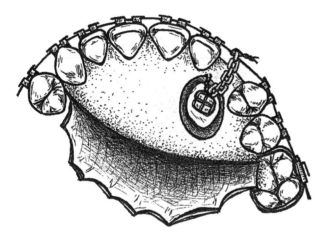

FIG. 8-9 Palatal flap retracted with bracket applied to cuspid crown and chain attached to orthodontic arch wire.

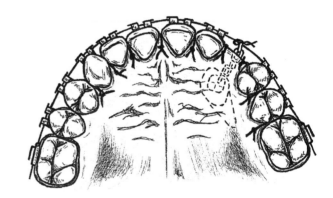

FIG. 8-10 Palatal flap closed with interrupted 3-0 black sutures. Note gold chain is under flap and sutured to orthodontic arch wire. Make certain area is hemostatic before closure to avoid hematoma formation.

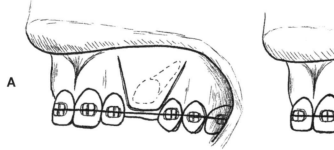
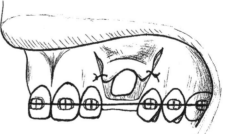

A **B**

FIG. 8-11 **A,** outlines trapezoidal incision used to expose underlying buccal impacted cuspid. Note how this incision maintains attached gingiva which is critical for periodontal long-term health of tooth. **B,** shows how buccal flap is vertically and apically repositioned and secured with interrupted 3-0 black sutures to maintain position and expose cuspid crown.

bonded and the flap replaced in its original position with the traction wire located beneath the mucosa (Fig. 8-12).

Surgical removal of impacted maxillary or mandibular canines is sometimes indicated and performed for orthodontic or patient management reasons. The surgical approach is similar to that involved in the exposure and bracketing of impacted canines. Diagnostic x-rays are essential as is the appropriate instrumentation. As in the extraction of all teeth, it should be done atraumatically with as little bone removed as possible. Lateral or vestibular impacted canines are somewhat easier to extract than their palatal counterparts. After retraction of the palatal soft tissue flap, special care must be taken when opening the bony window and exposing the full canine crown. If this is done too quickly, it can sometimes be difficult to differentiate enamel from sur-

rounding bone structure (Figs. 8-13 and 8-14). This is especially true when done on patients in their third decade or beyond and little or no follicular sac still remains associated with the impacted canine.

In an effort to conserve palatal bone and limit the surgical trauma the crown is sectioned horizontally slightly above the cementoenamel junction and delivered with an apical root teaser and then the remaining root is elevated and removed with an elevator (Figs. 8-15 and 8-16). Oftentimes, it is necessary to repeatedly section the crown in order to remove it in its entirety.

This procedure can be very difficult and frustrating at times, especially if a curved root is present or the tooth proves to be ankylosed.

When removing mandibular labially impacted canines special attention must be paid to the mental

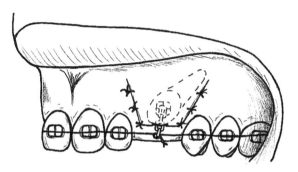

FIG. 8-12 Buccal mucosal flap closed with interrupted 3-0 black silk sutures. Note how gold chain lies under mucosal flap with chain secured to arch wire.

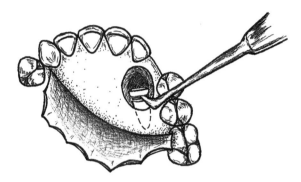

FIG. 8-14 Extraction of impacted palatal canines often proves to be a difficult procedure that requires patience. The cuspid crown may require multiple sectioning before its complete removal so as to avoid extensive palatal bone removal and possible injury to adjacent teeth. This technique has been referred to by some as the "Salami Procedure."

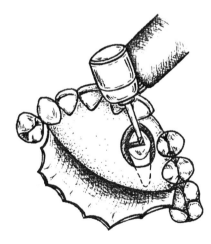

FIG. 8-13 High-speed surgical handpiece with side cutting carbide bur and copious irrigation sectioning exposed crown. Careful attention must be paid to adjacent teeth and roots.

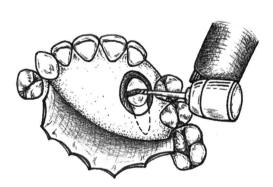

FIG. 8-15 Surgical sectioning of crown must be done carefully to avoid inadvertent damage to adjacent teeth and floor of nose. To avoid this happening, do not cut fully through the crown, but leave a small area that will allow easy fracture with elevator.

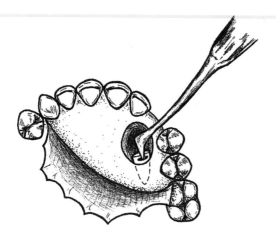

FIG. 8-16   After removal of cuspid crown, a hole can be drilled into root surface to allow the point of elevator to be engaged. Root should come up with controlled force. If no movement is perceived, the root may have curved apex or be hypercementotic; more bone may then have to be removed.

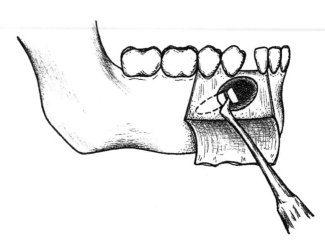

FIG. 8-18   As in the palatal impaction, the cuspid crown may require multiple sectioning in order to avoid large bony exposure and possible damage to adjacent vital structures. Note how the division of the tooth is done at the cemento-enamel junction but leaves a lip of root allowing for elevator engagement.

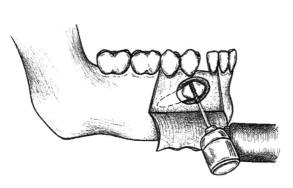

FIG. 8-17   The mandibular impacted cuspid is most frequently located in the labial position. The treating doctor should always be cognizant of the mental foramen that may be present in the surgical field. The underlying bone and cuspid are exposed through a vertical releasing incision and a posterior release if access is found to be restricted with only the one anterior release. The overlying bone is carefully removed and the crown sectioned.

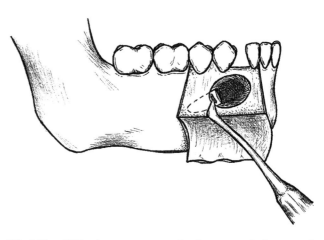

FIG. 8-19   With the crown completely removed the root is notched with a drill to allow an elevator to be engaged before its removal in the forward position.

foramen and its associated neurovascular bundle (Figs. 8-17 through 8-19). It should be identified and protected with a retractor at all times. Rarely is the lower impacted canine situated on the lingual aspect but if it is a lingual approach should be used if possible.

Patients should be discharged with a prescription for analgesics and antibiotics, depending on the extent of the surgical procedure. Penicillin is the preferred antibiotic, with erythromycin given for the penicillin-allergic patient.

POSSIBLE COMPLICATIONS ASSOCIATED WITH REMOVAL OF IMPACTED CANINES

1. After a large palatal flap is reflected for the bilateral removal of two maxillary palatal impacted canines a significant postsurgical hematoma can sometimes develop. Patients will return with the hard palate bulging down from the roof of the mouth as a result of a large hematoma collection contained therein. This complication can be easily prevented by having

a plastic maxillary acrylic splint fabricated before surgery and securing it with 30 gauge wires or 3-0 black silk sutures secured around the bicuspid teeth. If no stent has been prepared, gauze can be pressed into the palate and the bolster secured with cross arch sutures ligated to the opposing teeth. If hematoma formation does occur, remove some of the sutures and release the flap and suction the contents.

2. Perforation into the floor of the nose may occur with some postoperative nasal bleeding. If a small opening is seen during surgery it should be covered with a small layer of collagen membrane before the mucosal closure. Rarely does this lead to any permanent problem.

The patient should be seen for follow-up and suture removal in a week's time.

Key Surgical Tips

- For the periodontal long-term health of the maxillary impacted canine, an attempt should always be made to preserve attached gingiva during the surgical exposure procedure. Obviously, this does not apply to palatally impacted teeth as the entire palatal mucosa is of the attached dense variety.
- Surgical access and visibility is critical and one need not shy away from transecting the neurovascular bundle from the palatal incisive foramen when elevating a full thickness palatal flap, as the bleeding is minimal and no loss of sensitivity is appreciated by the patient.

- Make every effort to remove the remnants of the dental follicle surrounding the crown with a sharp periodontal curette as this will reduce the bleeding at the surgical site and make bonding of a bracket less difficult.
- Use a slow speed handpiece with moderate size round bur when removing bone to avoid cutting through to enamel.
- Rely more on your double x-ray buccal object rule in determining the position of the impacted maxillary canine rather than on your digital palpation.
- Hydrogen peroxide-soaked cotton pledgets applied to the crown can help in hemostasis before bracket application.
- After the bonded bracket is applied, pull chain or wire with a hemostat to be certain that bracket is well bonded (as you would like not to revisit the site in the near future).
- Use a throat curtain gently placed in the mouth to avoid any small items from possible aspiration.
- Local anesthesia works well with most young adults and children but be prepared to augment with nitrous oxide analgesia or intravenous sedation for patients unable to tolerate what may sometimes be a lengthy procedure.

REFERENCES

1. Peterson LJ: Principles of management of impacted teeth. In: *Contemporary oral and maxillofacial surgery*, ed 3, St. Louis, 1998, Mosby.
2. Koerner KR, Tilt LV, Johnson KR: Orthodontic brackets on unerupted teeth. In: *Color atlas of minor oral surgery*, London, 1994, Mosby-Wolfe.

ADVANCED
PROCEDURES

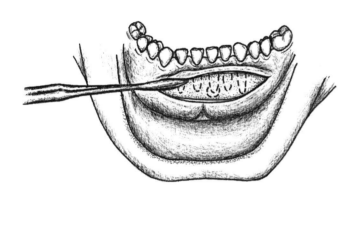

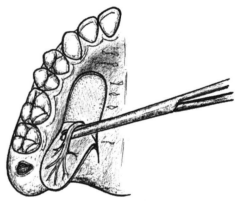

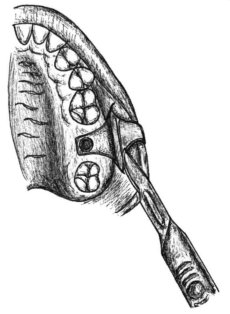

Endodontic Surgery

ORRETT E. OGLE, DDS

INDICATION

Endodontic surgery is performed to control or prevent inflammation at the apex of a tooth caused by toxins from nonvital teeth that cannot be managed by endodontic treatment. The aim of the surgery is to provide an adequate apical seal. The most common cause for endodontic surgery is incomplete obturation of the root canal system, with an apical seal that is not fluid tight, and therefore leads to percolation. It must be emphasized that endodontic surgery should not be the primary method of treating pulpless teeth, neither should it be a substitute for good instrumentation and obturation procedures. Endodontic surgery should almost always follow failed conventional root canal therapy, or iatrogenic problems, in which retreatment is difficult or impossible. One such instance is where it would be unwise to remove a large post.

Following endodontic failure, conventional retreatment (where possible) gives an average success rate of 73%, whereas surgical retreatment with retrofill gives a success rate of 60%.[1] Other studies, however, have also shown a 72% success rate with surgical retreatment.[2] Nevertheless, the surgical solution is never more successful than redoing the endodontics.

CAUSES OF ENDODONTIC FAILURE[3]

- Apical percolation   64%
- Operative errors   22%
- Errors in case selection   14%

The dentist should be fully aware that endodontic surgery done to correct technical errors from previous endodontic procedures often does not have a favorable prognosis.

STEPS

Endodontic surgery comprises five steps:
1. Soft tissue access via a mucoperiosteal flap
2. Cortical osteotomy to approach the root apex
3. Apical curettage
4. Apicoectomy
5. Retrofilling

INSTRUMENTATION

- Cartridge type aspirating dental anesthetic syringe and local anesthesia with vasoconstrictor
- #3 Bard Parker type blade handle and #15 surgical blade
- Molt periosteal elevator
- Seldin periosteal elevator (to be used as a retractor) or Cawood-Minnesota retractor
- Standard dental high speed hand piece
- Micro-head hand piece, or the Ultrasonic retrotip device
- #6 round bur
- #557 long fissure bur
- Micro inverted cone bur 33 2
- Lucas curettes: #1R-1L and 3R-3L
- Retro-filling amalgam carrier, small tip, dia. 3/64" (or Hu-Friedy mini-end amalgam carrier)
- Small amalgam pluggers: Behrman #1/Smith/Marquette #1-2, and #11-12 Back action
- Sterile dental cotton roll
- Needle holder: Hegar-Baumgartner or Mayo-Hegar
- Suture scissors
- Surgical dissecting scissors (optional): Dean
- 4-O silk suture on an F-S needle (This is, however, the choice of the operator.)

SURGICAL CONSIDERATIONS
Operating Field

The dental/surgical operatory should meet the requirements of the Occupational Safety and Health Administration (OSHA). The perioral soft tissues should be clean-washed and painted with povidone-iodine. Skin flora is primarily staphylococcus while the intraoral flora is streptococcus. Cleaning the perioral area minimizes the inoculum of staphylococcus that would contaminate the surgical wound. This risk, however, is very low, and possibly not clinically significant. It is also recommended that the intraoral tissues be painted lightly with an antiseptic solution such as povidone-iodine. Many surgeons, however, perform apical surgery without any preparation of the surgical site, and have not noted any significant increase in their infection rate.

Anatomy

Three anatomical structures are important in the performance of endodontic surgery. These are the maxillary sinus, the neurovascular bundle within the inferior alveolar canal, and the mental nerve as it emerges from the mental foramen. These anatomic features are a matter of concern only when doing surgery on posterior teeth. Occasionally, however, cystic lesions at the apex of anterior teeth can get very large and extend beyond its immediate apex to involve critical anatomical structures in the nose or the floor of the mouth.

SURGICAL PROCEDURE
Soft Tissue Access

Various soft tissue flap designs are available. Selection of the appropriate flap design should be based on the principles that will be presented here.

1. The incision should be planned so that it will be made on healthy bone and in such a position that the wound closure will be over solid bone, and not the pathological/surgical defect. Incisions closed over a dead space will break down.
2. The actual site of the incision must be influenced by the fact that wound healing is initiated by epithelial migration across the incision line, and that this migration is four times faster in attached gingiva than in alveolar mucosa. Horizontal incisions, therefore, should be placed in the attached gingiva so as to take advantage of the rapid epithelial migration that occurs in this area during wound healing.
3. The horizontal incision should extend at least one tooth on either side of the tooth having the apicoectomy. However, the extent of the pathology should determine the exact length of the horizontal incision. This length should be long enough to allow the operator sufficient room to be able to remove the periapical pathology. The flap must never be too small.
4. The incision should also be long enough to provide room for retraction, and to avoid damage to adjacent tissue, or bruising of the flap from forceful retraction in an attempt to increase surgical access. The flap must only be gently retracted, with the retracting instrument resting on bone

without unnecessary movements. The gentle handling of the soft tissues will minimize postoperative inflammation and pain, and will result in faster healing with less scarring.

5. The primary blood supply for the free alveolar mucosa is derived from the supraperiosteal vasculature that runs parallel to the long access of the teeth. Any horizontal incision in the unattached mucosa, therefore, will greatly compromise the blood flow during and after surgery. This will result in slower healing and more prominent scars.[4] Because of this only vertical incisions should be made in the alveolar mucosa.
6. The vertical component of the flap must intersect the horizontal incision at an angle greater than 90° so that the flap will have a broad base in order to ensure a proper blood supply to the raised tissue.
7. Periodontal health and the presence of prosthetic restorations are other important factors that must be considered. In advanced periodontal disease with excessive pocket depths and/or inadequate attached gingiva the horizontal incision should be modified, and in this situation it should not be placed on the attached gingiva. Attempting to do so would involve the flap with the periodontal pocket defects, and may result in postoperative problems ranging from fenestration to dehiscence. In this case the horizontal incision should be placed in the gingival sulcus (Fig. 9-1).
8. Both fixed and removable prostheses must be considered during flap design. In cases with porcelain restorations on maxillary anterior teeth the horizontal incision should be made in the attached gingiva (Fig. 9-2) and not in the sulcus. This will minimize postoperative scar contraction at the crown margin, and thus maintain proper esthetics. This principle should be applied to crowns on all maxillary teeth that are clearly visible during smiling. In the case of removable prostheses, the flap should be designed with the

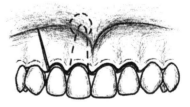

FIG. 9-1 Sulcular incision with vertical release for performing apicoectomy.

prosthesis in place so as to avoid placing any of the incisions under a clasp or at the border of the prosthesis.

9. Mandibular teeth require special considerations. In the lower anterior, a sulcular incision is best because of the narrow band of attached gingiva often found in this area. Vestibular incisions have a high incidence of dehiscence and should be avoided. Where crowns are present, and in the rare case where the margins may be seen during smiling, then the incision should be placed out in the lip, approximately 1 to 1.5 cm labial to the mucobuccal fold. This incision goes through the mucosa and about 2 mm into the orbicularis oris muscle. A myocutaneous flap is made, pedicled to the lingual gingiva. The periosteum is incised, and a superior flap elevated to expose the root apex (Fig. 9-3, *A* and *B*).

10. To access the mandibular premolars, the sulcular incision is indicated, with a vertical release placed in the region of the lateral incisor. The vertical incision should be long enough to allow wide exposure of the intended surgical site (Fig. 9-4). If crowns are present, and esthetics is a consideration, the horizontal incision can be placed in the attached gingiva at least 2 mm apical to the deepest level of the sulcus. The operator should be sure that the incision is not in the mandibular vestibule, and it should be at least 1 mm superior to the mucogingival line. The vertical will also be at the lateral incisor. For mandibular molars, sulcular incisions should always be done, and the vertical release placed at the canine. If additional access is needed a posterior vertical releasing incision may be made (see Fig. 9-4).

11. To access the palatal root of maxillary molars a palatal flap is used. This flap is made from a sulcular incision with a vertical release in the region of the canine (Fig. 9-5). This releasing incision should extend just short of the midline of the palate, and is tapered posteriorly. Surgical approaches to the palatal roots of the molars will require a large soft tissue flap to provide good visibility, and adequate surgical access through the dense bone of the palatal alveolar process. The vertical incision may involve the terminal branches of the palatine artery. If bleeding is

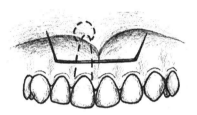

FIG. 9-2 A trapezoid incision for performing apicoectomy on maxillary anterior teeth with crowns or with advanced crestal bone loss. The horizontal incision is made in attached gingiva.

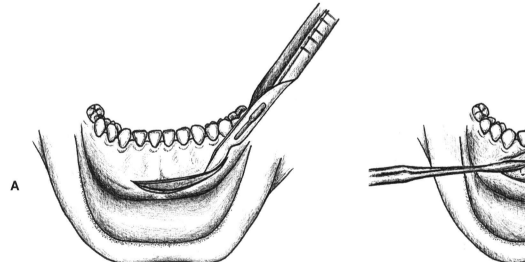
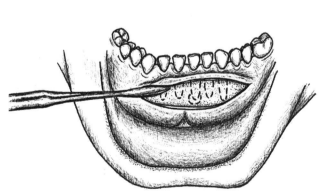

A

B

FIG. 9-3 **A,** An incision in the extended lip 5-7 mm from the lower vestibule. This incision is made through the labial mucosa and extends to a depth of 2-3 mm into the orbicularis oris muscle. **B,** A flap is developed and extended from the lip to the alveolus. On the buccal aspect of the mandible the periosteum is incised and elevated occlusally to expose the area where the apex of the lower incisors would be located.

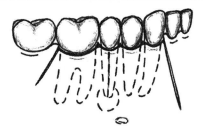

FIG. 9-4 A sulcular incision in the posterior mandible with vertical releases anteriorly and posteriorly. The vertical release in the anterior should be at the canine or lateral incisor area to avoid injury to the mental nerve.

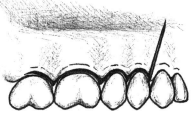

FIG. 9-6 A sulcular incision with a vertical release. The vertical release is done in the alveolar mucosa, and is tapered to provide a wide base for the flap that will be elevated from the bone. The vertical incision joins the sulcular incision in such a way so as to save the interdental papilla. This fixed papilla will provide a stable point onto which the repositioned flap may be anchored.

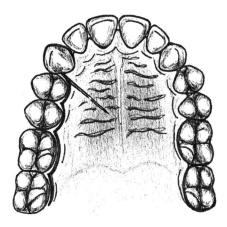

FIG. 9-5 An incision in the palatal sulcus of the molars and a release anteriorly. The flap will give wide exposure for performing apicoectomy of the palatal roots. A semicircular incision placed in the vicinity of the molars will injure the greater palatine vessels and cause a problem with visibility over the period of time necessary to complete the procedure.

brisk, the end of the vessel should be clamped, and the vessel either ligated, or controlled with cautery.

Technique

The horizontal incision is made first. It is made sharply to bone in a clean fashion, avoiding multiple incisions. The vertical arm or arms are added to the horizontal incision. When the horizontal incision is placed in the sulcus, the vertical incision meets it in a fashion that allows a sufficient quantity of the papilla to remain intact. This intact papilla will serve as an anchoring point for sutures (Fig. 9-6). The entire length of the incisions should be scored with the pointed end of the periosteal elevator so as to be sure that the incisions

are complete and down to bone. This will avoid accidental tearing of the flap.

The raising of the flap is started with the sharp end of the periosteal elevator. The entire horizontal incision is started first. Using the blunt end of the periosteal elevator, the entire flap is carefully reflected. With the sulcular incision, the elevation of the mucoperiosteal flap is started at the incised papillae farthest from the vertical release. If two vertical releases are used, the crestal gingiva is started first and taken to each vertical arm. At this point more extensive reflection is started from the intersections. The flap is reflected to expose the entire apical area of the intended surgery.

If there is a large cystic lesion adhering to the mucoperiosteal flap, a scissors should be used to dissect the flap from the cyst lining. (See Chapter 14 on cystectomy.) This may require blunt and sharp dissection. Often, a layer of thickened tissue will be present, this should be left attached to the cyst wall, and the free mucosa sharply dissected from it.

Bony Access (Cortical Ostectomy)

The purpose of the cortical ostectomy is to gain working access to the periapical area of the tooth being treated. The bony window should be large enough to allow total removal of the periapical pathology.

Three methods may be used to locate the apex of the tooth and thus the area for the ostectomy.

1. In the vast majority of cases, the cortical plate will be thin because of the underlying pathology, and fenestrations and fistulae may be present. In this situation a periosteal elevator or a curette may be used to start the access window.
2. In thicker bone, particularly over posterior teeth, the surgeon should establish the endodontic working length of the tooth. This can be done

from an accurate periapical film, or estimated from the Panorex. An endodontic file can be held against the radiograph to determine the working length. The premeasured file is placed in alignment over the axis of the involved tooth. This will place the tip almost directly over the apical area. A curette can also be used to transpose the measurement.

3. In the mandibular molar area it may be difficult for the clinician to properly determine the apical location by the above methods. If this is the case, a radiographic determination should be done. The steps are as follows:

   a. Using the round bur, drill a hole 2 mm deep into the buccal cortical plate as close to the estimated location of the apex as possible.

   b. Place a medium sized gutta-percha point into the hole. Cut the gutta-percha to protrude 5 to 7 mm.

   c. Take a well-aligned periapical x-ray. This radiograph will give the necessary orientation needed to approach the apex.

Once the apical region is determined, the overlying bone is wiped away with a bur in a high-speed handpiece under a lavage of a coolant (Fig. 9-7). An appropriate working window must be opened in the cortical plate. Most of the time the size of the opening will be determined by the preexisting pathology. Operations in the area of the posterior teeth and the palatal roots of the maxillary molars will require a larger field than do anterior teeth. Maxillary incisors will provide the easiest access. All unsupported bone must be removed because unsupported cortical bone has a poor vascular supply and will not heal well.

In cases of overfill or with small apical lesions, the surgeon need only prepare a small window with access to perform the required apical procedure. In this situation when the periapical lesion is not well demarcated it may be difficult to identify the apex of the intended tooth, and care must be taken not to injure adjacent roots. Sometimes lower incisors are very close, and the operator must be careful that surgery is not performed on the wrong tooth, or that adjacent teeth are not damaged. When no periapical lesion is present, it can sometimes be difficult to locate the root apex, particularly on lower molars.

Apical Curettage

For endodontic surgery to be successful, the surgeon must remove the periapical pathology and leave the surgical site in a state that will permit repair. Two types of pathosis are associated with endodontically involved teeth: granulation tissue or a radicular cyst.

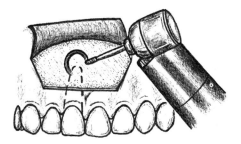

FIG. 9-7 Ostectomy to provide access to the root apex.

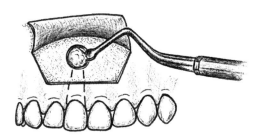

FIG. 9-8 Removal of granulation tissue with a curette from the apical region of the tooth.

Granulation tissue is removed by curettage. If the defect is small and radiographically locally confined to the immediate area, then 100% of the diseased tissue must be removed by the curettage (Fig. 9-8). With larger lesions, risks may be associated with attempted total enucleation. If the lesion is large, the surgeon should begin by carefully probing the bony walls of the lesion to identify its integrity. Communication with the nasal cavity, maxillary sinus, lingual plate defects, adjacent roots, or the inferior alveolar neurovascular bundle should be noted. If no apical or lateral communications are present, the area should be thoroughly curetted to remove all of the inflammatory tissues from the apex. If a communication exists, then only a partial removal of the pathosis is indicated to avoid morbid results.

Periapical cysts differ from granulation tissue in terms of tissue characteristics, organization, and structure. Cysts are well organized structures that the body uses to isolate the periapical infection. In general they should be removed in total as one unit. The bony–soft tissue border should be delineated. A curette is used to gently disengage the sac from the bone. To avoid perforation of the cyst, the curette is placed with the sharp edge against bone and the convex surface against the cystic membrane (Fig. 9-9). By careful dissection, the cyst can be separated from the bone and lifted out in toto.

Large cystic lesions that communicate with the inferior alveolar nerve should not be removed in toto if this would injure the nerve. If the etiology of the infection is removed by creating a good apical seal, and a portion of the cyst wall is disrupted, the cyst will resolve naturally.[5] Because both the cystic lesion and granulation tissue will resolve once the source of infection is removed, all portions of diseased tissues need not be removed if a more serious surgical complication will result. Remnants of tissue that are not accessible at this stage may be further removed once the root apex has been resected (Fig. 9-10).

All tissue removed from the periapical region should be submitted to an oral pathologist.

Apicoectomy

The purpose of an apicoectomy is to create an apical bevel to permit the operator access to the apex. Several studies have reported that the angle of apical resection influences root end leakage. The angle of the bevel should be kept to a minimum so as to minimize leakage through apical dentinal tubules.[6] Increasing the apical bevel increases apical leakage. As the bevel changes from 0° to the horizontal axis of the root to 30° and then to 45°, the apical leakage via dentinal tubules increases significantly[7] (Fig. 9-11). The ideal angle of resection is a flat (0°) cut because this minimizes apical leakage. However, the technical requirements for good surgical access to place a retrograde filling means that some bevel is necessary, but this bevel should be kept to the smallest angle possible.

Several factors will affect the inclination of the bevel. First is anatomy. To access posterior teeth, particularly the maxillary first premolar and the mandibular molars, the working access and surgical visibility is directly proportional to the bevel's inclination. Second will be the size of the instrument that will be used to prepare the root end for the retrograde fill. The larger the head of the instrument, the larger the angle of inclination will have to be.

The cut through the apex should bevel the root so that it gives a lateral/forward inclination toward the operator. This will permit an adequate view of the apical foramen. Care should be taken to prevent the bur from pulling or dragging the gutta-percha in the root canal by using high speeds and a gentle motion. As the apicoectomy is done, the surgeon should identify the filling material within the canal. Gutta-percha is very easy to identify.

Special consideration is required for the maxillary first premolar and the mandibular molars. These teeth have buccal and palatal/lingual canals which must be accessed from the buccal to complete the retrofill. The buccal root of the maxillary first premolar must be decreased significantly to be able to access the apex of the palatal root (Fig. 9-12). (Clinically, the palatal root of the maxillary first premolar will be anterior to the buccal root when viewed from the direct buccal.) The bevel on the mesial root of the mandibular molar must be very high toward the buccal so that the surgeon will be able to retroseal the apex of the mesiolingual canal (Fig. 9-13).

For the palatal root of the maxillary molar, the bevel should be large, and should be angled anteriormedially (Fig. 9-14).

Retrograde Filling

This is the step in which most of the endodontic problems are finally solved. The goal of the retrograde filling is to seal the canal system by a surgical approach, thereby preventing further communication

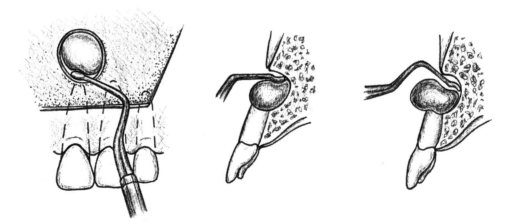

FIG. 9-9   Technique for removing a cyst from the apex of a tooth.

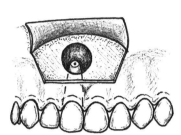

FIG. 9-10 Apical resection of a maxillary anterior tooth.

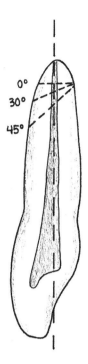

FIG. 9-11 A schematic to show the angles at which apical resections may be done. The greater the angle, the greater will be the risk for apical leakage.

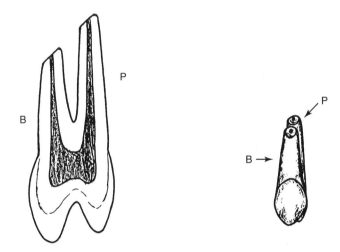

FIG. 9-12 Apical resection of a maxillary first premolar showing how the root resection should be done. The buccal root *(B)* has to be shortened so as to be able to access the palatal root *(P)*. This figure shows a sagittal and a lateral view.

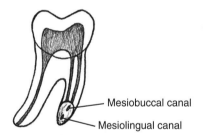

Mesiobuccal canal
Mesiolingual canal

FIG. 9-13 Mandibular first molar showing an apicoectomy on the mesial root. The root is beveled from buccal to lingual. The buccal cut is started high and tapered toward the lingual. The bevel is designed so that it faces anteriorly toward the incisors. This design will expose both the mesiobuccal and mesiolingual canals for retrofill.

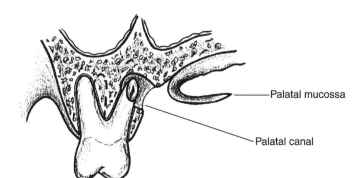

Palatal mucossa

Palatal canal

FIG. 9-14 Apicoectomy of a palatal root. The bevel should face anteriorly (toward the surgeon).

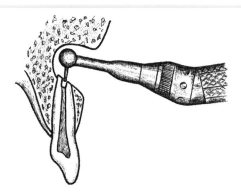

FIG. 9-15 An apex of a tooth being prepared with a microhead handpiece for retrofill.

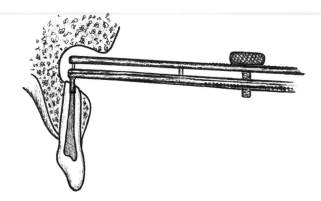

FIG. 9-16 Retrofill of the apex of a maxillary anterior tooth using a small amalgam carrier.

between the root canal system and the periapical tissues.

A small surface area of retrograde fill is desirable because of bioacceptance and future possible resorption of the filling material or chemical leeching. Using a micro head handpiece a cavity preparation is made into the apical portion of the canal (Fig. 9-15). The cavity preparation should be 2 to 3 mm in depth, and should follow the long axis of the tooth. Increasing the depth of the retrograde filling beyond 3 mm will not further reduce apical leakage. A cavity preparation made with a small round bur has been reported to give a better seal than one done with an inverted cone bur.[8] However, on several occasions I have noted dislodgement of the amalgam from the root apex when the undercut is not adequate to retain the amalgam. The slotted preparation done with a fissure bur gives the most leakage.[4,8]

The apex must be isolated after the retropreparation to ensure a dry field for a proper fill, and to prevent excess retrofill material from being lost in the adjacent bone. This can be achieved by packing the area around the apex with cotton from a sterile dental cotton roll, or with bone wax. The packing should be placed to cover all exposed marrow in the bony cavity, and packed tightly. Only the prepared apex should be exposed.

The retropreparation is sealed with amalgam using a microcarrier (Fig. 9-16). Although several materials have been suggested for root-end filling, amalgam still seems to be the best. Its advantages include: good apical seal, tissue compatibility, nonabsorbability, radiopacity, and familiarity of use.

Ultrasonic Apical Preparation. The ultrasonic root end tip when used to prepare the root apex for the retrofill offers several advantages.

1. Smaller bony access is required, therefore the size of the ostectomy can be minimized.
2. A 0° cut can be made. Because the head of the ultrasonic tip is smaller, and it comes with tips constructed at varying angles, it is capable of

preparing the canal within the long axis of the tooth with a minimal bevel.
3. A smaller preparation can be achieved, because the tip is smaller and it will follow the canal without removing excessive dentinal structure.
4. A smaller cavity preparation will require less filling material (Figs. 9-17 and 9-18).

If bone wax was used to isolate the area all of it must be removed before the wound is closed.

Closure and Postoperative Care

The wound should be thoroughly irrigated before it is closed. Copious irrigation will remove debris, remoisten the tissues, and will decrease the bacterial count by dilution. The first step is to reposition the flap by aligning the tissue at the point where the vertical incision or incisions meet the horizontal or crestal incision. Using 4-O silk, close the point where the vertical and horizontal incisions converge. Once this positional suture or sutures are in place, close the vertical incision or incisions (Fig. 9-19). Lastly, close the horizontal/crestal incision. The suture knots should not be too tight. Making them too tight will strangle the tissue and decrease the blood supply below the suture. This will cause hypertrophic scars with suture track marks. Tight sutures will also increase postoperative pain, and are more difficult to remove.

Pain. Pain medications should be started immediately postoperative, preferably before the local anesthesia has worn off. Preventing pain is a lot better than trying to treat pain. It is wise to manage pain very aggressively, and analgesics should be used routinely during the first 24 hours postoperatively rather than on a PRN basis. If there are no contraindications to their use, then the nonsteroidal antiinflammatory drugs (NSAIDs) are very effective and usually safe.

Antibiotics. This is not usually recommended, because the infection rate following endodontic surgery is

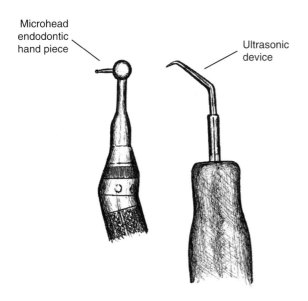

FIG. 9-17   A comparison of the microhead hand piece and the ultrasonic device, which are used for preparing the apex for retrofill. Several tips are available for the ultrasonic device to aid the surgeon in gaining access to the apex of a tooth.

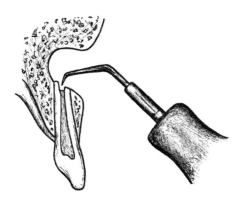

FIG. 9-18   The ultrasonic device being used to prepare the apex of the upper incisor for retrofill.

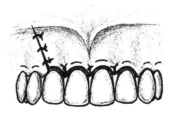

FIG. 9-19   Wound closure following completion of endodontic surgery.

low. However, the surgeon must decide whether or not to use antibiotics. The medical history, length of time that the wound was opened, surgical contamination, and clinical findings should be considered when making a decision to use antibiotics as an immediate postoperative medication.

Swelling. Slight to moderate swelling should be expected. Icepacks and NSAIDs may help. I do not routinely advocate the use of steroids for endodontic surgery.

Suture Removal. Mucoperiosteal tissue will reattach within 48 hours. Incisions in attached gingiva will heal very rapidly, and sutures can be removed in 4 to 5 days. However, clinical judgment should be used. For patient comfort 7 days may be adequate, because the soreness in the area is less and the patient more cooperative.

Follow-up Visits. Follow-up visits should be at 4 weeks post removal of sutures, then at 6 and 12 months.

ROOT RESECTION
Indications

Resection of a root is indicated (1) with localized periodontal destruction around one of the roots of a multi-rooted tooth; (2) when one canal of a multi-rooted tooth cannot be treated by either conventional or surgical endodontics; (3) when root resorption is limited to one root of a multi-rooted tooth; (4) with perforation of a root during endodontics or the placement of a post; (5) after subgingival fracture of one root of a molar; and (6) with a falling abutment within a large span bridge. The distobuccal root of the maxillary molar is the most commonly resected root.[9]

Sequence of Treatment

This is a multidisciplined procedure that requires careful attention to details. Endodontic therapy should be done first followed by the periodontal therapy, then the root resection.

The steps of the treatment sequencing are presented in Box 9-1.

Surgical Technique

Flap Design. A buccal sulcular incision is made with anterior and posterior vertical releasing incisions. The vertical incisions should be at least one tooth mesially and distally to the tooth being treated and should diverge so as to maintain a wide base for increased blood supply to the detached flap (Fig. 9-20). A palatal

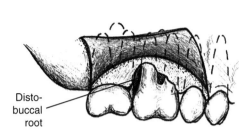

FIG. 9-20   Reflection of a buccal mucoperiosteal flap to expose the maxillary first molar for root resection.

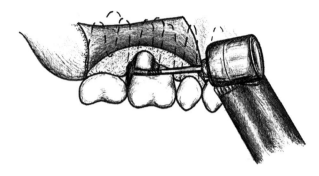

FIG. 9-21   Resection of the distobuccal root of the maxillary first molar.

BOX
Box 9-1   Sequential Endodontic and Periodontic Steps To Be Taken Prior to Root Resection

---

PRE-SURGICAL ENDODONTIC THERAPY

1. Conventional endodontics: pulpectomy and adequate instrumentation of all canals. The canal in the root to be resected should be instrumented to at least a size 45 or 50.
2. Obturation of canals with gutta-percha, excluding the root to be resected.
3. Preparation of dowel space immediately after canal obturation. The canal in which the post is to be placed should not be enlarged too much, as this will compromise the cross-sectional diameter of the root and lead to a predisposition toward coronal radicular fracture. The preparation for the post should never exceed 1/3 the root diameter.[10] The affected root may be further enlarged with a Peeso reamer* to about 7 mm below the orifice.
4. Place an amalgam plug in the affected root canal orifice to the level of the proposed resection. Make sure that the amalgam is tightly compacted into the canal. This will ensure a well-sealed stump. If there is adequate tooth structure, an amalgam core buildup can be continued. Otherwise, a post and core build-up is done.

PRE-SURGICAL PERIODONTAL THERAPY

1. Root planing and scaling to remove all calculus, and reduce inflammatory periodontal disease.
2. Thorough curettage of the furcal area.
3. Pocket depths should be reduced to a minimum through conservative periodontal therapy.

---

* Moyco/Union Broach Corp., Philadelphia, Pa. 19132.

---

sulcular incision is also made. The palatal incision should be longer than the buccal sulcular incision to allow for some retraction of the flap.

Buccal and palatal/lingual mucoperiosteal flaps are developed. The buccal flap should be extensive enough to expose the total length of the root to be resected as well as the total mesiodistal width of the affected tooth. The palatal flap should permit the placement of a Seldin elevator to protect the palatal mucosa.

Periodontal Curettage. Once the flaps are adequately developed, granulation tissue is curetted from the interdental and furcal areas. As much granulation tissue as possible should be removed at this stage. In the case where the root is being resected for other than periodontal defect, the buccal bone over the root to be resected should be removed. This will make visibility of the root easier, and will permit atraumatic removal of the root. Bone removal should be kept to a minimum however.

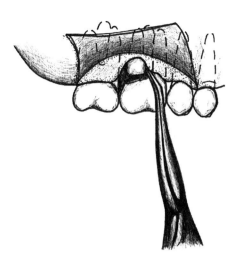

FIG. 9-22 The sectioned root being delivered with a Crane pick.

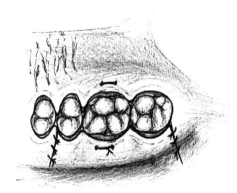

FIG. 9-23 Wound closure following root resection.

Root Resection. A long fissure bur is used to section the root under constant irrigation. The use of a 45% handpiece will make this part of the surgery easier, and will give a smoother cut (Fig. 9-21). The cut should start in the furca and proceed from that point. Care should be taken to resect the entire root as smoothly as possible, and to ensure that minimal residual subgingival root or furcal lips will remain after the resection. When the root moves independently from the tooth, it can be removed with small elevators or a Crane pick (Fig. 9-22). If difficulty arises in removing the root, a purchase point should be made into the root, and the Crane pick used to torque the root out. It may be necessary to shorten the root stump being removed. Once the root is removed all remaining granulation tissue can now be easily and completely curetted, and all exposed root surfaces should be root planed to remove all remaining calculus. This will allow for optimal healing. Sharp bony edges that would perforate or slice through the flap should be removed to permit good flap adaptation. Again, it must be emphasized that all bone removal be kept to a minimum.

Odontoplasty. This is done with a fine or medium diamond stone in a high speed handpiece and with copious irrigation. If a medium diamond is used for the gross removal, it should be followed with a fine diamond. The cut area is made as smooth as possible, being sure to reach all the way to the palate or lingual aspect. When working on the mandible, an instrument (Seldin elevator) should be placed to protect the soft tissues of the floor of the mouth. A gradual slope should now be made starting from deep on the palate to superficial on the buccal. This gradual slope will result in an area that will be easier to clean. The cut edges of the tooth should also be rounded off, but the contact should be preserved.

Wound Closure. An attempt should be made to bring the buccal flap to cover the bony defect, and to reach to the palatal mucosa. The flap is brought under the stump and secured with a horizontal mattress sling suture to the palate (Fig. 9-23).

Prosthetic restoration of the tooth may be done in about 8 to 12 weeks post root resection. This time will permit alveolar bone resorption, and tissue contraction to be at a relatively stable state.

When the root resection is being performed below an abutment in a long span bridge, the root(s) are resected and the canal retrosealed with amalgam. The area should be beveled to permit a sanitary type pontic, which will be easy to clean. The stump should be as smooth as possible to minimize the accumulation of accretions. The use of a water pick is acceptable as an oral hygiene device. Adequate periodontal follow-up is mandatory.

INTENTIONAL REPLANTATION

Intentional replantation involves the purposeful removal of a tooth and its reinsertion into the socket immediately after sealing the apical foramina.[11] It is a procedure of last resort, and the patient must be made aware that it is a "high risk" procedure. It is usually indicated for the mandibular or maxillary second molar teeth.

Indications for this procedure are:
■ A high risk of paresthesia with standard apicoectomy techniques because of approximation of the roots to the inferior alveolar canal
■ Thick external oblique ridge in the molar area making access difficult or impossible
■ Poor access for conventional apicoectomy—mouth size, a high vestibule, or a large bulging buccal fat pad

Contraindications are:
- Poor periodontal condition
- Furcation involvement
- Widely divergent or curved roots
- Litigious patients

When commenced, the procedure must be completed with an extraalveolar time of less than 20 minutes. The amount and extent of resorption in replanted teeth increases dramatically if they remain out of the mouth for more than 30 minutes.[12] Meeting this time restraint will require a well organized pretreatment arrangement of staff and material.

The success rate for intentional replantation was recently reported to be 72%.[13] Of the failures, 14% were for periodontal reasons, and 14% because of external root resorption.

Procedure

1. Extract the tooth with forceps as atraumatically as possible. Try to avoid injury to the buccal and lingual plates, and to the interradicular bone.
2. Following the extraction, immediately cover the tooth with gauze saturated with normal saline, leaving only the apex exposed.
3. The gauze should be frequently saturated during the procedure to keep the roots wet.
4. Resect the apical 3 to 5 mm with a new, sharp fissure bur under copious irrigation. This will provide an apical space for pooling of fluids in the postoperative phase.
5. Using a small round bur prepare a cavity 3 mm deep into the apical foramina.
6. Seal the cavity preps with zinc-free amalgam.
7. Curette the apical region of the socket to remove granulation tissue, and recently accumulated blood. Irrigate thoroughly with 0.9% saline.
8. Gently reinsert the tooth, pushing it back slowly into the socket so that pooled blood will escape from the socket.
9. Stabilize with wire or with composite if the tooth is mobile. If fixation is required it should be removed after 7 days.
10. Reduce occlusal surface of the opposing maxillary tooth to minimize occlusal trauma. The patient should be advised not to chew on the tooth for up to 2 weeks.

REFERENCES

1. Allen RK, Newton CW, Brown CE: A statistical analysis of surgical and nonsurgical retreatment cases. *J Endo* 15:261, 1989.
2. Grund B, Moven O, Halse A: Periapical surgery in a Norwegian county hospital: Follow-up findings of 477 teeth. *J Endodont* 16:411, 1990.
3. Ingle JL, Taintor JF: *Endodontics*, ed 3, Philadelphia, 1985, Lea & Febiger, p. 37.
4. Schoeffel GJ: Apicoectomy and retroseal procedures for anterior teeth. *Dent Clin North Am* 38(2):301-324, 1994.
5. Bhaskar SN: Non-surgical resolution of radicular cysts. *Oral Surg* 34:458-468, 1972.
6. Tidmarsh BG, Arrowsmith MG.: Dentinal tubules at the ends of apicected teeth: A scanning electron microscopic study. *Int Endodont J* 22:184-189, 1989.
7. Gilheany PA, Figdor D, Tyas MJ: Apical dentin permeability and microleakage associated with root end resection and retrograde filling. *J Endodont* 20(1):22-26, 1994.
8. Gulabivala K, Sayed AA, Wilson M: The effect of retrograde cavity design on microleakage of amalgam fillings. *Int Endodont J* 28(4):204-212, 1995.
9. Eastman JR, Beckmeyer J: A review of the periodontal, endodontic, and prosthodontic considerations in odontogenous resection procedures. *Int J Periodont Restorative Dent* 6(2):34, 1986.
10. Trabert KC, Cooney JP, Caputo AA, et al: Restoration of endodontically treated teeth and preparation for overdentures. In Ingle JI and Taintor JF, editors: *Endodontics*, ed 3, Philadelphia, 1985, Lea & Febiger, p. 822.
11. Grossman LI: *Endodontic practice*, ed 2, Philadelphia, 1988, Lea & Febiger, p. 334.
12. Andreason JO, Hjorting-Hansen E: Replantation of teeth: Radiographic and clinical study of 110 human teeth reimplantation after accidental loss. *Acta Odont Scand* 24:236, 1966.
13. Raghoebar GM, Vissink A: Results of intentional replantation of molars. *J Oral Maxillofac Surg* 57:240-244, 1999.

CHAPTER 10

Periodontal Surgery

HARRY DYM, DDS

Periodontal surgery is only a part of the overall complete periodontal treatment and it only follows after a thorough treatment planning and routine phase one therapy, consisting of root planing and curettage and home care instruction.

This chapter will address only the common periodontal surgical procedures seen routinely in a general practitioner's office. Basic knowledge of the normal morphology of the periodontal tissues is important for those involved in diagnosing and treating periodontal disease.

The gingiva begins at the mucogingival line and terminates at the free gingival margin. It is attached to the underlying calcified tooth structure by a specialized layer of cells referred to as the junctional epithelium. The mucogingival line marks the junction between the attached gingiva (keratinized tissue) and the free alveolar mucosa (Fig. 10-1).

Within the gingiva also course connective tissue fibers that connect and anchor it to both the alveolar bone, the cementum of the tooth, and each tooth to its neighbor (Fig. 10-2).

It is these gingival sites that can ultimately become infected and inflamed by bacterial infection as a result of plaque and debris accumulation. The spectrum of inflammation varies from mild gingivitis to severe periodontitis (Box 10-1 and Figs. 10-3, 10-4, and 10-5).

In the healthy gingival sulcus there should be no bleeding upon probing and a probe should normally penetrate to about 3 mm in depth. Clinical signs of advanced gingivitis include significant bleeding after sulcus probing, erythema and gingival swelling, and hypertrophy. Pocket formation occurs secondary to apical migration of the junctional epithelium and down the root surface and transformation of the junctional epithelium into a pocket epithelium.[1] Periodontitis is the condition in which pocket formation (greater than 3 mm) exists with loss of connective tissue attachment and inflammation (Fig. 10-6).

The activity of a pocket is of more importance than pocket depth with regard to treatment planning and prognosis.[2] Bleeding on probing and presence of exudate are signs of an active pocket.

Gingivitis need not progress to periodontitis and, unlike periodontitis, when adequately treated is reversible. The etiology of periodontitis is thought to be that of an opportunistic infection. If significant plaque and subgingival debris accumulate, an increased number of pathogenic organisms will result. The degree of damage to the surrounding bone and attachment will then be determined by the individual host response, as well as the rapidity with which the destruction of the periodontal tissue takes place. The underlying focus of all periodontal treatment is the elimination of gingival inflammation and reduction of periodontal pocket depth that represents potential sites for reinfection because of inability to adequately remove all subgingival deposits (Figs. 10-7 and 10-8).

Initial periodontal therapy is aimed at removing all supra- and subgingival plaque and debris along with the microorganisms that cause periodontal disease and the creation of a clean and smooth root surface through scaling and curettage (Table 10-1 and Box 10-2).

This along with a motivated patient following a regimen of good home care should decrease significantly the level of periodontal inflammation.

Each case is reevaluated 8 weeks following initial therapy by assessing pocket depths, gingival bleeding, and plaque accumulation. If persistent pocket depth remains (greater than 3 to 4 mm) a decision is made to perform some type of gingival surgical procedure.

It is at this time that reevaluation of the periodontium is performed by clinical probing. The type of bony defects are evaluated as well as the presence of furcation involvement in multirooted teeth (Box 10-3). This information will determine the prognosis of the teeth and also guide the clinician as to what type of surgical procedure is indicated (Figs. 10-9 and 10-10).

115

Gingivitis An inflammatory process limited to the gingiva with no loss of attachment.
Periodontitis This condition develops from a preexisting gingivitis and now includes pocket formation, bone resorption, and loss of attachment in addition to inflammation.
Recession A clinical condition in which the gingival tissues have retreated in an apical direction exposing root structure. In this condition the gingiva is inflammation free and usually involves only one or two teeth and only the facial aspect.

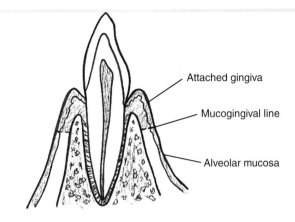

FIG. 10-1   Normal morphology of the periodontal tissues.

Attached gingiva
Mucogingival line
Alveolar mucosa

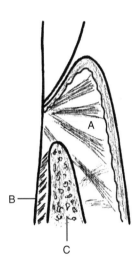

FIG. 10-2   Gingival and periodontal fibers. *A,* Gingival fibers. *B,* Periodontal ligament. *C,* Alveolar bone.

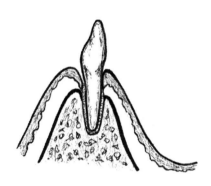

FIG. 10-3   A progression of periodontal disease. Normal healthy periodontium, normal junctional epithelium, no pocket depth, little plaque.

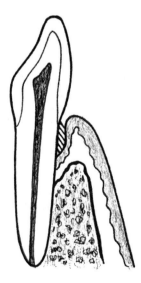

FIG. 10-4   Plaque accumulation with apical proliferation of the junctional epithelium and some collagen loss is present.

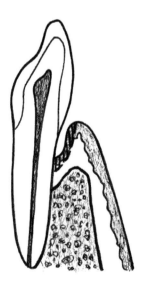

FIG. 10-5   Established plaque with mixed microbial flora (gram positive and negative organisms), true pocket formation, collagen loss, and loss of attachment and alveolar bone.

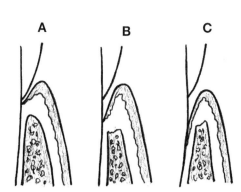

FIG. 10-6 Types of pockets. **A,** Normal sulcus—apical termination of junctional epithelium is at cementoenamel junction. **B,** Suprabony pocket. **C,** Infrabony pocket—extends beyond alveolar crest.

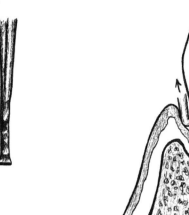

FIG. 10-7 The use of an instrument called a hoe for the removal of hard subgingival accretions in periodontal pockets.

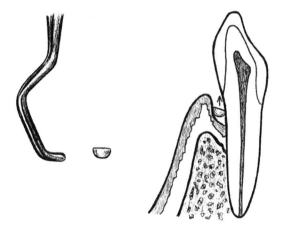

FIG. 10-8 A curette is the instrument of choice for removing both subgingival plaque and calculus as well as for root planing and gingival curettage.

BOX
10-2 Definitions

Scaling	Removal of both supra- and subgingival plaque and calculus
Root Planing	Removal of embedded root calculus and portions of cementum to produce a clean smooth root surface free of endotoxin
Gingival Curettage	Removal of the pocket epithelium and subepithelial connective tissue
Open Curettage	A surgical procedure in which the marginal gingiva is reflected and direct vision is used to perform a thorough scaling, root planing, and curettage.

TABLE
10-1 Sequence of Periodontal Treatment

Stage	Sequence	Procedure
I	Diagnosis	• History and clinical exam • Diagnosis • Patient education and oral hygiene instruction
II	Initial Therapy	• Supragingival plaque and calculus removal
III	Reevaluation	• Pocket evaluation
IV	Surgical Therapy	• Gingivectomy/Gingivoplasty • Modified Widman operation • Mucogingival surgery
V	Maintenance Therapy	• Periodic check ups • Plaque and calculus removal

Class 1: Furcation can be probed to a depth of 3 mm with a periodontal probe.
Class 2: Furcation can be probed to a depth of more than 3 mm but not through and through.
Class 3: Furcation involvement is through and through and can be probed completely. The prognosis for this type of defect is poor and root resection or hemisection of the tooth should be considered.

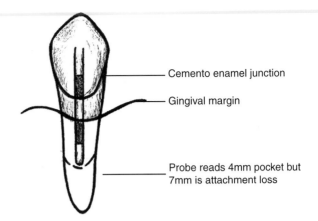

Cemento enamel junction

Gingival margin

Probe reads 4mm pocket but 7mm is attachment loss

FIG. 10-9   The measurement of probing depths provides information about attachment loss only when the gingival margin is at the cementoenamel junction. Consequently, true attachment loss must be measured from the cementoenamel junction and not from the gingival margin.

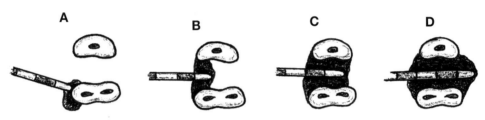

FIG. 10-10   Classification of furcation involvement. **A,** Pocket depth but no furcation involvement. **B,** Type 1—furcation can only be probed to 3 mm. **C,** Type 2—furcation can be probed deeper than 3 mm. **D,** Type 3—through and through furcation involvement.

GINGIVECTOMY AND GINGIVOPLASTY
(Figs. 10-11 through 10-15)

Gingivectomy (GV) refers to a surgical procedure in which gingival pockets are eliminated by removal of gingival tissue, whereas gingivoplasty (GP) refers to surgical recontouring of the mucosal surface.[3] Special instruments are used for gingivectomy (Kirkland knives), whereas fine electrosurgical tips are best used for performing gingivoplasties.

In most cases following gingivectomy a periodontal pack is applied for patient comfort. Only eugenol-free dressings are recommended and should be left in place for 7 to 10 days.

The GV/GP is indicated in cases of pronounced gingival enlargement or overgrowth and shallow suprabony pockets. This procedure is contraindicated for treatment of infrabony pockets and when attached gingiva is narrow or absent.

FLAP PROCEDURES
(Figs. 10-16 through 10-21)

This is the most common of all periodontal surgical procedures and consists of reflecting the entire soft tissue complex: gingival mucosa and periosteum. This is referred to as a full thickness flap whereas a split thickness flap refers to a technique in which the underlying periosteum is left attached to the underlying bone.

The basic purpose for a flap is to gain direct visual access to the deeper periodontal structures to allow for direct treatment which includes root scaling, soft tissue curettage, and the surgical elimination of infected granulation tissue, along with possible root resection. The modified Widman[4] flap is the most commonly used surgical periodontal technique. The original technique of Widman was modified by Ramfjord[5] in 1977 and is particularly indicated for the treatment of mild to moderate periodontitis (Box 10-4).

It is a technique that is conservative in nature and

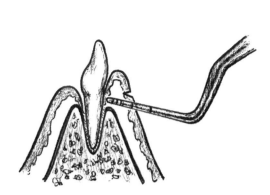

FIG. 10-11 A periodontal probe is inserted at a 45° angle to the tooth and is used to mark the gingivectomy incision by leaving a bleeding point.

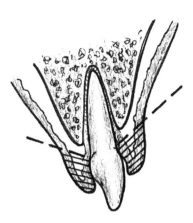

FIG. 10-12 Gingivectomy incisions performed labially and palatally. The labial incisions must be placed above the mucogingival line making certain to keep some attached gingiva surrounding the tooth structure.

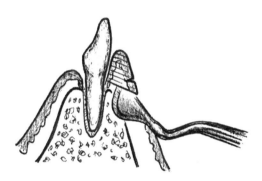

FIG. 10-13 Special gingivectomy knife (Kirkland) is used at a 45° angle to the tooth making certain to be above the mucogingival line.

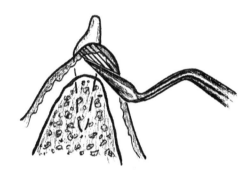

FIG. 10-14 Schematic showing the papilla knife utilized at a 45° angle to excise the interdental tissue.

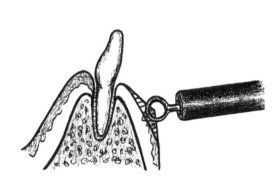

FIG. 10-15 Schematic showing an electrosurgical loop used in a sweeping fashion to sculpt and remove hyperplastic gingival tissue.

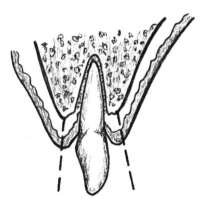

FIG. 10-16 Inverse bevel incision is made on both the labial and palatal sides of the tooth with a double-edged scalpel blade. The incision is made close to the gingival margin (1 to 2 mm away) and extends to the crestal bone.

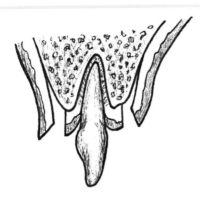

FIG. 10-17 A periosteal elevator is then used to raise a full thickness mucoperiosteal flap allowing for direct visualization of the crestal bone and root structure.

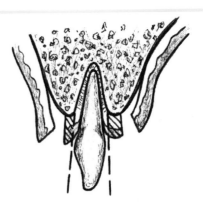

FIG. 10-18 Second incision is made between the tooth and the diseased remaining gingival pocket tissue.

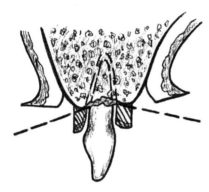

FIG. 10-19 Using a scalpel blade or a gingivectomy knife (Kirkland or papilla type), a horizontal incision is carried down to bone and then the infected tissue is removed, especially the interdental papilla.

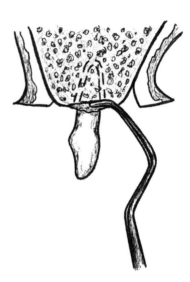

FIG. 10-20 With the flap fully reflected, fine periodontal curettes are now used to remove all remaining granulation tissue and to perform root planing, which is the most critical part of this procedure.

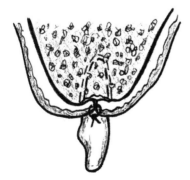

FIG. 10-21 The surgical site is irrigated and then the labial and palatal flaps are reapproximated and closed with 3-0 or 4-0 sutures.

BOX 10-4 Advantages of the Widman Flap versus Closed Curettage

1. Direct visual scaling of all deep subgingival pockets
2. Pocket epithelium can be removed by internal bevel incision
3. Following surgery, flap can be replaced at original location or be repositioned (coronally, apically, or laterally)
4. No open wound
5. Minimal pain and swelling

causes little postoperative pain and swelling. Basically a limited flap is raised and direct vision is then utilized to do thorough subgingival scaling and smoothing of the root surface as well as removing the diseased pocket tissue especially in the interdental area. No bone is removed and because of the scalloped initial incision, the flap closes easily with coverage of the interdental bone.

DISTAL WEDGE EXCISION
(Figs. 10-22 through 10-26)

Periodontal pockets distal to the last tooth in the arch are often difficult to eliminate by routine methods. The wedge excision is easily performed and offers the best surgical solutions.

MUCOGINGIVAL SURGERY
(Fig. 10-27)

In cases of progressive recession of attached gingiva around natural teeth or for aesthetic coverage of root surfaces denuded by gingival recession, mucogingival surgery can be performed. The most common mucogingival procedure is the gingival extension operation utilizing a free gingival graft. This procedure leads to creation of keratinized gingivae and has a most predictable outcome.

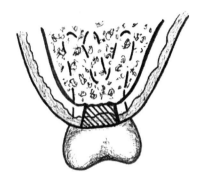

FIG. 10-22   Pocket depth distal to last tooth.

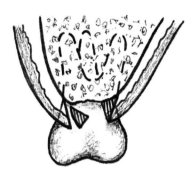

FIG. 10-24   Distal wedge excision is used to eliminate pockets.

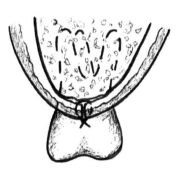

FIG. 10-25   Immediate appearance of distal tissue after closure with interrupted sutures.

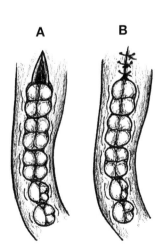

A   B

FIG. 10-23   **A,** A triangular-shaped wedge is excised to eliminate pocketing distal to the last tooth. **B,** Flaps are repositioned and closed with interrupted sutures.

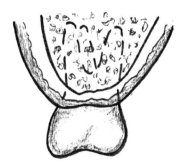

FIG. 10-26   3-month follow up showing pocket reduction.

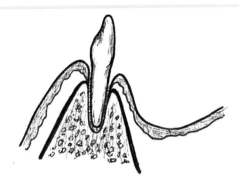

FIG. 10-27   Schematic showing gingival recession.

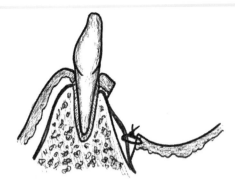

FIG. 10-29   The repositioned vestibular mucosa is fixed to the underlying periosteum in the new inferior position with 4-0 silk or Vicryl sutures.

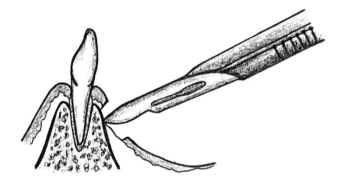

FIG. 10-28   Mucosal tissue has been sharply dissected away in an inferior direction, leaving only a periosteal recipient bed.

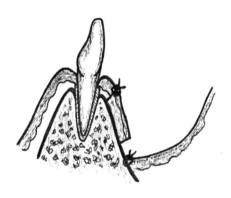

FIG. 10-30   Schematic showing how the repositioned vestibular free mucosa has been sutured inferiorly to the underlying periosteum and the free gingival graft has been placed on the recipient bed site and sutured to the coronal gingiva with 4-0 silk sutures.

SURGICAL PRINCIPLE OF THE FREE GINGIVAL GRAFT FOR INCREASING KERATINIZED ATTACHED GINGIVAL WIDTH
(Figs. 10-28 through 10-30)

First Phase (Box 10-5)

The first phase of surgery is to prepare the recipient bed apical to the area of gingival recession. A horizontal incision is made along the mucogingival line and 1 to 2 mm apical to the gingival margin if no keratinized mucosa exists. The incision is only through mucosa and submucosa but does not violate the underlying periosteum. The mucosal flap is then sutured to the periosteum at the most apical extent of the supraperiosteal dissection. Any extraneous tissue and muscle fibers are trimmed down from the exposed periosteum, and a moist gauze is placed over the recipient site. The graft is then harvested.

Second Phase (Box 10-6)

The most common area used as a donor site is the keratinized mucosa of the lateral palatal vault. The size of the donor tissue should be several millimeters larger than the recipient bed. The graft should be about 1 mm thick, which can be easily harvested with a #15 scalpel blade or a Paquette knife. The donor site may be either left undressed if small, covered with a periodontal pack, or sealed with a previously made plastic or acrylic stent. Be careful not to penetrate too deep into the mucosa so as to avoid injuring the palatal blood vessels, which can cause troublesome hemorrhage.

Third Phase

The graft is then placed over the recipient bed and sutured into place. Digital pressure over moist gauze is held on the graft for several minutes to eliminate hematoma formation underneath the flap that will inhibit healing. The site is then dressed with a periodontal pack.

Covering Areas of Recession

The free gingival graft can also be used to cover root dehiscences. It can be used to directly cover the denuded root surface only after the root has been prepared by root planing and burnishing with saturated citric acid for 5 minutes.[6] The cleft area is then debrided and a supraperiosteal graft bed is prepared and a slightly thicker graft is then harvested from the palate and sutured into place. Another technique that shows the most promise for covering root surfaces denuded by recession is *coronal repositioning* subsequent to free gingival grafting.

An initial surgical procedure is performed to position a free gingival graft just apical to the area of recession. A waiting period of at least 2 to 3 months follows. A second procedure is then performed to coronally reposition the band of attached gingiva to cover the denuded root (Figs. 10-31 through 10-36).

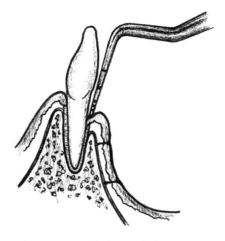

FIG. 10-31 Coronal repositioning technique, to cover denuded teeth after previously free gingival graft placement to increase width of attached gingiva has been performed.

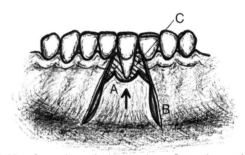

FIG. 10-32 Second surgical procedure: Coronal repositioning. Surgical plan: Incisions. *A,* Marginal: An arcurate incision is planned for the facial surface of #25. The "new papillae" are outlined by this initial incision. *B,* Vertical: The horizontal incision is carried vertically over teeth 24 and 26. *C,* Gingivectomy: Only the epithelium of the papillae coronal to the horizontal incision is excised to prepare a recipient bed.

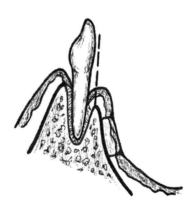

FIG. 10-33 Two vertical incisions are made bilaterally along with a horizontal incision at the cervix of the tooth.

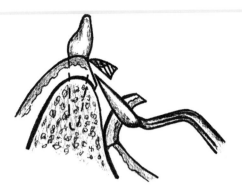

FIG. 10-34   After reflecting a mucoperiosteal flap, the epithelium of the papilla on either side of the involved tooth is excised.

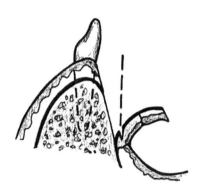

FIG. 10-35   The periosteum is then incised at the base of the flap to allow coronal repositioning of the attached gingiva without tension.

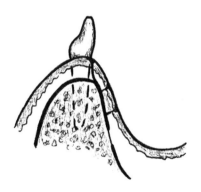

FIG. 10-36   Flap is then repositioned and sutured into place with interrupted Vicryl sutures.

Laterally Positioned Pedicled Graft

Another technique for covering areas of isolated denuded roots is the *laterally positioned pedicled graft.* It is highly predictable for covering isolated areas of denuded roots when there is adequate donor tissue laterally.

The technique basically consists of transposing a pedicled lateral tissue graft from an adjacent site whose vascularity is retained by virtue of the pedicled design.

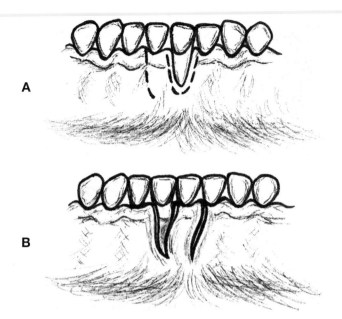

FIG. 10-37   Laterally positioned flap for coverage of denuded root. **A,** Incisions removing gingival margin around exposed root and outlining flap. **B,** After gingiva around exposed root is removed, flap is separated, transferred, and sutured.

Outline of Surgical Procedure (Fig. 10-37). An incision is made resecting the periodontal pocket or gingival margin around the exposed roots. It should be extended to the periosteum and include a border of 3 mm of bone mesial, distal and apical to the root to provide a connective tissue base to which the flap can attach. Remove the resected tissue without disturbing the periosteum around the tooth and scale and plane the root surface.

A vertical incision is then made lateral to the recipient site. The flap should be wider than the recipient site to cover the root and provide a margin for attachment to the tissue around the root. Carefully incise the flap away from the underlying periosteum to the desired depth in the vestibule. Slide the flap laterally onto the adjacent root and suture the flap to the adjacent gingiva. Cover the surgical site with a soft periodontal pack and remove both pack and sutures in one week.

Subepithelial Connective Tissue Graft

Finally, Langer and Langer have described a technique that uses a connective tissue graft to cover denuded roots and is referred to as the *subepithelial connective tissue graft procedure.*[7] It can be used to cover single and multiple denuded root surfaces. The predictability of the procedure is excellent.

Outline of Subepithelial Connective Tissue Graft Technique

1. Denuded root is thoroughly root planed and area is free of inflammation.
2. Horizontal incision is made slightly coronal to cementoenamel junction in the interdental papillae adjacent to the denuded root, making certain to be 2 mm away from the tip of the papilla.
3. Sulcular incision is then made to connect the interdental incisions.
4. Vertical incisions are then made 1 to 2 mm away from the gingival margin.
5. The flap is elevated as a partial thickness flap, making certain to retain periosteum on the underlying bone.
6. A connective tissue-free graft is harvested from the palate and placed over the denuded root 1 mm apical to the cementoenamel incision and sutured to the underlying periosteum with 5-0 resorbable sutures.
7. Cover the graft with the previously raised partial thickness flap and suture it with 3-0 silk sutures.
8. Cover area with thin foil and surgical pack.

POSTSURGICAL PROTOCOL

As with any alveolar surgical procedure, patients undergoing extensive periodontal surgical procedures should be given a prescription for pain medication along with an antibiotic. Penicillin or erythromycin or azitromycin (a newer synthetic macrolide antibiotic which causes less gastrointestinal irritation than erythromycin) for the penicillin-allergic patient are the commonly prescribed antibiotics. There are some who recommend clindamycin or amoxicillin and clavulanate potassium (Augmentin) alone or the combination regimen of metronidazole/Augmentin or metronidazole/ciprofloxacin (for the penicillin-allergic patient) for the treatment of adult and juvenile periodintitis that has proved refractory to mechanical debridement and previous periodontal surgery.[8] Topically applied rinsing solutions that contain chlorhexidine are most useful in the perioperative setting to control plaque formation and to reduce the overall quantitative number of oral microbial flora.

Some patients following therapy for their periodontal disease will complain of sensitivity in areas of exposed root surfaces. A commercially available dentrifice, Sensodyne, containing strontium chloride has proven to be effective therapy. There are also many commercially available solutions that desensitize the root surfaces by sealing the dentinal tubules through a one step paint-on process. Another technique sometimes used is ionization of the exposed root surfaces with a fluroide solution through commercially available apparatuses. If hypersensitivity is severe despite all available treatments, the involved tooth can be treated endodontically.

It is also not uncommon for some patients to experience increased tooth mobility following periodontal flap surgery, due to the loss of gingival and periosteal support. Initial reattachment and tightening may be evident in 10 to 14 days, but it may take as much as 30 to 45 days to firm up.

REFERENCES

1. Muller-Glauser W, Schroeder HE: The pocket epithelium: a light and electron microscopic study, *J Periodont* 53:133, 1982.
2. Rateitschack KH, Wolf HF, Hassel TM: *Color atlas of periodontology,* New York, 1985, Thieme.
3. Sullivan HC, Atkins JH: Free autogenous gingival grafts, *Periodontics* 6:121, 1968.
4. Widman L: The operative treatment of pyorrhea alveolaris. A new surgical method, *Svensk tandläk.-T,* Dec, 1918.
5. Ramfjord SP: Present status of the modified Widman flap procedure, *J Periodont* 48:558, 1997.
6. McGuire MK: Coverage of the denuded root surface using the free soft tissue auto graft, *JADA* 121:277-279, 1990.
7. Langer B, Langer L: Subepithelial connective tissue graft technique for root coverage, *J Periodont* 56:715-720, 1985.
8. Rams TE, Slots J: Antibiotics in periodontal therapy: an update. *Compendium* 13:1130, 1132, 1134, 1992.

11

Closure of Oral Antral Communications and Treatment of Sinus Infections

PAUL R. BAKER, DDS

ANATOMY OF THE MAXILLARY SINUS

The bilateral maxillary sinuses, which are air-filled cavities within the maxillary bone, lie superior to the dental alveolus and inferior to the orbits. The superior aspect of each sinus makes up a significant portion of the orbital floor. Through the orbital floor bone runs the inferior orbital nerve, a terminal branch of the second division of the trigeminal nerve, which gives sensation to the upper lip, ala of the nose, and the inferior eyelid. The medial wall of the sinus is the lateral wall of the nose. The maxillary sinus drains from the middle meatus via the maxillary os or ostium. This is located high on the medial wall. Drainage is accomplished by the presence of healthy respiratory epithelium. The size of the maxillary sinus is approximately 34 mm in an anterior–posterior direction, 33 mm in height, and 23 mm in width, with a mean capacity of 15 milliliters.[1,2] The sinus' primary function is to help humidify the inspired air and to decrease the weight of the osseous facial skeleton. A secondary function of the sinuses is thought to be resonance and voice modulation[3] (Fig. 11-1).

Its close proximity to the oral cavity makes the sinus vulnerable to odontogenic infection, neoplasm, and iatrogenic injury. Injury to the sinus epithelium can occur with large periodontal defects, endodontic procedures, and dental extractions. Conversely, disease processes within the sinus may first present with odontogenic-like symptoms. A clear understanding of morphology and function will help the dental practitioner make a diagnosis while evaluating a sometimes confusing set of symptoms.

Much has been written about maxillary sinusitis causing dental pain (Box 11-1). A good medical history and discussion of the patient's symptoms may help elucidate the proper diagnosis. Maxillary sinusitis of dental origin is generally described as a unilateral pain, usually vague in origin, involving one or more teeth on the affected posterior maxillary quadrant. When the patient bends over the pain seems to increase. Extraorally, the midface area lateral to the nose is tender to touch. Intraorally, the vestibule over the molar/premolar area is tender to palpation and percussion and it may have an erythematous appearance. Vital teeth may be sensitive to percussion and there may be unilateral nasal drainage. If the patient presents with these symptoms with no remarkable dental etiology, special imaging may be useful. Panoramic x-rays and the Water's view are two of the most commonly used radiographic views. Panoramic radiographs may show a "mass-effect" within the sinus. This can best be seen and evaluated by comparing it to the contralateral side. An increase in density may be mucosal thickening or evidence of a fluid level within the sinus. A mucous retention cyst may present itself as a dome-shaped lesion within the confines of the sinus. Its pathology represents a fluid accumulation within the Schneiderian membrane. The membrane consists of a layer of pseudostratified, ciliated, columnar epithelium, a loose connective tissue layer containing goblet cells, and finally a mucoperiosteum. The collection is believed to be contained in the loose connective tissue layer.[4]

As clinicians working in the maxillofacial region, dental practitioners must be cognizant of pathologic conditions that may arise in the maxillary sinus. We must also be aware of the possible effects of our procedures to this complex region. Good clinical exam and an understanding of the anatomic and physiologic structures can lead to a timely diagnosis and intervention. Dental origins of maxillary sinus diseases (Box 11-2) are pathologic conditions that can be attributed to teeth or their embryonic precursors.[5] Diseases may include those of iatrogenic origin such as the creation of a sinus communication caused by extraction or overfill of endodontic therapy material. Also included in these

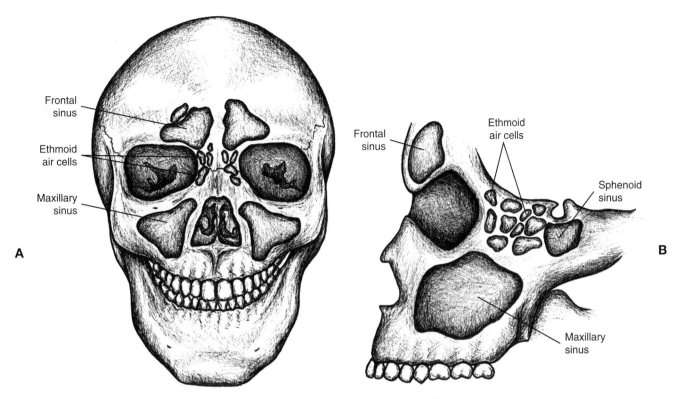

FIG. 11-1 Bony anatomy of the facial skeleton.

BOX 11-1 Unilateral Symptoms Caused by Dental Sinusitis

- Nasal secretion, with erythema of the external nares
- Purulent exudate in the pharynx
- Pressure sensitivity of the maxillary sinus
- Reddening of the skin on the affected side
- Percussion sensitivity of even vital teeth
- Diffuse swelling of the vestibular soft tissues
- Nonvital testing tooth (or teeth), especially the molars
- Communication between oral cavity and the maxillary sinus, a contiguous periodontal pocket
- Abscess formation, vestibular or palatal

BOX 11-2 Causes of Dental Sinusitis

- Oroantral communication: This may be created accidentally during tooth extraction or an oroantral fistula may be unrecognized
- Apical osteitis
- Radicular cyst or residual cyst
- Periodontal pockets
- Impacted teeth
- Foreign bodies in the sinus (root canal filling, aspergillosis)

conditions are tumors that may arise from the remainders of the embryonic origins of the teeth.

The most common complication of the maxillary sinus is the oral-antral communication. This commonly occurs during the extraction of upper molars or premolar teeth. A well-pneumatized sinus can contribute to this situation. Careful clinical evaluation and analysis of radiographs can help predict the possibility of this occurrence prior to extraction. Periapical radiographs should be of good quality and show the complete root structure. Identification of the sinus membrane is easily done. The size of the tooth and its configuration must

be evaluated. Severely dilacerated or divergent roots in close proximity to the maxillary sinus have a high potential of creating a sinus opening during extraction. Improper surgical technique can lead to fracture of the buccal plate and interradicular bone loss. This bone loss can then lead to large openings into the sinus. Those teeth identified to be high risk for oral-antral communication should be removed via a surgical approach with multiple sectioning. Figs. 11-2 and 11-3 illustrate the technique for surgical removal of the upper molars.

The crown, if present, is sectioned at the cemento-enamel junction at the level of the trifurcation (Fig. 11-2). Care should be taken not to enter the antrum with rotary cutting instruments during cutting proce-

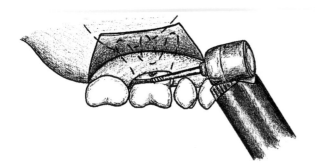

FIG. 11-2 Section at trifurcation with high speed surgical handpiece.

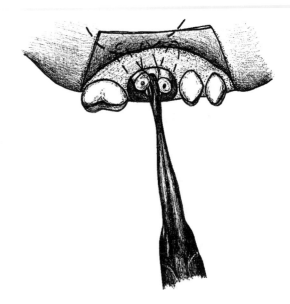

FIG. 11-3 Careful elevation of root segments.

dures. The remaining root structure is then sectioned, first in a sagittal direction isolating the palatal root, which is then extracted. The buccal roots are then also sectioned and removed; this procedure is shown in Fig. 11-3.

Extraction of maxillary root tips can be complicated by the use of improperly vectored forces. The fragment of a root, root tip, or entire tooth can be displaced into the maxillary antrum. During an extraction it is important not to place upward vertical forces into the socket of a maxillary tooth. This could have the effect of driving the root tip through the fragile remaining alveolar bone into the sinus. Small, uninfected root tips (2 to 3 mm in size) may be displaced beneath the antral membrane and sinus floor and no attempt should be made to remove these. Generally, these small root fragments will fibrose and cause no further problems.[6] The patient should, however, be made aware of this and placed on the appropriate antibiotics. If signs and symptoms of infection develop, the patient should be referred to the oral and maxillofacial surgeon.

Maxillary sinusitis of dental origin occurs when congestion leads to narrowing or obstruction of the sinus opening called the os. The result is decreased drainage and accumulation of fluids and debris within the sinus cavity. Over time bacterial invasion can occur leading to infection and a maxillary sinusitis. Acute disease is characterized by pain over the lateral sinus wall, pain when bending over, and discharge from the ipsilateral nares. There may also be a change in sensation in the posterior molar area of either generalized pain or a "peg-like" feeling.

The pathogens commonly isolated from the acutely infected maxillary sinus are *Haemophilus influenzae* and *Streptococcus pneumoniae*, both gram-positive organisms.[7,8,9] *Moraxella catarrhalis* is also commonly isolated in the acute infection.[10,11,12] The microbiology of the chronically infected sinus is somewhat different. The sinusitis is considered chronic if it is resistant to treatment and has recurred or has been present greater than 3 months.[13] As the disease progresses and the drainage

is reduced, oxygen concentration and the pH decrease. The resulting conditions are ideal for the support of anaerobic growth. Anaerobic bacteria and the facultative anaerobes are frequently isolated in the chronically infected maxillary sinus. Bacteria commonly found are the porphymonas (*Bacteroides*) species, *Veillonella*, and *Corynebacterium*. The facultative anaerobes present may include alpha-hemolytic *Streptococcus*, *Staphylococcus*, and *Streptopyogenes*.[14]

Medical management of sinusitis is imperative prior to and in conjunction with surgical intervention. It generally consists of prescribing an antimicrobial agent to reduce the bacterial load along with a decongestant to promote drainage of the sinus and to help change the bacterial environment from that of an anaerobic promoting one to an aerobic one. Finally, an analgesic may be required for pain management.

Penicillins are effective against many of the organisms associated with acute maxillary sinusitis. One must be cognizant of the fact that most infections exist as a mixed bacterial population. Therefore antimicrobial therapy should be directed at the spectrum of organisms most commonly involved: *Haemophilus influenzae*, *Streptococcus pneumoniae*, and *Moraxella catarrhalis*. Infections of dental origin should be considered a mixed bacterial flora because of the nature of the gingival crevice and periradicular lesions. These organisms include *Prevotella* and *Porphyromonas*. Most authors suggest antimicrobial therapies to run a course of 10 days. However, treatment should be tailored to the patient's response to local measures and medications.[15] Patients resistant to therapy should have a sinus aspiration and microbial cultures done.

Patients allergic to penicillin should be given either

a second-generation cephalosporin or trimethoprim-sulfamethoxazole, a sulfa-based bacteriostatic antibiotic. Patients with penicillin allergy should be questioned carefully regarding their hypersensitivity reaction. Those with a history of edema, shortness of breath, and anaphylaxis should not be given any penicillin-type drug. If the history is questionable the patient should be prescribed an alternative antibiotic.

Systemic decongestants are of great importance in treating maxillary sinusitis. One must promote drainage of the sinus contents and thus cause a change in the oxygen environment of the sinus cavity. The systemic decongestants commonly used are a combination of medications with either an antihistamine or sympathomimetic, which may produce side effects that can be distressing to the patient. Antihistamines produce varying degrees of sedation in most patients, whereas sympathomimetics can elevate blood pressure and pulse rate. This can be alarming to some patients and detrimental to cardiac patients. These medications should be prescribed with the patient's systemic health in mind. Systemic medications commonly used are Dimetapp (brompheniramine, phenylephrine, and phenylpropanolamine) and Entex (phenylpropanolamine and guaifenesin). Dimetapp is thought to have a drying effect on the nasal secretions and Entex is thought to be an agent that thins the nasal secretions.[16]

Topical decongestants may be used but should be limited to no more than 7 days, as a rebound edema or "rhinitis medicamentosa" may occur with chronic use.[16] Afrin (oxymetazoline hydrochloride) is an example of a topical decongestant. It is a sympathomimetic amine and has the effect of shrinking nasal mucosa by acting on the vascular smooth muscle. Topical corticosteroids have been used with good effect in those patients thought to have an allergic component to their congestion. The effect of corticosteroids is to stabilize mast cells in the nasal mucosa and reduce the overall numbers of these cells and eosinophils and basophils.[17,18,19,20]

ORAL-ANTRAL COMMUNICATION

Occasionally even with proper evaluation of clinical presentation, a perforation into the sinus may occur during extraction. Acute perforations into the maxillary sinus are termed oral-antral communications (OAC). Those that persist and develop an epithelium lined tract are termed oral-antral fistula (OAF).

If a perforation is suspected, examination of the socket should be done with irrigation, suction, and a good light source. Instruments should not be placed deep in the socket to "sound" for openings. Some authors advocate having the patient hold their nostrils closed and blow against the obstruction. The operator

views the socket for movement of the membrane or displacement of socket debris. Others condemn this practice as a method to tear a membrane which may be the last tissue boundary crossing the osseous defect. Treatment of the perforations is based upon the patient's sinus history prior to the procedure and the size of the opening.

The operator should question the patient concerning a history of allergy, sinus disease, and any previous sinus procedures. Any periapical pathology should be noted preoperatively. Generally those patients with healthy sinuses preoperatively tolerate sinus perforations better than those with a history of sinus inflammation. If a patient with no history of sinus disease has a perforation under 4 to 5 mm the chance for spontaneous healing is excellent.[21,22]

Simple closure without mobilization of flaps with figure-8 suture is suggested. Stabilization of the blood clot is critical and placement of clot-stabilizing medicaments may be beneficial. Examples of these include Gelfoam, oxidized cellulose, and collagen dressings. Those sinuses with a history of disease with openings greater than 4 to 5 mm should be considered for closure. The most common initial treatment for an oral-antral communication is the buccal sliding flap. It is critical, prior to extraction, to have considered the possible need for tissue mobilization to close a perforated sinus. Mobilization of mucosal flaps and development of a watertight closure rely on a tension-free closure and maintenance of a blood supply to the flap. If tension-free closure is not obtained, flap failure and possible tissue loss may result. The buccally placed flap is trapezoidal in nature and can be advanced with periosteal releasing incisions (Fig. 11-4). Prominent buccal ledges should be smoothed down to allow the flap to lie passively. The closure is performed over bone, and if at all avoidable, never over "dead space" (Figs. 11-5 through 11-7). An advantage to this type of flap is that a Caldwell-Luc procedure can be done through this incision if foreign body removal is required. The disadvantage of the technique is that buccal vestibule height is lost, which could be significant if the patient requires multiple closure procedures or if the patient wears a prosthesis. Some authors report a 50% loss in vestibular height.

Another flap design used to close lateral defects in the edentulous patient is the buccal finger flap developed by Mozcair.[23] Little loss of vestibular height is reported with this flap design. The flap is based anteriorly and slides horizontally in a posterior direction (Fig. 11-8). Regardless of flap design the practitioner should not place the suture line over "dead space." All suture lines are best placed over bone to decrease chance of wound breakdown.

All patients suspected of having a sinus perforation, a small perforation, or a closed perforation should be

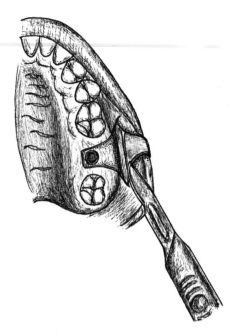

FIG. 11-4 Trapezoidal flap raised with two vertical releasing incisors.

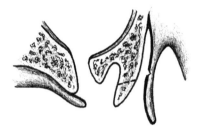

FIG. 11-5 Bone edges smoothed prior to closure.

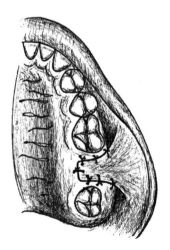

FIG. 11-6 Buccal flap closed with vertical mattress sutures.

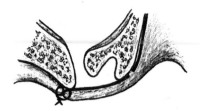

FIG. 11-7 Closure away from dead space over the bone.

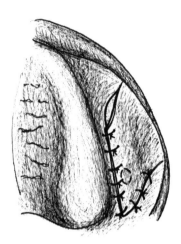

FIG. 11-8 Sliding buccal flap to close lateral defect.

placed on "sinus precautions." These precautions consist of an antibiotic to manage the microbes of the antral environment and a decongestant to help shrink inflamed sinus mucosa and promote sinus drainage. The patient is asked to refrain from nose blowing and closed mouth sneezing to reduce any sudden increase in antral pressure. The patient should refrain from tooth brushing in the area for 2 weeks. The sutures are left in place for 2 weeks. Smoking cessation is highly recommended. Chronic opening of the maxillary sinus that is persistent for greater than 48 hours is considered to have become a fistula.[24] Patients with an OAF require removal of the fistula (fistulectomy), and closure of the sinus opening. Before this procedure the patient will require medical management of the resultant sinusitis.

An antibiotic and decongestant should be prescribed in conjunction with frequent sinus irrigation to clear the chronic infection. OAF should be evaluated via imaging and clinical examination. Those patients with discharge from the fistula and nasal discharge require sinus irrigation. Maxillary sinus irrigation should never be done under pressure, as excessive pressure can cause distribution of infected material into neighboring tissue planes, including the orbit. Irrigation should be done at 48-hour intervals and all affluent discharge evaluated for clarity and odor. No closure should be attempted before the resolution of the sinus infection.

After the sinus disease has been controlled, a surgical closure can be planned. A critical part of the procedure is the removal of any residual chronic diseased mucosa. The size of the oral-antral defect is usually considerably greater than the fistula itself.[25,26] The Caldwell-Luc operation is used to gain access to the antrum to perform the necessary debridement. Access is done high in the vestibule in the canine eminence and a dime-size opening is made and antral curettes are used to remove diseased mucosa. Nasal packing is usually placed with antibiotic impregnated ribbon gauze to control bleeding within the sinus and encourage healing of the mucosa. Attention is then directed to the removal of the fistula and closure of the defect. Fistulectomy is performed and the defect is visualized (Figs. 11-9 through 11-11).

Many methods are used to close the residual defect. Awang has divided closure sources for oral-antral communication into local flaps, distal flaps, and grafts.[27] Local flaps include those whose tissue origin is adequate to cover the defect. Sliding buccal flaps have been discussed earlier. Palatal tissue flaps are another alternative but these are usually reserved for larger and persistent defects. Palatal flaps are composite flaps that consist of either full thickness mucosa or split thickness.[27,28] Split thickness flaps consist of periosteum and submucosa. Both of the flap variations are based on the greater palatine artery and great care must be tailored to preserve the blood supply. The palatal flaps are raised and rotated to cover the defect[29] (Figs. 11-12 through 11-15).

Large defects with chronic disease may be difficult to close and failure of the initial closure attempt may occur. If there is inadequate tissue for a second operation a distant flap is used. A tongue flap is an example of a distant flap.[30,31] These flaps are trapezoidal in nature, may be posteriorly or anteriorly based, and include elements of mucosa and muscle. Closed reduction is usually required to decrease tongue mobility.

Graft materials that may be used to close OAFs include gold foil and allograft bone graft material.[32,33,34] This graft material is found in sheets or cores. Methylmethacrylate in a soft sheet has also been advocated.[8] Generally most defects are closed via a soft tissue approach only. The major indication for bone grafting is ridge reconstruction with OAF closure.[16]

A clear understanding of the morphology and pathophysiology of the maxillofacial region is crucial for clinicians practicing in this area. Careful evaluation and treatment planning can avoid many adverse outcomes. Those situations that arise requiring such treatment can be diagnosed early and treated to a successful outcome with an understanding of the multiple factors involved.

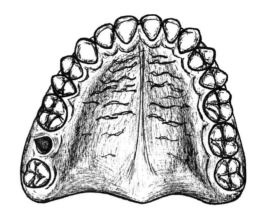

FIG. 11-9   Fistula presentation.

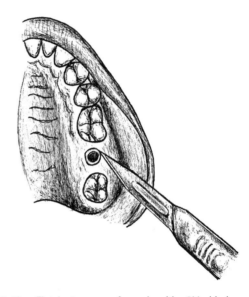

FIG. 11-10   Fistulectomy performed with #11 blade prior to closure.

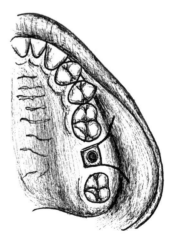

FIG. 11-11   Oral antral bony defect is always clinically larger after soft tissue fistula is removed.

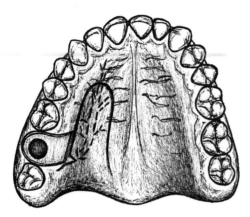

FIG. 11-12 An outline of the flap is carefully measured prior to outlining incision. Note, be careful to place incisions lateral and medial to artery.

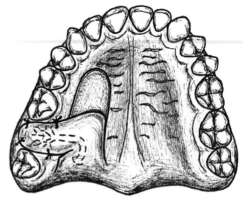

FIG. 11-14 Palatal island flap rotated into antral opening site and closed.

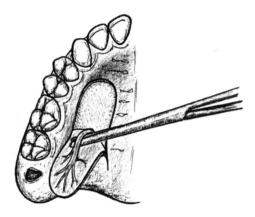

FIG. 11-13 The palatal flap should be a full thickness one in order to avoid injuring the artery that travels above the periosteum. The artery is not to be violated if possible.

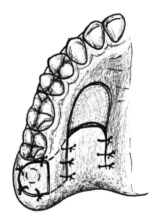

FIG. 11-15 Rotated palatal flap is then closed with multiple interrupted 3-0 or 4-0 sutures. The denuded palatal bone can be left open or covered with a collagen pad for patient comfort.

Referrals for the situations requiring specialist care should be identified early to avoid the sequelae of iatrogenic maxillary sinus injury.

REFERENCES

1. Schaefer JP: *The nose, paranasal sinuses, nasolacrimal passageways, and olfactory organs in man,* Philadelphia, 1920, Blaskiston's Son and Co.
2. Clemente CD, Gray H: *Anatomy of the human body,* ed 30, Philadelphia, Lea & Febiger, 1984.
3. Alberti PW: Applied surgical anatomy of the maxillary sinus, *Otolaryngol Clin North Am* 9:12, 1979.
4. Van Nostrand AW, Goodman WS: Pathologic aspects of mucosal lesions of the maxillary sinus, *Otolaryngol Clin North Am* 9:21-34, 1976.
5. Schow SR: Infections of the maxillary sinus, *Oral Maxillofac Clin North Am* 3(2):343, 1991.
6. Peterson L: Prevention and management of surgical complications. In Peterson L, Ellis E, Hupp JR, Tucker MR: *Contemporary oral and maxillofacial surgery,* ed 3, St. Louis, 1988, Mosby.
7. Van Cauwenberge P, Verschraegen G, Van Rentergghem L: Bacteriological findings in sinusitis, *Scand J Infect Dis* 9:72, 1978.
8. Jousimies-Somer HR, Salvolainen S, Ylikoski JS: Bacteriological findings of acute maxillary sinusitis in young adults, *J Clin Microbiol* 26:1919, 1988.
9. Evans FO, Sydnor JB, Moore WEC, et al.: Sinusitis of the maxillary antrum, *N Engl J Med* 293:735, 1975.
10. Schurin PA: Etiology and antimicrobial therapy of paranasal sinusitis in children, *Ann Otol Rhinol Laryngol* 90(84):72, 1981.
11. Nelson JD: Changing trends in the microbiology and management of acute otitis media and sinusitis, *Pediatr Infect Dis* 5:749, 1986.
12. Wald ER, Milmoe GJ, Bowen DA, et al.: Acute maxillary sinusitis in children, *N Engl J Med* 304:749, 1981.
13. Melen I, Lindahl I, Andreasson L, Rundcrantz H: Chronic maxillary sinusitis, *Acta Otolaryngol* 101:320, 1986.
14. Brooke I: Bacteriology of chronic maxillary sinusitis in adults, *Ann Otol Rhinol Larygol* 98:426, 1989.
15. Evans FO, Sydnor JB, Moore WEC, et al.: Sinuitis of the maxillary antrum, *N Engl J Med* 293:735, 1975.
16. Gonty AA: In Peterson L: Diagnoses and Management of Sinus Disease. *Oral and maxillofacial surgery,* Philadelphia, 1997, Lippencott Raven vol 1, p 240.
17. Kapp JF: Use of corticosteroids in management of rhinitis. In Settipane GA: *Rhinitis,* Providence, RI, 1984, New England Regional Allergy Proceedings. pp. 108-115.

18. Elwany S, Talaat M, et al.: Allergic nasal mucosa following treatment with beclomethasone dipropionate, *J Laryngol Otol* 97:165, 1983.

19. Viegas M, et al.: Effects of corticosteroids on mast cells in nasal mucosa, *J Allergy Clin Immunol* 79:197, 1987.

20. Kastrup EK: *Drug facts and comparisons*, Philadelphia, 1990, JB Lippincott, p. 184.

21. Martensson G: Operative method in fistulas of the maxillary sinus, *Acta Otolaryngol* 48:253, 1957.

22. Schuchardt K: Treatment of oro-antral perforation and fistulae, *Int J Oral Surg* 5:157, 1955.

23. Moczair L: Nuovo methodo operatopela chisura della fistole del seno massella se di origina dentale, *Stomatol* 28:1087, 1930.

24. Von Wowern N: Closure of oroantral fistula with buccal flap: Behrmann versus Moczair, *Int J Oral Surg* 11:156, 1982.

25. Von Wowern N: Correlation between the development of an oroantral fistula and size of the corresponding bony defect, *J Otolaryngol* [supp] 31:98, 1973.

26. Anderson M: Surgical closure of oroantral fistula: report of a series, *J Oral Surg* 27:862, 1969.

27. Awang M: Closure of oroantral fistula, *Int J Oral Maxillofacial Surg* 17:110, 1988.

28. Ito T, Hara H: A new technique for closure of oroantral fistula, *J Oral Surg* 38:509, 1980.

29. Gullane P, Arena S: Palatal island flap for reconstruction of oral defect, *Arch Otolaryngol* 103:598, 1977.

30. Vaughan E, Brown A: The versatility of the lateral tongue flap in the reconstruction of defects of the oral cavity, *Br J Oral Surg* 21:1, 1983.

31. Guerrero-Santos J, Altamirano J: The use of lingual flaps in the repair of fistulas of the hard palate, *Plast Reconstr Surg* 38:123, 1966.

32. Skolnik E, O'Neill J, Baim H: Closure of oroantral fistula, *Laryngoscope* 89:844, 1979.

33. Goldman E, Stratigos G, Arthur A: Treatment of oroantral fistula by gold foil closure: report of a case, *J Oral Surg* 27:875, 1969.

34. Meyerhoff W, Christiansen T, Rontal E, Boerger W: Gold foil closure of oroantral fistulas, *Laryngoscope* 83:940, 1973.

INFECTIONS

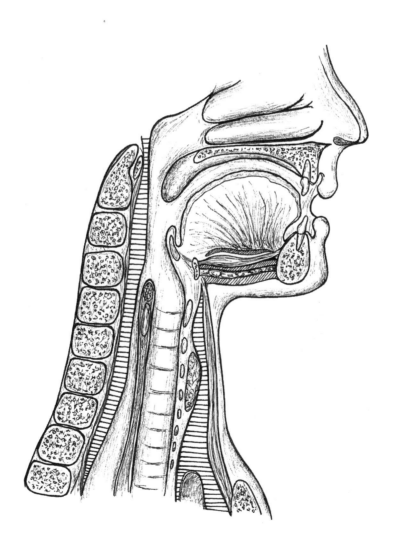

12 Odontogenic Infections: Anatomy and Surgical Management

DUDLEY S. JACKMAN, DMD
J. HAMIL WILLOUGHBY, DDS

Despite the development of new technology in dentistry, and the introduction by the pharmaceutical industry of antibiotics that are more specific and powerful, modern dentists will still be faced with patients who will require surgical management of dentoalveolar infections. To properly manage these patients the dentist must have an adequate knowledge of the causes of inflammation, the regional anatomy, applied pharmacology, bacteriology, and immunology. The management of dentoalveolar infections will often involve the use of pharmaceutical agents as well as surgical interventions. In order to best understand the dissemination of dental infections and their surgical management the dentist must have reasonable knowledge of the anatomy of the muscles of facial expression, the muscles of mastication, structures within the floor of the mouth, facial spaces, the significance of alveolar bone architecture, and the position of the root apices to adjacent muscle attachments (Fig. 12-1).

ASSESSMENT OF THE PATIENT WITH AN ODONTOGENIC INFECTION

A thorough history and physical examination is essential in the evaluation of any patient with a suspected maxillofacial infection. This thorough history can only be obtained by good interviewing techniques, as the information obtained will only be as good as the questions asked. During the initial interview the dentist should gather information related to the present problem as well as information from the medical history that may influence or affect the outcome of therapy.

Important historical data that should be gathered during the initial interview include:

- A history of dental pain prior to the appearance of the swelling.
- Dental trauma (pulpal necrosis can be the result of trauma to the teeth sustained years previously).

- The length of time that the swelling was evident—acute vs. chronic.
- Changes in the nature of the swelling and how fast this change is occurring. Did the swelling begin as a soft mass, or was it consistently firm?
- Is pain associated with the swelling?
- Is this an episodic swelling, or is it associated with a specific event such as eating?
- The nature of the pain. Is it increased in intensity? Does the pain feel like more than one tooth is involved?

The medical history should be aimed at identifying systemic diseases or local conditions that may influence the management decisions. Some common and important systemic factors are:

- *Diabetes mellitus:* These patients may have significant changes in microvascular circulation throughout the body, and their host response to invading bacteria will be diminished. Consequently, the ability for antibiotics to reach the area of increased inflammatory activity will be reduced. The infected diabetic patient will require aggressive medical (antihyperglycemic agents and antibiotics) and surgical management. Infection will tend to make the diabetes worse.
- *Systemic steroids:* Steroids will decrease the inflammatory response including the flow of white blood cells to the infected area. The effects of steroids will be to mask the infection and allow it to become more widespread.
- *Immunosuppressive medications:* These patients are often organ transplant patients and will be at a great disadvantage in mounting the appropriate defense to bacterial invasion.
- *Leukocyte disorders or hematologic malignancies:* Nonfunctional or poorly functional white cells.
- *Bleeding disorders:* Poor control of bleeding may lead to hematoma formation and a more rapid spread of the infection.

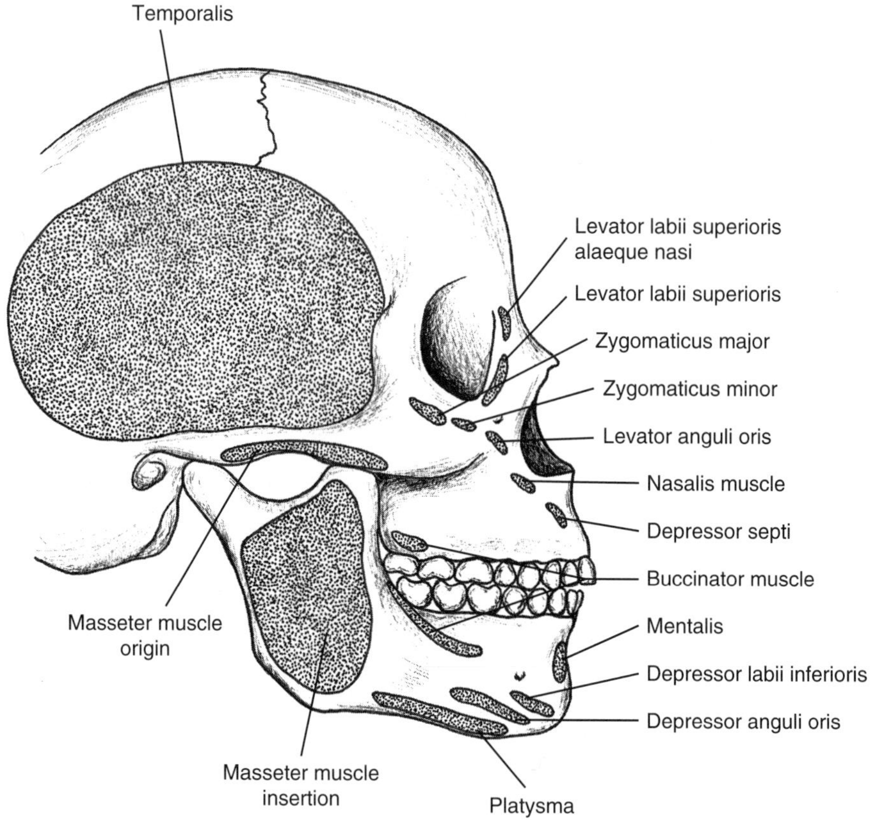

Temporalis

Levator labii superioris alaeque nasi

Levator labii superioris

Zygomaticus major

Zygomaticus minor

Levator anguli oris

Nasalis muscle

Depressor septi

Buccinator muscle

Mentalis

Depressor labii inferioris

Depressor anguli oris

Masseter muscle origin

Masseter muscle insertion

Platysma

FIG. 12-1 Muscle attachments to the facial bones. The position of the root apex to these muscles will determine the path of spread of infection and where an abscess will localize.

- *Renal dialysis and patients on long term antibiotic therapy:* These patients may develop resistant strains of organisms and may require special consideration in antibiotic selection.
- *Hepatic dysfunction and alcoholism:* Patients may have alterations in the ability to produce proteins, and eliminate and conjugate drugs and toxins. Their immune systems will also be compromised and they may have coagulation problems. Alcohol also affects the function of white blood cells.
- *Pregnancy:* Timing of treatment, choice of antibiotic and analgesics must be made in consultation with the obstetrician.
- *The elderly:* Vascularity and the immune system may be impaired, and their ability to metabolize drugs may be decreased. They may also be less likely to comply with therapy.

EXAMINATION

The examination should begin with a good visual examination of the head and neck, and conclude with a comprehensive intraoral survey, including dental and nondental structures. Palpation is another important part of this physical examination. The nature of the swelling should be assessed through digital palpation, first with one finger and then in a bimanual mode to

determine fluctuance. To examine for fluctuance, one finger is pressed against the swelling while the other remains passive to register any fluid impulse (Fig. 12-2).

It should be emphasized that all pertinent data—including negative ones—must be accurately recorded in the patients' records. Vital signs should also be obtained and recorded.

DENTOALVEOLAR INFECTIONS

Infection of the dentoalveolar structures may present to the clinician as a cellulitis or as an abscess. A cellulitis is a diffuse, hard, erythematous swelling, resulting from the spread of microorganisms through soft tissue planes. An abscess is a localized cavity lined by fibrous connective tissue that contains pus.[1] In general, cellulitis is treated with antibiotics, and abscesses by surgical intervention. The area of localization of the swelling and the path of spread of a dentoalveolar infection is related to the anatomic position of the root apex of the tooth from which the infection originated.

In the maxilla, the lateral cortical bone is thin and porous, and the anterior teeth (with the exception of the maxillary lateral incisors), the buccal root of the premolars, and the buccal roots of the molars are in close proximity to it. Infections from these maxillary

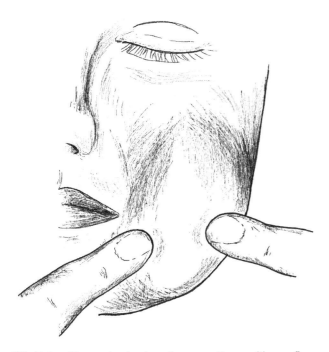

FIG. 12-2 Bimanual palpation of a mass. Press with one finger against the mass, while the finger of the other hand remains passive to detect any fluid pulse movement.

teeth will therefore take the path of least resistance and spread toward the buccal. The palatal shelf is thicker and because of its architecture and the position and angulation of the maxillary teeth within, the practitioner will not very often see a dentoalveolar infection on the palate. Abscesses on the palate will originate from the lateral incisors or from the palatal roots of the molars. The dentist should be cognizant of the fact that tooth position, through rotation or inclination, may cause the root of any tooth to come in close proximity to one cortex and change the usual expected clinical picture.[1,2]

In the mandible both cortices of bone are relatively thick and an infection will take longer to spread out of its bony confines. Where the infection becomes clinically evident in the soft tissue depends on the position of the roots in relationship to the bony insertion of the various muscles of the maxillofacial region. Infections associated with a specific tooth will usually be localized a short distance from the anatomic origin. A general rule is that most dentoalveolar infections will spread by the path of least tissue resistance through the medullary bone and through the soft tissues (Fig. 12-3).

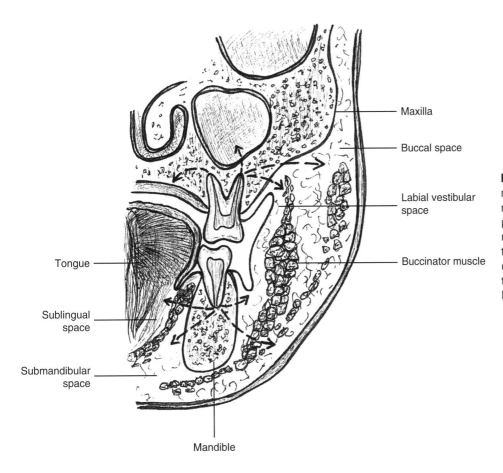

Maxilla

Buccal space

Labial vestibular space

Buccinator muscle

Tongue

Sublingual space

Submandibular space

Mandible

FIG. 12-3 A coronal view of the molar region in the maxilla and the mandible diagramming possible paths for infection to spread from root apices, through bone, to soft tissue. Muscle attachments will determine where a clinical presentation of an abscess will be localized.

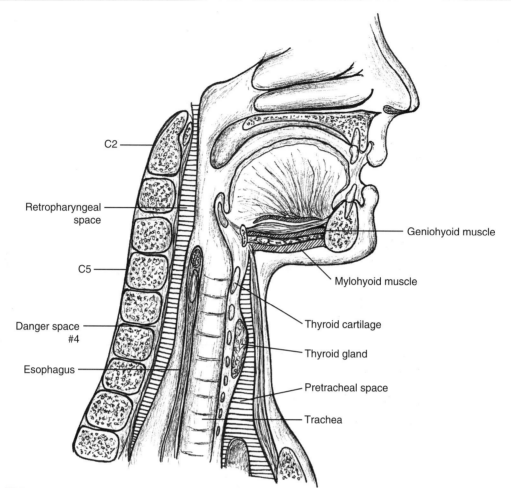

FIG. 12-4 Sagittal view of the spaces of the neck. Horizontal lines indicate retropharyngeal space, situated posterior to the esophagus, and the pretracheal space anterior to the trachea.

FASCIA OF THE HEAD AND NECK

Although most dental infections remain localized, they can spread from the immediate dental area along fascial planes and cause serious morbidity to the patient, and may even become life-threatening. Because of the possibility of spread along with increased morbidity the dentist must have an in-depth knowledge about the fascial planes along which the infection may spread.

Fascia is the loose connective tissue associated with muscle bundles that allows an individual muscle to perform its specific action and slide against adjacent muscles.[3] An odontogenic infection can travel along the fascia and may eventually organize, producing pus, in one of the specific fascial spaces of the head and neck. These fascial spaces exist only as potential spaces, but become "real spaces" when created by the spread of odontogenic infection that dissects into deeper adjacent tissues rather than exiting superficially through mucosa

or skin. The fascia provides an effective pathway for infection to spread from its dentoalveolar origin to deep parts of the face, head, and neck (Fig. 12-4).

Fascia of the head and neck can be divided into three parts: superficial, prevertebral, and visceral fascia. The superficial fascia (superficial investing fascia) is just deep to the subcutaneous tissue of the skin, surrounding the muscles of facial expression, and covering the platysma. The undersurface of the muscles of facial expression is covered by the deep layer of the superficial fascia. This layer descends from the hyoid bone to follow the great vessels of the neck into the mediastinum. Prevertebral fascia envelops the vertebral column and its muscles and contributes a portion of the carotid sheath, which contains the internal jugular, the common carotid, and the vagus nerve. The visceral fascia envelops the pharynx and continues downward to include the esophagus and trachea[2,3] (Fig. 12-5).

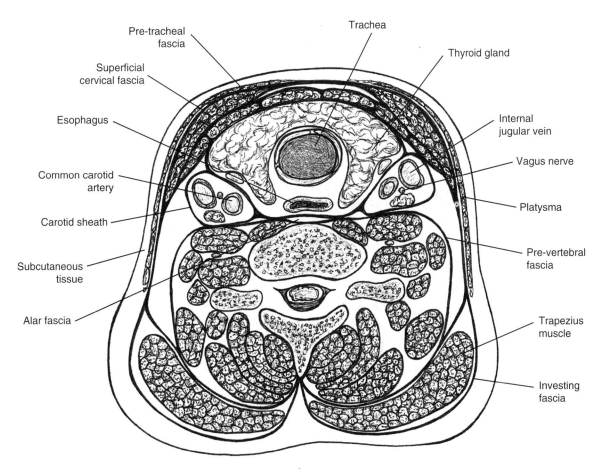

FIG. 12-5 Superficial and deep layers of the fascia of the neck. The superficial layer of investing fascia encircles the neck deep to the subcutaneous layer of the skin.

SPACES OF THE HEAD AND NECK

Infections may spread into several potential spaces within the head and neck. Lateral to the visceral fascia are the paired parapharyngeal spaces. The lateral pharyngeal space is shaped like an inverted cone with its apex at the hyoid bone.[4] The base of this cone is formed by the lateral pterygoid muscle and the base of the skull. The lateral extent of this space is the medial surface of the medial pterygoid muscle, whereas the medial border is the muscle of the superior pharyngeal constrictor. The lateral pharyngeal space contains the carotid artery, the internal jugular vein, and the vagus, glossopharyngeal, and hypoglossus nerves. This space is divided into anterior and posterior compartments by the styloglossus and stylopharyngeus muscles.[2] Infections in this area can be the result of: tonsillitis, pharyngitis, odontogenic infections, otitis, or mastoiditis. Infections involving the anterior compartment will have clinical symptoms that include fever, chills, dysphagia, medial bulging of the lateral pharyngeal wall, and pain and swelling at the angle of the mandible. Patients with infections in the posterior compartment will not have

trismus or swelling at the angle of the mandible. Clinical signs of posterior compartment abscess include: respiratory difficulties, fever, formation of septic thrombosis of the jugular vein, erosion of one of the great vessels of the neck, ipsilateral Horner syndrome, and palsies of the ninth through twelfth cranial nerves. The lateral pharyngeal space is continuous with the submandibular, sublingual, and pterygomandibular spaces.[1]

The *retropharyngeal* space is a potential space that exists between the buccopharyngeal fascia and the alar fascia. It has its superior limit at the base of the skull and extends to the level of C-6 and T-4 of the cervical spine (Fig. 12-6). It contains the retropharyngeal lymphatic chain that drains the nose, nasopharynx, middle ear, and paranasal sinuses. Infections in this area are usually the result of upper respiratory and pharyngeal infections.[4] However, odontogenic infection can spread to this space via the lateral pharyngeal space. Infections within the retropharyngeal space can be observed in a lateral neck soft tissue radiograph. The thickness of the soft tissue shadow between the vertebral column and

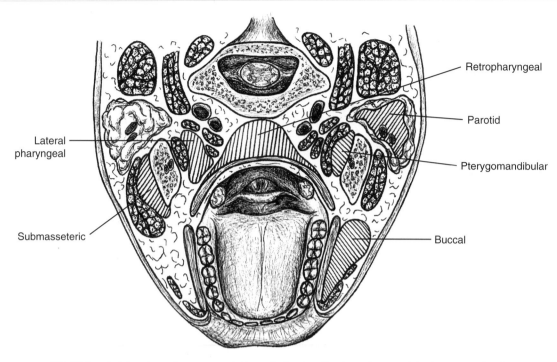

FIG. 12-6 Axial schematic representation of the localization of potential abscesses in the submasseteric, lateral pharyngeal, retropharyngeal, pterygomandibular, and parotid spaces.

the oropharynx will be increased. CT scans should also be obtained for management of serious infections.

A potential space exists between the vertebral column and the posterior visceral fascia. This potential space follows the spinal column into the mediastinum and is known as space 4, or the danger space. The management of odontogenic infections involving these fascial spaces will require hospitalization and management by a qualified oral and maxillofacial surgeon in consultation with an infectious disease specialist and an otorhinolaryngologist.

DENTOALVEOLAR STRUCTURES AND THEIR FASCIAL SPACES
Labial Vestibular Space

The labial vestibular space (LVS) is continuous with the buccal gingivae and vestibule of the maxilla and mandible. Involved teeth will usually have their roots in close approximation to the buccal cortex of bone. Mandibular and maxillary central, mandibular lateral incisor, and cuspid teeth of both arches most frequently have an odontogenic infection localized to this space. An abscess that is pointing will usually organize the pus between the involved root apex and the elevators of the upper lip or the depressors of the lower lip. Spread of infection from the LVS in the maxilla can cause deformity at the alar base of the nose, and spread to the

buccal space, canine space, or other contiguous spaces (Figs. 12-7, *A* and *B*). In the mandible the spread of infection may also include the buccal, mental, and sublingual spaces. Infections of the mandibular anterior teeth, with presentation in the LVS, may spread across the midline of the mandible because of a lack of midline soft tissue barriers. The position of the mentalis and depressor labii muscles and the lack of barriers in the midline to restrict spread of infection can result in rapid dissemination of infection to the mental and adjacent spaces.[2,4]

Canine Space

Canine space infections are the most rare of dentoalveolar infections and are usually associated with the maxillary canine tooth. Periapical infection from the canine tooth will spread through buccal cortical bone into the soft tissues. Most often we see it as an LVS swelling adjacent to the maxilla. If the apex of the root of the canine tooth is above the origin of the levator labii superioris muscle, flocculence lateral to the alar base may be present. This abscess may be best approached from an intraoral route with a sharp incision, blunt dissection, and placement of a drain. On rare occasions when the clinical presentation is on the skin, an extraoral incision may be necessary. Incisions made parallel and close to the

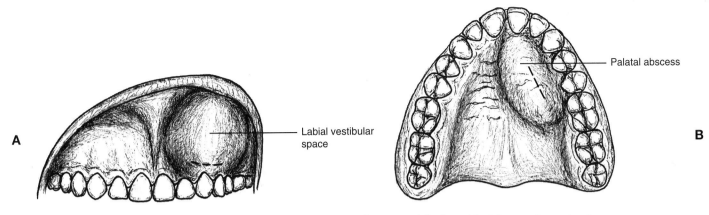

FIG. 12-7   A, Maxillary labial vestibular space abscesses. A horizontal incision can be made at the mucogingival junction. Blunt dissection is used to enter and explore all pockets within the abscess pocket to obtain drainage. **B,** A palatal abscess is usually related to infection within a lateral incisor tooth or the palatal root of a molar or bicuspid tooth. Incisions for drainage should be made only through mucosa, parallel to the course of any blood vessels in the area, then blunt dissection to obtain drainage.

nasolabial skin crease will heal with minimum cosmetic deformity.

Cavernous sinus thrombosis may be a sequela of a canine space abscess. Infections of the canine space may spread through the anterior facial vein to the superior ophthalmic vein, and rarely the inferior ophthalmic vein, into the orbit. These veins have no valves, allowing retrograde flow through the orbit where the thrombophlebitis is finally transmitted to the cavernous sinus through the superior orbital fissure.[2] (Infections may also spread to the cavernous sinus via the pterygoid plexus of veins (Fig. 12-8). Clinical signs of cavernous sinus thrombosis are: proptosis, fever, altered level of consciousness, ophthalmoplegia, paresis of the oculomotor, trochlear, abducens nerves, and bilateral periorbital edema. This is a life-threatening event requiring immediate neurosurgical consultation.[1,4]

When dentoalveolar abscess is present in the posterior maxilla the dentist must be careful not to track infectious material from the area of abscess formation into the deeper temporal spaces, through the injection of local anesthetic solutions by an infiltration technique. A second division block of the trigeminal nerve through the greater palatine foramen should be used to provide local anesthesia in these cases.

Buccal Space

Infections in the buccal space are usually the results of periapical pathology in the bicuspid and molar teeth. The presentation of a buccal space abscess can usually be determined by the position of the root apices to the origins of the buccinator muscle along the alveolus in the mandible or the maxilla. In the mandible, if the apex of the tooth is above the origin of the buccinator muscle, the infection will spread to the labial vestibular space. Infections that spread below the origin of these muscles will ultimately find their way into the buccal space. In the maxilla, if the roots of the infected tooth are below the origin of the buccinator muscle, pointing of the abscess will be in the labial vestibular space. Root apices that are above the attachment of the buccinator muscle will make their clinical presentation in the buccal space (Fig. 12-9).

It is suggested that a buccal space abscess is best managed through cutaneous incision and drainage, yet intraoral approaches should be considered to avoid scarring. Profound local anesthesia or a general anesthetic is required.

When an abscess is to be drained from a cutaneous approach it must be examined with bimanual palpation to locate the point of maximal flocculence. The incision is placed in healthy tissues where dependent drainage can be obtained. One should avoid making an incision in the center of flocculence, where the abscess is pointing. The skin is thinnest in this area, with a diminished blood supply. Incisions placed in this area will be compromised by poor wound healing and excessive scar formation. The incision is made through skin into the subcutaneous tissue, then blunt dissection with a small hemostat is continued into the center of flocculence. Once inside the abscess, the hemostat is opened, and withdrawn through the incision while open to break up any compartments within the abscess pocket. Local anatomy must be respected as the mental nerve, facial nerve, parotid duct, and other significant structures occupy the buccal space.[2]

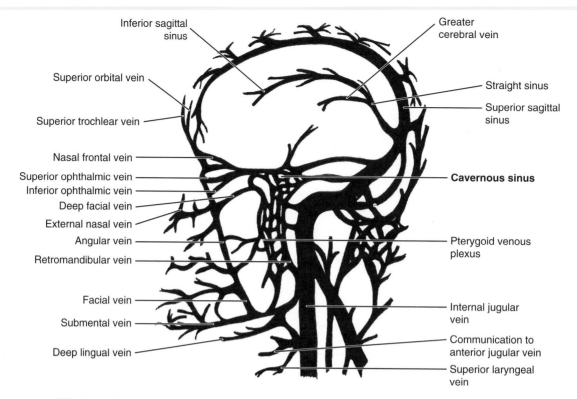

FIG. 12-8 Venous drainage of the head and neck. The facial vein connects to the cavernous sinus through the ophthalmic vein, pterygoid plexus of veins, and the pharyngeal plexus of veins. Infection can spread rapidly through this valveless, venous system.

FIG. 12-9 Path of spread of infection into the buccal space. An abscess will point (red and shiny area) and attempt to spontaneously drain. Incisions for drainage should be made in healthy skin.

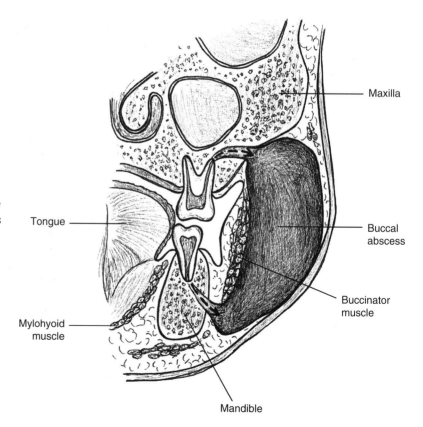

Masticator Space

The masticator space is defined by the muscles that insert onto the mandible and are responsible for its movement: the masseter, medial and lateral pterygoid, and temporalis muscles. The masticator space communicates with the buccal space anteriorly, the submandibular and lingual spaces medially, the lateral pharyngeal space posteriorly, and the temporal space superiorly (see Fig. 12-6). The masticator space is divided into the masseteric and pterygoid compartments.

The masseteric compartment is formed by the lateral surface of the ramus of the mandible and the medial aspect of the masseter muscle. Infections within the masseteric compartment may not exhibit significant swelling because of the integrity of the masseter muscle.

The pterygoid compartment is a well-defined space between the medial surface of the mandibular ramus and the lateral surface of the medial pterygoid muscle. Infections within this compartment will usually present symptoms of trismus. Swelling or drainage may be noted below the base of the tongue in the region of the mandibular third molar.[1]

Masticator space infections are usually the result of pericoronitis or infected third molar teeth. These infections are frequently associated with trismus, which will often present the greatest obstacle to the surgical management of these infections. Local anesthesia techniques will challenge the dental surgeon when confronted by a patient with severe trismus. The Akinosi injection technique may be helpful in these patients with trismus. (See Chapter 3, "Techniques of Local Anesthesia," for details of the technique.) Intraoral drainage of this abscess may be obtained through incisions made lateral to the pterygomandibular raphe, followed by blunt dissection into the center of flocculence. An extraoral incision, made below the angle of the mandible, in a skin crease, can be used to approach both compartments of the masticator space for drainage. It is important to remember that the surgeon should first approach the bony structure of the mandible before exploring various compartments. By this method one is aware of starting from a known position and can use this as a guide to complete the drainage of various spaces (Fig. 12-10 and see Fig. 12-6).

Temporal and Parotid Spaces

Temporal space infections are usually the result of direct spread of infection from a tooth, but have often been found as an extension of a needle tract infection. Temporalis fascia descends from the temporal crest to join the zygomatic arch, as temporalis muscle fibers pass deep to the arch to insert on the coronoid process of the mandible. The temporalis muscle divides the temporal space into a deep and superficial compartment.[3] An abscess within the deep temporal space can be approached from an intraoral incision which we have found to be fairly difficult. To accomplish this, the incision is made high in the posterior maxillary vestibule, adjacent to the second molar tooth. Dissection is carried in a superior direction, medial to the coronoid and up to the temporal bone. Placement and securing of a drain in this area is accomplished with some difficulty. We do not advocate this approach, as the cutaneous approach is predictable and the incision is in a cosmetic area. For extraoral drain placement, the incision is made superior and parallel to the zygomatic arch and kept within the hairline. The incision is

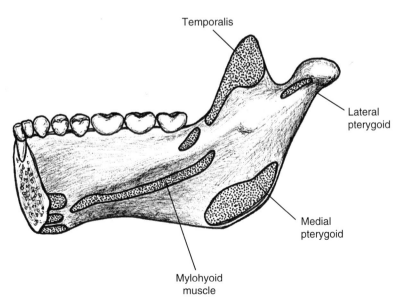

FIG. 12-10 Lingual view of the mandible showing position of muscle attachment. Infection from adjacent teeth will spread into the submandibular space if the root apex and the path of spread of the infection is below the mylohyoid muscle.

through skin into adjacent subcutaneous tissue. Blunt dissection with a hemostat is used to enter the appropriate compartment, and a drain is placed.

Parotid Space

The parotid space is formed by the anterior layer of deep cervical fascia (see Fig. 12-6). This layer splits to encompass the parotid gland and is continuous with the temporalis fascia. Infections in this area are usually not of dental origin. Abscess formation in this area is best managed through skin incisions. The incision is placed in a skin crease at the angle of the mandible. Blunt dissection with a curved hemostat is used to identify the bony angle of the mandible, and then to enter the abscess. Parotid abscess not localized to the tail of the parotid gland is beyond the scope of this atlas and these patients should be referred to an oral and maxillofacial surgeon experienced in managing this type of infection.

Submandibular, Lingual, and Mental Spaces

The submandibular and sublingual spaces are two contiguous spaces that communicate with each other at the proximal border of the mylohyoid muscle. The submaxillary space is a synonym for the sublingual and submandibular spaces. Each space has distinct anatomic borders. The sublingual space is bounded by the floor of the mouth above, and the mylohyoid muscle below. It contains the sublingual gland, the submandibular duct, the lingual nerve, and sublingual artery. The body of the mandible is lateral, with the muscles of the tongue defining the medial limits. The submandibular space consists of a roof formed by the mylohyoid muscle, with its floor composed by the skin and subcutaneous tissues. The submandibular space contains the submandibular gland, facial artery, and vein. The sublingual space lacks a well-defined midline barrier to the spread of infection from one space to the contralateral space. This fact becomes clinically evident when a dentoalveolar infection spreads rapidly through the submaxillary spaces.[1,2,3]

The mental space separates the left submandibular space from the right. The mental space is formed by the left and right anterior bellies of the digastric muscles, and their attachment to the hyoid bone and the symphysis. The mylohyoid muscle forms the roof of this space, the skin the floor of the space, and the digastric muscles the lateral walls. The anterior jugular veins are found in this space.

The position of root apices in relationship to the mylohyoid muscle will determine the clinical presentation of a dentoalveolar infection in the submaxillary

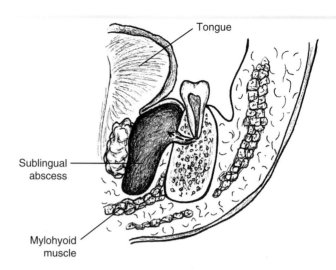

FIG. 12-11 Spread of infection into the sublingual space. There are no barriers to the spread of infection to the contralateral space or to the proximal submandibular and pterygomandibular spaces.

space. Often the roots of the lower bicuspid teeth and the first molar tooth will have their root apices above the mylohyoid muscle. Infections from these teeth may present as a flocculent swelling in the floor of the mouth. Submandibular space infections are usually related to second and third molar teeth, which have their root apices below the insertion of the mylohyoid muscle into the mylohyoid ridge, located on the lingual aspect of the body of the mandible[2] (Fig. 12-11 and see Fig. 12-10).

Anteriorly, the sublingual space and the mental space communicate along the lingual periosteum and the insertion of the genioglossus and geniohyoid muscles. Infected mandibular anterior teeth may cause a flocculent swelling in the anterior floor of the mouth between the plica of the sublingual gland and the alveolus. This abscess formation may cause elevation of the tongue, swelling in the mental area, and may occupy both sides of the midline (Fig. 12-12). The submandibular space communicates with the lateral pharyngeal space at the proximal edge of the mylohyoid muscle. It is at this junction that the masticator, parotid, submaxillary, and lateral pharyngeal spaces are contiguous.

Ludwig's Angina

Ludwig's angina is a firm, indurated, acute, fulminating cellulitis of bilateral submandibular and sublingual spaces, and the mental space. Before the advent of antibiotic therapy this toxic infection caused great fear among surgeons because it could rapidly kill through airway obstruction or overwhelming sepsis. Ludwig's

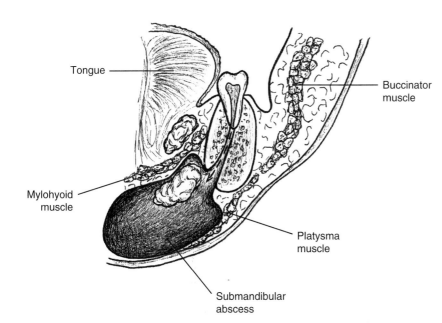

Tongue

Buccinator
muscle

Mylohyoid
muscle

Platysma
muscle

Submandibular
abscess

FIG. 12-12 Submandibular space abscesses usually require extraoral incisions for drainage. Infections can spread to the contralateral submandibular space, mental space, and sublingual spaces. Dependent drainage is always advisable.

angina was first observed and described by the physician Wilhelm Friedrich von Ludwig in 1836. He described the manifestation of "angina," a symptom of airway obstruction or choking that was observed in patients with a brawny hard swelling of the deep spaces of the neck, cellulitis spreading through all of the spaces of the floor of the mouth. Patients often presented with other symptoms that included: trismus, odontalgia, dysphagia, fever, dysphonia, and elevation of the tongue.[1] The sublingual swelling causes the tongue to become elevated, occupying the full volume of the oral cavity, and to be pushed backward to put pressure on the epiglottis, causing airway obstruction. The authors have observed in the clinical setting that the patient would find that a recumbent position would increase any breathing distress. When observed in the emergency room these patients are usually sitting up, using all of the accessory muscles of the neck and chest to help in air exchange.

Ludwig's angina is still a life-threatening emergency that requires hospitalization, high dose antibiotic therapy covering gram negative anaerobic rods and gram positive facultative cocci, supportive care, and early incision and drainage. Early incision and drainage is indicated as this rapidly spreading cellulitis may not have organized any pockets of pus. Incisions will assist in reducing high tissue tension pressure and establishing pathways for drainage of purulent material.

Incisions are usually generous and made in a skin crease, below both angles of the mandible. It is important when performing the blunt dissection that the inferior border of the mandible be touched by the curved hemostat. This will provide you with orientation to further dissection, and is a starting point for deeper dissections. Through and through drains may be placed. All involved spaces must be explored. A third incision is made in the mental region, with exploration into the floor of the mouth and sublingual spaces. Maintaining a patent airway is a challenge to the doctor. Intubation, cricothyroidotomy, tracheostomy, or other adjuncts to maintaining an open airway may be required early in the management of this patient (Fig. 12-13).

TECHNIQUES FOR INCISION AND DRAIN

The spread of infection and the development of an abscess is the result of factors pertaining to host resistance and microbial influences. Host resistance is described by local defenses, cellular, and humoral immunity. Microbial factors are determined by virulence and number of invading organisms. The pathogenic potential changes as the aforementioned factors change. When the microbial factors dominate and the host's resistance cannot contain the invading microorganisms, the spread of infection will prevail.[1] The inflammatory reaction is then initiated and phagocytic cells and lymphocytes are called into action. Polymorphonuclear leukocytes eliminate bacteria through phagocytosis. Inflammatory mediators such as histamine, serotonin, leukotrienes, prostaglandins, and lysosomal components are released. Mononuclear phagocytes, monocytes, and macrophages will next become involved in the inflammatory process and are involved in removing

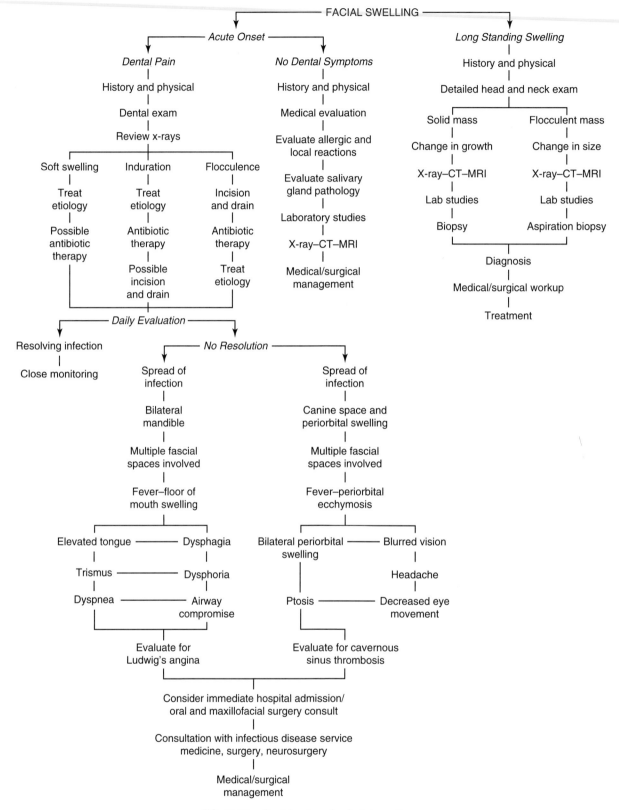

FIG. 12-13 Decision tree for facial swelling.

resistant microorganisms and dead cellular debris. When pus accumulates and swelling ensues as the result of a dental infection, surgical drainage is indicated. Intra- and extraoral techniques for the draining of maxillofacial abscesses should be a part of the armamentarium of the modern dentist.

Guidelines for Successful Incision and Drainage

1. Use block injection techniques to obtain profound anesthesia.
2. Incisions are made in healthy tissue and not in the center of the height of flocculence.
3. Stab incisions to bone or in soft tissues are never indicated.
4. Make all incisions through skin or mucosa into connective tissue, then use a blunt hemostat to open and explore any compartments within the abscess pocket.
5. Obtain dependent drainage whenever possible.
6. The same drain must not remain in place for more than 72 hours.
7. Suture drains in place.
8. Leave a drain in place only as long as it is productive.
9. Irrigate the drain daily with normal saline or an antibiotic solution.
10. Patients with a drain in place should be examined daily.
11. Most infections will not drain through an extraction site or a root canal preparation.
12. When performing extraoral incisions the inferior border of the mandible must be palpated with the curved hemostat as a starting point for orientation to then begin to explore additional spaces.
13. All loculations of the abscess must be explored.
14. When the source of the infection has been removed, drainage obtained, and antibiotic therapy instituted, the infection should begin to resolve within 3 to 4 days. After this time period reevaluation of your therapy must be considered.

Instrument Tray Setup for Incision and Drainage

1. Aspirating syringe for local anesthesia
2. #15 blade and blade holder
3. Curved and/or straight mosquito hemostat
4. Gauze director
5. Needle holder, suture material, and scissors
6. One-quarter inch Penrose drain
7. Culture bottle and/or a syringe to aspirate pus to send for culture
8. Gauze dressing, bandage, tape, etc.
9. Skin scrub preparation, alcohol sponge, disinfectant

REFERENCES

1. Topazian RG, Goldberg MH: *Oral and maxillofacial infections,* ed 3, Philadelphia, 1993, WB Saunders.
2. Sicher H: *Oral anatomy,* ed 6, St. Louis, 1975, Mosby.
3. Hollinsfead WH: *Anatomy for surgeons, 1: The head and neck,* ed 2, Hagerstown, MD, 1968, Harper & Row.
4. Piecuch JF, Joseph, F and Flynn TR: Infection section, *Oral and maxillofacial surgery knowledge update (1),* Chicago, 1994, AAOMS.

13 Antibiotics and Their Use in Oral and Maxillofacial Infections

FRANCIS D. CHIONCHIO, DDS

One of the most difficult problems to manage in dentistry is an odontogenic infection. These infections may range from low-grade, well-localized infections that require only minimal treatment to a severe, life-threatening fascial space infection. The basic principles of infection management are: 1) incision and drainage, 2) appropriate usage of antibiotics, 3) optimizing medical conditions, and 4) supportive treatment.

The primary purpose of this chapter is to review:
1. Principles of antibiotics
2. Common pathogenic organisms of soft and hard tissues of the oral region
3. Selection of antimicrobial drugs
4. Prophylactic antibiotics for the practicing clinician

Some of the things to be considered when antibiotics are given are efficacy, toxicity, cost, dosage, route of administration, duration of antibiotic treatment, and the use of combination therapy. When discussing efficacy of the drug it is important to understand absorption, distribution and excretion characteristics of the selected antibiotic. If the drug can reach the site of the infection and be active against the pathogenic organisms, it has good efficacy.

Toxicity relates to immediate allergic reactions, idiosyncratic reactions, and dose-dependent end organ damage. The antibiotics should maintain broad effect of antimicrobial action with minimal risk to the patient.

Cost involves price of the agent, frequency of the doses, and duration of treatment.

Dosages should maintain serum levels within wide or narrow margins between therapeutic and toxic levels. Usually those drugs with narrow margins of safety are calculated on the basis of the patient's weight. Route of administration is dependent on the patient's condition and severity of the infection. Oral therapy is more indicated for low to moderate-grade infections whereas parenteral therapy should be considered in compromised patients or in more serious infections as blood serum levels and tissue levels are more rapidly achieved.

Duration of treatment is dependent on type and severity of infection, organism sensitivity, and patient's clinical improvement and typically is continued for 5 to 14 days.

Combination therapy is usually indicated for more severe life-threatening infections to achieve appropriate antibiotic therapy. The advantage of multiple antibiotic therapy results from the synergistic nature among antibiotics. The drawbacks are increased side effects, development of superinfections, and alteration of normal flora. Combinations of antibiotics are indicated in infections caused by *Pseudomonas*, enterococcal group D streptococci, resistant pathogens, and life-threatening infections.

In the initial therapy of life-threatening infections in which a bacterial cause is suspected, the emphasis should be on extended-spectrum antibiotic coverage. Definitive antibiotic coverage should be initiated after organisms are isolated, identified, and when indicated in vitro susceptibility tests are obtained.

MICROBIOLOGY OF ODONTOGENIC INFECTIONS

The bacteria that cause infection are typically those that live on or in the host, and oral infections are no exception, because the bacteria that cause odontogenic infections are normal oral flora: those that comprise the bacteria of plaque, those found on mucosal surfaces, and in the gingival sulcus. These usually involve anaerobic and aerobic gram-positive cocci, and anaerobic gram-negative rods. These bacteria cause a variety of common diseases such as gingivitis, periodontitis, dental caries, and when introduced into deeper tissues via necrotic pulp or deep periodontal pockets, can lead to odontogenic abscess or infection.

Almost all of these odontogenic infections are caused by multiple bacteria, and in most cases, the lab will identify an average of five species of bacteria. The polymicrobial nature of these infections makes it important for the clinician to understand the variety of bacteria likely to cause the infection. Another factor is the aerobic–anaerobic characteristic of the bacteria causing odontogenic infections. Infections caused only by aerobes comprise only 5%, those caused only by anaerobic bacteria comprise 35%, and those of mixed anaerobic and aerobic origin are approximately 60% of all oral maxillofacial infections[1,2,3,4,5] (Table 13-1).

Of the aerobic bacteria, the most common causative organisms are streptococci comprising 70%, staphylococci accounting for 6%, and a large population of miscellaneous bacteria contributing 1% (Table 13-2). Rarely found bacteria include Group D streptococci, *Neisseria* species, *Corynebacterium*, and *Haemophilus* species. The anaerobic bacteria that cause infections include two major groups, anaerobic gram-positive cocci such as *Streptococcus, Peptostreptococcus,* and *Peptococcus* accounting for 11% of infections and gram-positive rods comprising 15% of the anaerobic bacteria. The gram-negative anaerobic rods are cultured in about 2% of the infections. The *Bacteroides* species account for 34% and *Fusobacterium* for 13% (Table 13-2) of these gram-negative organisms.

The method by which mixed aerobic and anaerobic bacteria cause infections begins with initial inoculation into the deeper tissues by more invasive organisms with higher virulence (aerobic *Streptococcus* species). This begins the infection process, initiating a cellulitis-type infection. The anaerobic bacteria will then also multiply, becoming more prominent as the local reduction-oxidation potential becomes lower. As the infection reaches a more chronic, abscess stage the anaerobic bacteria begin to predominate and eventually become the exclusive causative organism. As a result, early infections appearing initially as cellulitis are characterized as streptococcal infections, and late, chronic abscess may be characterized as anaerobic infections.

ODONTOGENIC INFECTIONS

These infections have two major origins: periapical, as a result of pulpal necrosis and subsequent bacterial invasion into periapical tissue and periodontal, as a result of deep periodontal pocketing allowing inoculation of bacteria into underlying soft tissues. The periapical source is the most common cause in odontogenic infections. Once the tissue is inoculated with the bacteria an active infection is established. The infection will spread equally in all directions following the least resistant path. The infection spreads through cancellous bone until it encounters the cortical plate. If the cortical plate is thin, the infection will erode through into soft tissue. When the infection does erode through the cortical plate of the alveolar process, it appears in predictable anatomic locations. The location of the infection from a specific tooth relies on two major

TABLE 13-1 Bacteria Responsible for Odontogenic Infections

Aerobic Bacteria	Frequency	Anaerobic	Frequency
GRAM-POSITIVE COCCI			
Streptococcus spp.			
Alpha hemolytic	VC	*Streptococcus* spp.	C
Beta hemolytic	U	*Peptostreptococcus*	C
Group D	R	*Peptococcus* spp.	C
Staphylococcus spp.	R		
GRAM-NEGATIVE COCCI			
Neisseria spp.	R	*Veillonella* spp.	U
GRAM-POSITIVE BACILLI			
Corynebacterium spp.	R	*Eubacterium* spp.	U
		Lactobacillus spp.	U
GRAM-NEGATIVE BACILLI			
Haemophilus influenzae	R	*Bacteroides*	
Eikenella corrodens	R	oralis	VC
		melaninogenicus	VC
		gingivalis	VC
		fragilis	R

VC, Very common; *C,* common; *U,* uncommon; *R,* rare.

TABLE 13-2 Microorganism Causing Odontogenic Infections

Organism	Average Percentage Per Study
AEROBIC	
Gram-positive cocci	78
Streptococcus spp.	70
Streptococcus (group D) spp.	1
Staphylococcus spp.	6
Eikenella spp.	1
Gram-negative cocci *(Neisseria)*	1
Gram-positive cocci (*Corynebacterium* spp.)	1
Gram-negative rods (*Haemophilus* spp.)	1
Miscellaneous and undifferentiated	19
ANAEROBIC	
Gram-positive cocci	34
Streptococcus spp.	11
Peptococcus spp.	11
Peptostreptococcus spp.	12
Gram-negative cocci (*Veillonella* spp.)	4
Gram-positive rods	15
Eubacterium spp.	7
Lactobacillus spp.	6
Actinomyces spp.	1
Clostridium spp.	1
Gram-negative rods	47
Bacteroides spp.	34
Fusobacterium spp.	13

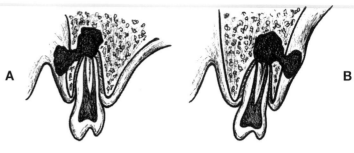

FIG. 13-1 When infection erodes through bone, it will enter soft tissue through thinnest bone. **A,** Tooth apex is near thin labial bone, so infection erodes labially. **B,** Apex is near palatal aspect, so bone will be perforated.

factors: thickness of bone overlying the apex of the tooth and the relationship of the site of perforation of bone to the muscle attachments of the maxilla and mandible.[6]

Fig. 13-1 illustrates how infections perforate through bone into overlying soft tissue. In Fig. 13-1 *A,* the labial bone overlying the apex of the tooth is very thin compared with the palatal bone. Therefore, as the infection spreads, it will go into the labial soft tissues. In Fig. 13-1 *B,* the labial bone is much thicker with a thinner palatal bone. In this situation, as the infection spreads through the bone into the soft tissue, the infection manifests as a palatal abscess. As the infection has eroded through the bone and exited below the attachment of the buccinator muscle the result is a vestibular abscess. On occasion a long maxillary canine tooth will erode through bone superior to insertion of the levator anguli oris muscle and will cause a canine space infection. Most maxillary teeth erode through the labial cortical plate and cause vestibular abscesses. Maxillary posterior teeth infections generally erode through superior to the insertion of the buccinator muscle resulting in a buccal space infection. In the mandible, incisors, canines, and premolars usually erode through the labial plate and above the associated musculature, resulting in vestibular abscesses. Some exceptions are noted in Table 13-3. Most posterior infections perforate buccally or lingually; and most third molar infections perforate lingually. The mylohyoid muscle determines the level of infection and whether the sublingual or submandibular space is involved.

Sometimes the abscess establishes a chronic sinus tract that drains into the oral cavity. As long as the sinus tract continues to drain, the patient will experience no pain. Antibiotics usually cause cessation of drainage, but when antibiotics are stopped, the drainage recurs. Definitive treatment by root canal therapy or extraction is necessary.

TREATMENT OF ODONTOGENIC INFECTIONS

Chemotherapeutic agents for odontogenic infections should be an adjunct to adequate surgical drainage and removal of causative factors. Antibiotic protocol for "non–life-threatening" and "life-threatening" odontogenic infections were developed by Finn and Karas assuming effective surgery.[2] They advocate use of penicillin G or penicillin V in non–life-threatening infections, the alternative being erythromycin or clindamycin for allergic patients. Amoxicillin with clavulanic acid may be used for aerobic infections when penicillin V has failed or sinus infection is present. Second generation cephalosporins, such as cefaclor, are also effective for non–life-threatening anaerobic infections. For infections with evidence of anaerobes addition of clindamycin or metronidazole is indicated (Table 13-4).

Protocol for life-threatening infections indicates triple antibiotic therapy involving the use of penicillin, clindamycin or metronidazole, and gentamicin for situations when the patient's condition does not improve. Addition of gentamicin reduces minimum inhibitory

TABLE 13-3 The Spread of Infection from the Teeth

Involved Teeth	Usual Site of Perforation of Bone	Relation of Perforation to Muscle Attachment	Determining Muscle	Site of Localization
MAXILLA				
Central incisor	Labial	Below	Orbicularis oris	Labial vestibule
Lateral incisor	Labial	Below	Orbicularis oris	Labial vestibule
	(Palatal)	—	—	(Palatal)
Canine	Labial	Below	Levator anguli oris	Oral vestibule
	Labial	(Above)	Levator anguli oris	(Canine space)
Premolars	Buccal	Below	Buccinator	Buccal vestibule
Molars	Buccal	Below	Buccinator	Buccal vestibule
	Buccal	Above	Buccinator	Buccal space
	(Palatal)	—	—	(Palatal)
MANDIBLE				
Incisors	Labial	Above	Mentalis	Labial vestibule
Canine	Labial	Above	Depressor angulioris	Labial vestibule
Premolars	Buccal	Above	Buccinator	Buccal vestibule
First molar	Buccal	Above	Buccinator	Buccal vestibule
	Buccal	Below	Buccinator	Buccal space
	Lingual	Above	Mylohyoid	Sublingual
Second molar	Buccal	Above	Buccinator	Buccal vestibule
	Lingual	Below	Buccinator	Buccal space
	Lingual	Above	Mylohyoid	Sublingual space
	Lingual	Below	Mylohyoid	Submandibular space
Third molar	Lingual	Below	Mylohyoid	Submandibular space

concentration of penicillin V, clindamycin, and metronidazole against *Bacteroides*.[6] Another alternative to triple antibiotics is the use of a single broad spectrum agent such as Timentin (ticarcillin/clavulanic acid) or Unasyn (ampicillin/sulbactam); note that these drugs are only used parenterally.

Peri-implantitis

The long-term stability of osseous integrated implants can be compromised with the progressive loss of peri-implant bone.[8] Pathologic changes of peri-implant tissues are referred to as peri-implant mucositis for the associated soft tissue whereas the term peri-implantitis is used for bone loss associated with inflammatory changes of the surrounding soft tissue.[8] Occlusal forces from functioning and parafunctional loading can combine with inflammatory and infectious factors to compromise the implant and lead to failed osseous integration. Oral hygiene measures and debridement with plastic instruments are the first line of treatment. Failing implants with pocket depths of 6 mm or more were found to have moderate levels of *Actinobacillus, Actinomycetem comitans, Prevotella intermedius,* and *Porphyromo-*

nas gingivalis by DNA probe analysis.[9] Another report of 19 failing implants found *Fusobacterium nucleatum, Porphyromonas gingivalis,* and *Prevotella intermedin* as the prevalent bacteria involved in the infection.[5]

In cases of peri-implantitis, local microbial factors are controlled with topical chlorhexidine .12% along with one of the following medications: amoxicillin/clavulanate, clindamycin, minocycline, or doxycycline.[10] Amoxicillin with metronidazole is also useful for the treatment of periimplantitis, with selection based on susceptibility results.

Osteomyelitis

Osteomyelitis of the jaws occurs primarily in elderly, malnourished, immunosuppressed, noncompliant patients, in patients with congenital or acquired disruption of microvascular perfusion of the bone, or in patients with lack of access to health care.[11] Contemporary studies indicate that anaerobic bacteria and *Streptococcus viridans* are the major etiologic agents involved in jaw osteomyelitis as opposed to earlier *Staphylococcus aureus* bacterium.[12] Anaerobic species recovered from positive cultures include *Bacteroides, Fusobacterium, Acti-*

TABLE 13-4 Antibiotic Administration Regimens for Oral Infections

Antibiotic	Route	Mechanism	Dosage and Frequency	Indication
Aminoglycosides		Bactericidal		
Gentamicin	IM or IV		3 mg/kg/day in equal doses q 8 hours	Component of bacterial endocarditis prophylaxis for patients at high risk
Cephalosporins		Bactericidal		
Cefaclor	PO		250-500 mg q 8 hours	Useful when broader spectrum is needed
Cefadroxil	PO		500 mg to 1 g q 12 to 24 hours	
Cephalexin	PO		250-500 mg q 6 hours	
Penicillins		Bactericidal		
Amoxicillin	PO		1 gm initially, then 250-500 mg q 6 hrs	Bacterial endocarditis prophylaxis
Cloxacillin	PO		250-500 mg q 6 hours	Staphylococcus infection
Dicloxacillin	PO		125-250 mg q 6 hours	Drug of choice for serious infections
Penicillin G	IM or IV		600,000-1,200,000 units q 12-24 hours	Drug of choice for most infections
Penicillin V	PO		500 mg initially, then 250-500 mg q 6 hours	
Macrolides		Bacteriostatic		
Erythromycin Stearate Ethylsuccinate	PO		250-500 mg q 6 hours	Useful for mild infection and bacterial endocarditis prophylaxis if patient is penicillin allergic
Azithromycin	PO		10 mg/kg up to 500 mg initially followed by 5 mg/kg up to 250 mg qd to complete 5 days.	
Clarithromycin	PO		250-500 mg PO bid. Peds: 7.5 mg/kg PO bid	
Tetracycline		Bacteriostatic		
Doxycycline	PO		Initially 100 mg q 24 hours or 50 mg q 12 hours	Mild infections when need broad spectrum, periodontal disease
Oxytetracycline	IM		250 mg q 24 hours	
Tetracycline	PO		500 mg q 6 hours	
Clindamycin	IV or PO	Bactericidal and bacteriostatic	150 mg q 6 hours	Instead of metronidazole for penicillin allergic patients with serious infections, or endocarditis prophylaxis if cannot use penicillin or erythromycin
Metronidazole	IV or PO	Bactericidal	500 mg q 6 hours	Second line of therapy for odontogenic infections, ANUG, HIV periodontitis
Vancomycin	IV	Bactericidal	1 gm infused over 1 hour before procedure	Component of bacterial endocarditis prophylaxis for patients at high risk

nomyces, Peptococcus, Peptostreptococcus, Veillonella, and *Eubacterium.*[13]

Treatment for osteomyelitis can involve multiple treatment regimens including evaluation and correction of host defenses, imaging studies to rule out bony tumors, removal of involved teeth and sequestrated bony fragments, placement of irrigating drains or antibiotic beads, as well as debridement of the region, resection of the jaws, reconstruction, and use of hyperbaric oxygen.[11]

Empiric therapy for acute osteomyelitis is penicillin G 2 million units intravenously (IV) every 4 hours until the patient is asymptomatic for 72 hours, then penicillin VK 500 mg every 4 hours for 2 to 4 weeks. If the Gram stain initially shows predominance of clusters of cocci suggestive of *Staphylococcus,* a penicillinase-resistant antibiotic is added to the regimen. Two choices are oxacillin 1 g every 4 hours IV until asymptomatic for 72 hours, followed by dicloxacillin 500 mg orally for 2 to 4 weeks. For penicillin-allergic patients, clindamycin may be given 600 mg every 6 hours IV, then oral therapy 300 to 450 mg every 6 hours for 2 weeks. Allergic patients can receive clindamycin or cefazolin IV followed by Keflex (cephalexin) or erythromycin.[12]

Wound Infections

Wound infections following oral surgical procedures are generally a result of invasion of normal host bacteria, with a similar microbiology to that found in odontogenic infections. Usually, there is a higher rate of infection by penicillin-resistant bacteria, so cultures and sensitivities should be taken to determine whether exogenous bacteria are present.[14]

Compound fractures of the maxilla and mandible usually have higher rates of contamination by bacteria within the oral cavity initially. Unstable fractures have higher rates of infection as the bacteria migrate into the fracture line during the motion of the jaw and splaying of the fracture site.

Animal bites from dogs and cats most commonly carry the organisms *Pasteurella multocida* (25%), *Staphylococcus* (10%), α-hemolytic *Streptococcus* (40%), *Bacteroides* (20%), and *Fusobacterium* (20%).[3] Antibiotic coverage is best accomplished through the use of amoxicillin with clavulanic acid 875 mg twice daily or clindamycin 300 mg three times daily when *Pasteurella multocida* and *Staphylococcus aureus* are the suspected organisms.[15]

Human bites result in a higher rate of infection than do animal bites. The common organisms seen here are *Streptococcus viridans, Bacteroides, Peptostreptococcus, Fusobacterium,* and *Eikenella corrodens.*[16] In the acute setting, thorough exploration, irrigation (with peroxide, saline, Dakins solution), and debridement of the human bite

is necessary. The bacterial count of human saliva is 10^7 to 10^8 bacteria per ml and sometimes this high titer of inoculum precludes closure of these wounds. Deep bites of the face should be debrided, irrigated, and dressed until the bacterial level is reduced to a level compatible with successful delayed treatment. Superficial bites of the face can usually be closed primarily with a few sutures provided adequate debridement has been performed.

Infections in the Immunocompromised Patient

Radiation therapy is used for the management of malignant disease. Its primary purpose is to eradicate tumors without adversely affecting the surrounding tissues. However, many tissues in the body are sensitive to the effects of radiation, depending on the stage of the cell cycle.[17] Marx and colleagues reported that cellular damage exists in all irradiated tissues to varying degrees and can lead to cell death. Radiation therapy induces hypovascularity, hypocellularity, and hypoxia. The reduced vascularity limits the concentrations of nutrients and available oxygen reaching the diseased area.[18] The reduced vascularity in the bone and surrounding tissues promotes bacterial, fungal, and/or viral infections. Necrotic tissue also promotes microbial proliferation.

Radiation-induced injury also causes mucocutaneous changes, accelerates dental caries, causes a reduction in salivary function, osteoradionecrosis of the jaws, and acute and chronic osteomyelitis. Candidiasis (*Candida albicans*) is seen commonly in these patients because of the change in quantity and composition of the saliva.[19]

Management of candidiasis includes oral antifungal agents such as topical nystatin ointment (100,000 units per g) applied four times daily to the affected area; nystatin oral suspension (100,000 units per ml), dispense 120 ml, rinse with 5 ml 2 minutes and swallow four times daily; nystatin troches (100,000 units), dispense thirty tabs, use one tab twice daily. For more severe cases systemic antifungal therapy should be applied (such as ketoconazole, fluconazole, and amphotericin B).

HIV-Infected Patients

The human immunodeficiency virus (HIV-1) subjects the patient to a great variety of opportunistic infections. The diagnosis of AIDS (acquired immune deficiency syndrome) must meet the criteria of the CDC (Centers for Disease Control) and includes a large number of opportunistic infections, neoplasms, or both, indicating a deficit in cellular immunity. Development of one of these conditions, with a positive HIV finding, constitutes the diagnosis of AIDS.[20]

The human immunodeficiency virus attacks the CD4 + helper T lymphocytes, gradually depleting these cells and reducing the absolute lymphocyte count. Antigen-presenting cells (such as macrophages and Langerhans cells) for T-lymphocytes are also affected by HIV.[21] HIV is of the lentivirus subfamily and considered a retrovirus. This virus codes for the enzyme reverse transcriptase, allowing transcription of viral RNA into proviral DNA with subsequent integration into the host's cellular genome (Box 13-1) resulting in opportunistic infections associated with acquired immunodeficiency syndrome.

Currently no curative treatment modalities are available, but a great deal of research is being conducted for an effective vaccine. Infection control procedures are recommended to protect healthcare workers and other patients. Drugs approved by the FDA for treatment of HIV include the antiviral drugs zidovudine (AZT) and didanosine (DDI). These two drugs interfere with viral replication. Zidovudine prolongs survival of the host, decreases the frequency of opportunistic infections, and decreases AIDS-associated morbidity and mortality.

Zidovudine is given orally in a dosage of 100 mg five times per day, or 200 mg every 8 hours. Common side effects of this drug include nausea and vomiting, headache (usually resolving in a few weeks), and bone marrow toxicity (anemia, neutropenia). Didanosine (Videx or DDI) is a purine nucleoside active against HIV-1, and HIV-2 in vitro, including zidovudine-resistant isolates. DDI is 10 to 100-fold less potent than AZT with regard to both antiviral activity and cytotoxicity in activated peripheral blood mononuclear cells (PBMC) but appears more active in quiescent cells and human monocyte/macrophages.[22,23] In vitro DDI is much less toxic for hematopoietic precursor cells or lymphocytes than AZT.[24] Combinations of DDI and AZT synergistically inhibit HIV-1 replication including zidovudine-resistant strains.[25,26]

Didanosine is taken up intracellularly and metabolized by other cellular enzymes to its active derivative DDATP. DDATP functions as a competitive inhibitor of viral reverse transcriptase with respect to dATP and as a chain terminator of viral DNA synthesis.[22,27]

Toxicity related to DDI includes both painful peripheral neuropathy and pancreatitis, which are dose limiting.[28,29,30,31,32] Both usually develop in the first 3 to 6 months of dosing but may occur later. Neuropathy usually involves the lower extremities beginning acutely with paresthesia, numbness, and/or pain, which usually resolves with cessation of therapy. The risk of pancreatitis, which can be fatal, is increased by a history of prior pancreatitis (up to sixfold), exposure to intravenous pentamidine, and higher doses greater than 750 mg per day.[33] At recommended doses, pancreatitis occurs in 7% of patients. Glucose intolerance has been associated

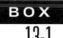

BOX 13-1 The Opportunistic Infections Associated with AIDS

BACTERIAL INFECTIONS
- *Mycobacterium avium-intracellulare, Mycobacterium kansasii* (disseminated)
- *Mycobacterium tuberculosis* (extrapulmonary)
- *Salmonella, Enterobacter cloacae, Klebsiella pneumoniae*

FUNGAL INFECTIONS
- *Candida albicans*
- *Cryptococcus* (disseminated)
- *Histoplasma* (disseminated)
- *Coccidioides* (disseminated)

VIRAL INFECTIONS
- Herpes simplex (HSV) (chronic >1 month)
- Cytomegalovirus (CMV) any organ except liver, spleen, lymph node
- Epstein-Barr (EBV) associated with oral hairy leukoplakia

PROTOZOAN INFECTIONS
- *Pneumocystis carinii* pneumonia
- Toxoplasma (disseminated)
- Chronic *Cryptosporidium enteritis* (>1 month)

with didanosine and may precede the onset of pancreatitis. Other side effects include skin rash, headache, seizures, and optic neuritis.[34]

The majority of treatment is aimed at the management of specific clinical manifestations of immunodeficiency, including opportunistic infections (bacterial, fungal, viral. and protozoan). Recurrent perioral herpes simplex virus (HSV) infection usually responds to oral acyclovir. Acyclovir-resistant HSV strains may require intravenous foscarnet. *Candida albicans* infections respond to clotrimazole troches, ketoconazole, and/or fluconazole (Diflucan). Disseminated fungal infections may require intravenous amphotericin B. Patients infected with *Pneumocystis carinii* are treated with trimethoprim-sulfamethoxazole and pentamidine.

Bacterial Endocarditis

Endocarditis is a life-threatening disease, although it is relatively uncommon. Substantial morbidity and mortality can result from this infection, despite improvement in outcome as a result of the advances in antimicrobial therapy and enhanced ability to diagnose and treat complications. Primary prevention of endocarditis, whenever possible, is therefore very important.

Bacterial endocarditis usually develops in individuals with underlying structural cardiac defects who develop bacteremia with organisms likely to cause endocarditis.

Bacteremia may occur spontaneously or may complicate a focal infection (such as a urinary tract infection, pneumonia, or cellulitis). Some surgical and dental procedures and instrumentations involving mucosal surfaces or contaminated tissue cause transient bacteremia that rarely persists for more than 15 minutes. Blood-borne bacteria may lodge on damaged or abnormal heart valves or on the endocardium or the endothelium near anatomic defects, resulting in bacterial endocarditis or endarteritis. Although bacteremia is common following many invasive procedures, only certain bacteria commonly cause endocarditis. It is not always possible to predict which patients will develop this infection or which particular procedure will be responsible.

There are currently no randomized and carefully controlled human trials in patients with underlying structural heart disease to definitively establish that antibiotic prophylaxis provides protection against development of endocarditis during bacteremia-inducing procedures. Furthermore, most cases of endocarditis are not attributable to an invasive procedure. The incidence of endocarditis following most procedures in patients with underlying cardiac disease is low. A reasonable approach for endocarditis prophylaxis should consider the following: the degree to which the patient's underlying condition creates a risk of endocarditis, the apparent risk of bacteremia with the procedure, the potential adverse reaction of the prophylactic antimicrobial agents to be used, and the cost-benefit aspects of the recommended prophylactic regimen. Failure to consider all these factors will result in excessive cost, risk of adverse drug reaction, and overuse of antimicrobial agents.

Certain cardiac conditions are associated with endocarditis more often than others.[35] When endocarditis develops in individuals with underlying cardiac conditions, the severity of the disease and the ensuing morbidity can be variable. Prophylaxis is recommended in individuals who have a higher risk for developing endocarditis than the general population and for individuals in whom endocardial infection is associated with high morbidity and mortality (Box 13-2). Box 13-2 stratifies cardiac conditions into high- and moderate-risk categories primarily on the basis of potential outcome if endocarditis occurs.

Individuals at highest risk are those who have prosthetic heart valves, a previous history of endocarditis (even in the absence of other heart disease), complex cyanotic congenital heart disease, or surgically constructed systemic pulmonary shunts or conduits.[35,36] These individuals are at greatest risk for developing severe endocardial infection and often are associated with high mortality and morbidity.

Certain patients with other underlying cardiac defects are at moderate risk for severe infection.[37] Congenital

---

BOX 13-2 Cardiac Conditions Associated with Endocarditis

ENDOCARDITIS PROPHYLAXIS RECOMMENDED

High-Risk Category
- Prosthetic cardiac valves, including bioprosthetic and homograft valves
- Previous bacterial endocarditis
- Complex cyanotic congenital heart disease (e.g., single ventricle states, transposition of the great arteries, tetralogy of Fallot)
- Surgically constructed systemic pulmonary shunts or conduits

Moderate-Risk Category
- Most other congenital cardiac malformations (other than above and below)
- Acquired valvar dysfunction (e.g., rheumatic heart disease)
- Hypertonic cardiomyopathy
- Mitral valve prolapse with valvar regurgitation and/or thickened leaflets

ENDOCARDITIS PROPHYLAXIS NOT RECOMMENDED

Negligible-Risk Category (No Greater Risk Than the General Population)
- Isolated secundum atrial septal defect, ventricular septal defect, or patent ductus arteriosus (without residual beyond 6 mo)
- Previous coronary artery bypass graft surgery
- Mitral valve prolapse without valvar regurgitation
- Physiologic, functional, or innocent heart murmurs
- Previous Kawasaki disease without valvar dysfunction
- Previous rheumatic fever without valvar dysfunction
- Cardiac pacemakers (intravascular and epicardial) and implanted defibrillators

---

cardiac conditions noted in the moderate-risk category include the following uncorrected conditions: patent ductus arteriosus, ventricular septal defect, atrial septal defect, coarctation of the aorta, and bicuspid aortic valve. Acquired valvular dysfunction (for example, as a result of rheumatic heart disease or collagen vascular disease) and hypertrophic cardiomyopathy are also moderate-risk conditions. Mitral valve prolapse (MVP) is common and the need for prophylaxis is controversial. Only a small percentage of patients with documented MVP develop complications at any age.[38] Mitral valve prolapse represents a spectrum of valvular changes and clinical behavior. In view of the controversy surrounding the need for prophylaxis of the individual patient with MVP a detailed description of the spectrum of mitral valve prolapse is warranted.

Normal mitral valve leaflets close at or below the plane of the mitral annulus. This closure position is controlled by the lengths of the leaflets, their attached chordae and papillary muscles, and the systolic size of the ventricle. The closure position will shift beyond the annular plane toward the left atrium or prolapse if the lengths of the valve apparatus become too large for the size of the end-systolic ventricle, which is variable and dynamic. Dehydration and tachycardia are common causes of intermittent MVP. Abnormal motion of normal mitral valves are found on echocardiographic exam in a small percentage of the adult and adolescent ambulatory population. The high prevalence of such motion abnormalities in young adults underscores that mitral valve prolapse is often an abnormality of volume status, adrenergic state, or growth phase and not of valve structure or function. When normal valves prolapse without leaking, as in patients with one or more systolic clicks but no murmurs and no Doppler-demonstrated mitral regurgitation, the risk of endocarditis is not increased above that of the normal population.[39] Antibiotic prophylaxis for bacterial endocarditis is therefore not necessary. This is because it is not the abnormal valve motion but the jet of mitral insufficiency that creates the shear forces and flow abnormalities that increase the likelihood of bacterial adherence on the valve during the bacteremia. The regurgitation that occurs with structurally normal but prolapsing valves originates from larger regurgitant orifices and creates broader areas of turbulent flow. Patients with prolapsing and leaking mitral valves, evidenced by audible clicks and murmurs of mitral regurgitation or Doppler-demonstrated mitral insufficiency, should receive prophylactic antibiotics.[40]

Negligible Risk

Although endocarditis may develop in any individual, including persons with no underlying cardiac defect, the negligible-risk category lists cardiac conditions in which the development of endocarditis is not higher than in the general population. Whereas in pediatric patients innocent heart murmurs may be clearly defined on auscultation, in the adult population other studies such as the echocardiogram may be necessary to confirm that a murmur is innocent. Individuals with innocent heart murmurs have structurally normal hearts and do not require prophylaxis.

Bacteremias commonly occur during activities of daily living such as routine toothbrushing. With respect to endocarditis prophylaxis, significant bacteremias are only those caused by organisms commonly associated with endocarditis and attributed to identifiable procedures. Poor dental hygiene and periodontal or periapical infections may produce bacteremia even in the absence of dental procedures. The incidence and magnitude of bacteremias of oral origin are directly proportional to the degree of oral inflammation and infection.[41] Individuals who are at risk for developing bacterial endocarditis should establish and maintain the best possible oral health to reduce potential sources of bacterial seeding. Optimal oral health is maintained through regular professional care.[42] Oral irrigator or air abrasive polishing devices used inappropriately or in patients with poor oral hygiene have been implicated in producing bacteremia, but the relationship to bacterial endocarditis is unknown.[43,44,45] Antiseptic mouth rinses applied immediately before dental procedures may reduce the incidence or magnitude of bacteremia. Agents include chlorhexidine hydrochloride and povidone iodine. All at-risk patients can be given 15 ml of chlorhexidine via gentle oral rinsing for about 30 seconds prior to dental treatment; gingival irrigation is not recommended. Sustained or repeated frequent interval use is not indicated as this may result in selection of resistant microorganisms.[41]

Antibiotic prophylaxis for at-risk patients is recommended for dental and oral procedures likely to cause bacteremia (Box 13-3). In general, prophylaxis is recommended for procedures associated with significant bleeding from hard or soft tissues, periodontal surgery, scaling, and professional prophylaxis. Edentulous patients may develop bacteremia from ulcers caused by ill-fitting dentures. Denture wearers should be encouraged to have periodic examinations or to return to the

BOX 13-3 Dental Procedures and Endocarditis Prophylaxis

ENDOCARDITIS PROPHYLAXIS RECOMMENDED
- Dental extractions
- Periodontal procedures including surgery, scaling and root planing, probing, and recall maintenance
- Dental implant placement and reimplantation of avulsed teeth
- Endodontic (root canal) instrumentation or surgery only beyond the apex
- Subgingival placement of antibiotic fibers or strips
- Initial placement of orthodontic bands but not brackets
- Intraligamentary local anesthetic injections
- Prophylactic cleaning of teeth or implants where bleeding is anticipated

ENDOCARDITIS PROPHYLAXIS NOT RECOMMENDED
- Restorative dentistry (operative and prosthodontic) with or without retraction cord
- Local anesthetic injections (nonintraligamentary)
- Intracanal endodontic treatment; post placement and buildup
- Placement of rubber dams
- Postoperative suture removal
- Placement or removal prosthodontic or orthodontic appliances
- Taking of oral impressions
- Fluoride treatments
- Taking of oral radiographs
- Orthodontic appliance adjustment
- Shedding of primary teeth

practitioner if discomfort develops. When new dentures are inserted, it is advisable to have the patient return to the practitioner to correct any problems that could cause mucosal ulceration.

If a series of dental procedures are required, it may be prudent to observe an interval of time between procedures to both reduce the potential for emergence of resistant organisms and allow repopulation of the mouth with antibiotic-susceptible flora. If possible a combination of procedures should be planned within the same period of prophylaxis.

Prophylaxis Regimens

Prophylaxis is most effective when given preoperatively in doses that are sufficient to assure adequate antibiotic concentrations in the serum during and after the procedure. To reduce the likelihood of microbial resistance, it is important that prophylactic antibiotics be used only during the perioperative period. They should be initi-

ated shortly before a procedure and should not be continued for an extended period (no more than 6 to 8 hours). Practitioners must exercise their own clinical judgment in determining the choice of antibiotics and number of doses that are to be administered in individual cases or special circumstances. Furthermore, because endocarditis may occur in spite of appropriate antibiotic prophylaxis, physicians should maintain a high index of suspicion regarding any unusual clinical events (such as unexplained fever, night chills, weakness, myalgia, arthralgia, lethargy, or malaise) following dental or other surgical procedures in patients who are at risk for developing bacterial endocarditis.

Streptococcus viridans (α-hemolytic streptococci) is the most common cause of endocarditis following dental or oral procedures and procedures involving the respiratory mucosa. Prophylaxis should be specifically directed against these organisms. The same regimens are recommended for all these procedures (Table 13-5). The antibiotics amoxicillin, ampicillin, and penicillin V

TABLE 13-5 High-Risk Category Patients

Situation	Agents	Regimen
Standard general prophylaxis	Amoxicillin	Adults: 2.0 g; children: 50 mg/kg orally 1 h before procedure.
Unable to take oral medications	Ampicillin	Adults: 2.0 g intramuscularly (IM) or intravenously (IV); children: 50 mg/kg IM or IV within 30 min before procedure.
Allergic to penicillin	Clindamycin	Adults: 600 mg; children: 50 mg/kg orally 1 h before procedure.
	Cephalexin or cefadroxil	Adults: 2.0 g; children: 20 mg/kg orally 1 h before procedure.
	Azithromycin or clindamycin	Adults: 500 mg; children: 50 mg/kg orally 1 h before procedure.
Allergic to penicillin and unable to take oral medications	Clindamycin	Adults: 600 mg; children: 10 mg/kg IV within 30 min before procedure.
	Cefazolin	Adults: 1.0 g; children: 25 mg/kg IM or IV within 30 min before procedure.
High-risk patients	Ampicillin plus gentamicin	Adults: amphicillin 2.0 g intramusculary (IM) or intravenously (IV) plus gentalmicin 1.5 mg/kg (not to exceed 120 mg) within 30 min of starting the procedure; 6 h later, ampicillin 1 g IM/IV or amoxicillin 1 g orally. Children: ampicillin 50 mg/kg IM or IV (not to exceed 2.0 g) plus gentamicin 1.5 mg/kg within 30 min of starting the procedure; 6 h later, ampicillin 25 mg/kg IM/IV or amoxicillin 25 mg/kg orally.
High-risk patients allergic to ampicillin/amoxicillin	Vancomycin plus gentamicin	Adults: vancomycin 1.0 g IV over 1-2 h plus gentamicin 1.5 mg/kg IV/IM; (not to exceed 120 mg); complete injection/infusion within 30 min of starting the procedure. Children: vancomycin 20 mg/kg IV over 1-2 h plus gentamicin 1.5 mg/kg IV/IM; complete injection/infusion within 30 min of starting the procedure.
Moderate-risk patients	Amoxicillin or ampicillin	Adults: amoxicillin 2.0 g orally 1 h before procedure, or ampicillin 2.0 g IM/IV within 30 min of starting the procedure. Children: amoxicillin 50 mg/kg orally 1 h before procedure, or ampicillin 50 mg/kg IM/IV within 30 min of starting the procedure.
Moderate-risk patients	Vancomycin	Adults: vancomycin 1.0 g IV over 1-2 h; complete infusion within 30 min of starting the procedure. Children: vancomycin 20 mg/kg IV over 1-2 h; complete infusion within 30 min of starting the procedure.

are equally effective in vitro against α-hemolytic strep-tococcus, however amoxicillin is recommended because it is better absorbed from the gastrointestinal tract and provides higher and more sustained serum levels. A 2 g dose results in adequate serum levels for several hours and causes fewer adverse gastrointestinal effects.[46] The newly recommended dose for moderate-risk patients is 2.0 g of amoxicillin (pediatric dose is 50 mg per kg, not to exceed the adult dose) 1 hour before the procedure. A second dose is not necessary, both because of pro-longed serum levels above the minimum inhibitory concentration of most oral streptococci[46] and the pro-longed serum inhibitory activity induced by amoxicil-lin against such strains (6 to 14 hours).[47] For individu-als who are unable to take or absorb oral medications a parenteral agent may be given. Ampicillin sodium is recommended because parenteral amoxicillin is not available in the United States. Penicillin-allergic patients should be treated with the provided alterna-tive oral regimens. Clindamycin hydrochloride is one recommended alternative. Those who could tolerate first generation cephalosporins (cephalexin or cefa-droxil) may receive these agents provided they have not had an immediate local or systemic IgE-mediated ana-phylactic allergic reaction to penicillin. Azithromycin or clarithromycin are also acceptable alternative agents for the penicillin-allergic individual[48] although they are more expensive than other agents. Azithromycin dosing for adults is 500 mg 1 hour before the procedure and children should have 15 mg per kg orally, not to exceed the adult dose. Clarithromycin dosing for adults is 500 mg 1 hour before and dosing for children is 15 mg per kg orally. Clindamycin dosing for adults is 600 mg orally or IV and for children, 20 mg per kg. When parenteral administration is needed in a penicillin-allergic patient, clindamycin phosphate is first choice; cefazolin may be used if the individual does not have a history of immediate-type local or systemic anaphylac-tic hypersensitivity to penicillin. Erythromycin previ-ously was an alternative but is no longer used because of gastrointestinal upset and complicated pharmacoki-netics of the various formulations.[49]

Occasionally, a patient may be taking an antibiotic when coming to the dentist. If the patient is taking an antibiotic normally used for endocarditis prophylaxis, it is prudent to select a drug from a different class rather than increase the dose of the current antibiotic. In particular, antibiotic regimens used to prevent the re-currence of acute rheumatic fever are inadequate for the prevention of bacterial endocarditis. Individuals who take an oral penicillin for secondary prevention of rheumatic fever or for other purposes may have viridans streptococci in their oral cavities that are relatively resistant to penicillin, amoxicillin, or ampicillin. In such cases, the physician should select clindamycin phosphate, azithromycin, or clarithromycin for endo-carditis prophylaxis (Table 13-5). If possible, one could delay treatment until 9 to 14 days after completion of the antibiotic. This will allow the usual oral flora to be reestablished.

REFERENCES

1. Fleming A: On the bacterial action of cultures of a penicillin, with special reference to their use in the relation of *B. influenza, Br J Exp Pathol* 10:226, 1929.
2. Finn R, Karas N: Maxillofacial infections: part 1, *Selected Readings in Oral and Maxillofacial Surgery* 2(3):1, 1992.
3. Peterson LJ: Microbiology of head and neck infections, *Oral Maxillofac Surg Clin North Am* 3:247, 1991.
4. Finegold SM: Anaerobic infections. In: *Humans*, London, 1989, Academic Press.
5. Laskin, DM: Anatomic considerations in diagnosis and treatment of odontogenic infections, *JADA* 69:308, 1964.
6. Brook I, Coolbaugh JC, Walker RI, Weiss E: Synergism between penicillin, clindamycin, or metronidazole and gentamicin against species of the *Bacteroides fragilis* groups, *Antimicrob Agents Chemother* 25:71, 1984.
7. Janovic S: Recognition and treatment of peri-implantitis. In: Block MS, Kent JN, editors: *Endosseous implants for maxillofacial reconstruction*, Philadelphia, 1995, WB Saunders, p. 591.
8. Becker W, Becker BE, et al: Clinical and neurobiological features that may contribute to dental implant failure, *Int J Oral Maxillofac Implants* 5:31, 1990.
9. Shordone L, Barone A, Ramalgia L, Ciaglia RN: Antimicrobial susceptibility of periodontopathic bacteria associated with failing implants, *J Periodontol* 66(1):69, 1995.
10. Cavanagh NJ: Infections of grafts and implants. In: Topazian RG, Goldberg MH, editors: *Oral and maxillofacial infections*, Philadel-phia, 1994, WB Saunders, p. 451.
11. Hudson JW: Osteomyelitis of the jaws: A 50-year perspective, *J Oral Maxillofac Surg* 51:1294, 1993.
12. Topazian RG: Osteomyelitis of the jaws. In: Topazian RG, Goldberg MH, editors: *Oral and maxillofacial infections*, ed 3, Philadelphia, 1993, WB Saunders, p. 251.
13. Chow AW, Roser SM, Brady, FA: Orofacial odontogenic infec-tions, *Ann Intern Med* 88:392, 1978.
14. Brook I, Hirokawa R: Microbiology of wound infection after head and neck cancer surgery, *Ann Otol Rhinol Laryngol* 98:323, 1989.
15. Sanford JP, Gilbert DN, Sande MA: *The Sanford guide to antimicro-bial therapy*, Vienna, Va. , 1996, Antimicrobacterial Therapy, Inc., p. 35.
16. Mandell GL, Douglas RG Jr, et al: *Mandell, Douglas, and Bennett's principles and practice of infectious diseases*, ed 5, New York, 2000, Churchill Livingstone, p. 61.
17. Marx RE, Johnson RP: Studies in the radiobiology of osteoradio-necrosis and their clinical significance, *Oral Surg Oral Med Oral Pathol* 64:379, 1987.
18. Mercuri LG: Aute osteomyelitis of the jaws, *Oral Maxillofac Surg Clin North Am* 2:355, 1991.
19. Silverman S: Diagnosis. In: Silverman S, editor: *Oral cancer*, New York, 1985, American Cancer Society, p. 37.
20. Centers for Disease Control: AIDS and human immunodeficiency virus infection in the United States—1988 update, *MMWR* 38 (suppl 4), May 1989.
21. Miyasaki SH, Perrot DH, Kaban LB: Infections in immunocom-promised patients, *Oral Maxillofac Surg Clin North Am* 2:393, 1991.
22. McLaren C, Datema R, Knupp CA, et al: Review: Didanosine, *Antiviral Chem Chemother* 2:321-328, 1991.

23. Chu CK. Schianazi RF, Ahn MK, et al: Structure-activity relationships of pyrimidine nucleosides as antiviral agents for human immunodeficiency virus type 1 in peripheral blood mononuclear cells. *J Med Chem* 32:612-617, 1989.

24. Molina JM, Groopman JE: Bone marrow toxicity of dideoxyinosine. *N Engl J Med* 321:1478, 1989.

25. Johnson VA, Merrill DP, Videler JA, et al: Two-drug combinations of zidovudine, didanosine, and recombinant interferon-alpha A inhibit replication of zidovudine-resistant human immunodeficiency virus type 1 synergistically in vitro, *J Infect Dis* 164:646-655, 1991.

26. Dornsife RE, St.Clair MH, Huang AT, et al: Anti-human immunodeficiency virus synergism by zidovudine (3'-azidothymidine) and didanosine (dideoxyinosine) contrasts with their additive inhibition of normal human marrow progenitor cells, *Antimicrob Agents Chemother* 35:322-328, 1991.

27. Johnson MA, Fridland A: Phosphorylation of 2', 3'-dideoxyinosine by cytosolic 5'-nucleotidase of human lymphoid cells, *Mol Pharmacol* 36:291-295, 1989.

28. Yarchoan R, Pluda JM, Thomas RV, et al: Long-term toxicity/activity profile of 2', 3'-dideoxyinosine in AIDS or AIDS-related complex, *Lancet* 336:526-529, 1990.

29. Lambert JS, Seidlin M, Reighman RC, et al: 2', 3'-Dideoxyinosine (ddI) in patients with the acquired immunodeficiency syndrome or AIDS-related complex. A phase I trial, *N Engl J Med* 322:1333-1340, 1990.

30. Cooley TP, Kunches LM, Saunders CA, et al: Once-daily administration of 2', 3'-dideoxyinosine (DDI) in patients with the acquired immunodeficiency syndrome of AIDS-related complex. Results of a phase I trial, *N Engl J Med* 322:1340-1345, 1990.

31. Butler KM, Husson RN, Balis FM, et al: Dideoxyinosine in children with symptomatic human immunodeficiency virus infection, *N Engl J Med* 324:138-144, 1991.

32. Pike IM, Nicaise C: The didanosine expanded access program: Safety analysis, *Clin Infect Dis* S63-68, 1993.

33. Kahn JO, Lagakos W, Richman DD, et al: A controlled trial comparing continued zidovudine with didanosine in human immunodeficiency virus infection, *N Engl J Med* 327:581-587, 1992.

34. Abrecht H, Arasteh K: Didanosine induced disorders of glucose tolerance (Letter), *Ann Intern Med* 119:1050, 1993.

35. Steckelberg JM, Wilson WR: Risk factors for infective endocarditis, *Infect Dis Clin North Am* 7:9-19, 1993.

36. Saiman L, Prince A, Gersony WM: Pediatric infective endocarditis in the modern era, *J Pediatr* 122:847-853, 1993.

37. Gersony WM, Hayes CJ, Driscoll DJ, et al: Bacterial endocarditis in patients with aortic stenosis, pulmonary stenosis, or ventricular septal defect, *Circulation* 87(suppl I):121-126, 1993.

38. Carabello BA: Mitral valve disease, *Curr Probl Cardiol* 7:423-478, 1993.

39. Boudoulas H , Wooley CF: Mitral valve prolapse. In Emmanouilides GC, Riemenschreider TA, Allen HD, Gutgesell HP, editors: *Moss and Adams heart disease in infants, children, and adolescents including the fetus and young adult,* ed 5, Baltimore, 1995, Williams & Wilkins, pp.1063-1086.

40. MacMahon SW, Roberts JK, Kramer-Fox R, et al: Mitral valve prolapse and infective endocarditis, *Am Heart J* 113:1291-1298, 1987.

41. Pallasch TJ, Slots J: Antibiotic prophylaxis and the medically compromised patient, *Periodontol 2000* 10:107-138, 1996.

42. Guntheroth WG: How important are dental procedures as a cause of infective endocarditis? *Am J Cardiol* 54:797-801, 1984.

43. Roman AR, App GR: Bacteremia, a result of oral irrigation in subjects with gingivitis, *J Periodontol* 42:757-760, 1971.

44. Felix JE, Rosen S, App GR: Detection of bacteremia after the use of oral irrigation device on subjects with periodontitis, *J Periodontol* 42:785-787, 1971.

45. Hunter KD, Holborrow DW, Kardos TB, Lee-Knight CT, Ferguson MM: Bacteremia and tissue damage resulting from air polishing, *Br Dent J* 167:275-277, 1989.

46. Dajani AS, Bawdon RE, Berry MC: Oral amoxicillin as prophylaxis for endocarditis: what is the optimal dose? *Clin Infect Dis* 18:157-160, 1994.

47. Fluckiger U, Francioli P, Blaser J, et al: Role of amoxicillin serum levels for successful prophylaxis of experimental endocarditis due to tolerant streptococci, *J Infect Dis* 169:397-400, 1994.

48. Rouse MS, Steckelberg JM, Brandt CM, et al: Efficacy of azithromycin or clarithromycin for the prophylaxis of viridans streptococcal experimental endocarditis. *Antimicrob Agents Chemother,* 41:1673-1676, 1997.

49. Sande MA, Mandell GL: Antimicrobial agent-tetracyclines, chloramphenicol, erythromycin, and miscellaneous antibacterial agents, In Gilman AG, Rall TW, Nies AS, Taylor P, editors: *Goodman and Gilman's pharmacological basis of therapeutics,* ed 8, New York, 1990, Pergamon Press, pp. 1117-1145.

PATHOLOGY

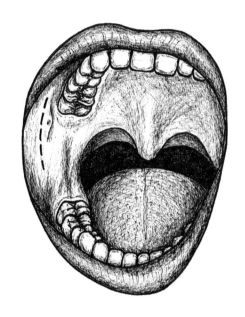

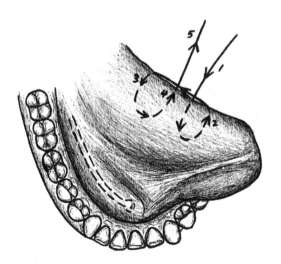

CHAPTER 14

Cysts and Their Management

MANAF SAKER, DMD
ORRETT E. OGLE, DDS

A cyst is a cavity that contains a liquid, a semisolid material (sebum, keratin, or cholesterol), or air. It is surrounded by a definitive connective tissue wall or capsule and usually has an epithelial lining.[1] Cysts in the oral and perioral region can be congenital, developmental, or of the retention type. They may develop from odontogenic or nonodontogenic sources and in either soft or hard tissue. Odontogenic cysts are by far the most common, and are usually associated with teeth. Cysts in the jaws are usually the result of an inflammatory process, an embryogenic defect, or trauma. They do not tend to cause pain unless they become secondarily infected.

Cysts are expansile lesions that are locally destructive when they occur in the jaws, sometimes even causing pathologic fractures of the mandible. The expansion of these lesions tends to be in a buccal-lingual/palatal direction, except in the posterior mandible where they can extend up into the ramus, and where lingual expansion is the rule (because of the thick external oblique ridge). The growth of the cyst will cause resorption and thinning of adjacent bone, occasionally causing the cortical bone to become so thin that it takes on a "parchment" like appearance, and the area will then become fluctuant or rubbery. It may even grow through the bone to become contiguous with other structures such as the floor of the nose, the sinus mucosa, the floor of the mouth, or neural structures medial to the mandibular ramus.

CLASSIFICATION (Box 14-1)
Diagnosis

Jaw Cysts. The vast majority of jaw cysts are diagnosed from radiographic imaging, and it is not unusual for the patient not to be aware of a problem. Jaw cysts will cause bony changes that will be readily evident on a routine intraoral complete series of radiographs, or on a panographic radiograph (panorex). To make the diagnosis, and to plan treatment for the case, good radiographs are required, and the surgeon should take care to analyze various radiographic parameters. Some specific radiologic criteria that should be examined are:

1. *The degree of lucency manifested by the lesion:* A cyst is a well-defined radiolucency that may have varying appearances—circular, unilocular, or multilocular configuration, and fingerlike projections between the teeth.
2. *Location of the lesion within the jaws:* Cysts of the jaw will either be in the maxilla or the mandible (symphysis, body, angle, or ramus).
3. *Relationship of the cysts to dental or other anatomic structures:* The cysts may be associated with a root apex, the crown of an impacted/unerupted tooth, or be unrelated to dental structures. It may also expand to involve the nose, maxillary sinus, or inferior alveolar canal.
4. *The border of the lesion:* Cysts are well delineated, and will frequently show a hyperostotic line that represents a sclerotic reaction or new bone formation adjacent to the cysts.

Using these radiographic criteria, the practitioner should be able to make an educated guess as to the likelihood of the entity being cystic, and how extensive the surgery will be. It should be noted that several pathologic conditions may also have the same radiographic appearance as a cystic lesion, and should therefore be considered in the differential diagnosis. These include: ameloblastoma, hemorrhagic bone cyst, aneurysmal bone cyst, Stafne bone "cyst," giant cell lesion, fibrous dysplasia, ossifying fibroma, central hemangioma of bone, histiocytosis, and metastatic or primary carcinoma.

To further assist in the diagnosis of the radiolucency an aspiration should be done (see Chapter 15 on biopsy techniques for details of aspirating lesions in bone). Indeed, every large radiolucency of the jaw should be aspirated before opening into it surgically, so as to avoid the disaster of opening into a vascular cavity. The aspirant obtained from the radiolucency should give a fairly good idea if the lesion is a cystic one. The diagnosis of any large radiolucent lesion in the jaw,

BOX 14-1   Classification of Cysts

CYSTS IN BONE	CYSTS IN SOFT TISSUE
Radicular	Eruption cysts
Dentigerous	Nasolabial cysts
Periodontal cysts	Dermoid and epidermoid cysts
Residual	Sebaceous cysts
Primordial (follicular)	Mucocele
OKC	Ranula
Calcifying odontogenic cysts	
Globulomaxillary cysts	
Nasopalatine cysts	
Cystic ameloblastoma	

however, should be made from biopsy, and one should be done even when the aspirant yields a straw-color fluid. Large ameloblastomas can be filled with straw-color fluid, and may appear as cysts on radiograph. Simple enucleation may be inappropriate treatment.

The odontogenic keratocyst (OKC) deserves special mention because of its aggressive nature and high recurrence rate. These cysts occur from changes that take place in the nature of the epithelial lining of a small percentage of all types of odontogenic and some fissural cysts.

The characteristics of the OKC are:

1. A thin epithelial lining, usually less than 2 mm in thickness, which is evenly uniform and devoid of rete pegs. This epithelium is covered by a thin layer of orthokeratin.
2. A cyst lumen that contains keratin scales.

There is up to a 50% recurrence rate following removal of the OKC, as a result of the thinness of the lining epithelium and the multilocularity of the cysts which prevents complete enucleation.[2] These cysts are almost impossible to enucleate in their entirety, because the thin lining is very friable and it tears easily. This means that fragments of the lining may be left behind attached to the bony wall, where they develop into a recurrent cyst. Simple enucleation will not, therefore, be adequate treatment for this cyst.

In planning a cystectomy, clinical and radiographic findings should be considered.

Clinical Examination. This is traditionally divided into several well-known components.

- Visualization. The surgeon should survey the oral cavity, its mucosa, and the surrounding dentition for any pathologic changes of color either of the teeth or of the mucosa, the presence of fistula, swelling, and distortion of natural anatomic landmarks. The involved side should be compared with

the noninvolved side of the oral cavity. Buccal-lingual or palatal expansion should be ascertained.

- Palpation. This is done to determine expansion of the lesion, if the cyst has perforated its bony borders, or if the cortical plates are very thin and have a fluctuant or rubbery feeling. Bony expansion could feel hard and continuous with the surrounding natural bony structure, which is the usual indication of a slow growing intrabony process. Or it could sometimes feel like a solid bone expansion that would change to a softer, rubbery consistency at certain spots indicating a possibly fast growing lesion that has broken out of its bony boundaries.

- Aspiration. This is critical in the differential diagnosis of bony radiolucencies. A cystic lesion would yield a blood-tinged fluid, a straw-color fluid, or a thick cheesy material. The aspiration should be done with an 18-gauge hypodermic needle attached to a 5 or 10 cc syringe. The technique is described in Chapter 15.

Radiographic Examination. Panoramic radiography is the most useful imaging method for evaluating maxillofacial pathology. It will provide a survey of the entire mandible and its dentition (including condyles and coronoid processes), the maxilla and its dentition, the maxillary sinuses, inferior orbital rims, and nasal cavity. Radiographic characteristics of cystic lesions have been described previously.

With a radiograph of high clarity and resolution, one should be able to discern the inferior alveolar canal, mental foramen, maxillary sinus, nasal cavity, along with the entire cystic lesion.

- CT scan. This will only be required in selected cases, mostly where the cyst has extended beyond the bony cortex into the adjacent soft tissues, or into the mandibular ramus, maxillary sinus, or nasal cavity. Both axial and coronal sections should be obtained, and should include bone and soft tissue windows.

- MRI. This has limited application for most jaw lesions, however, it may provide information on the type of fluid within a cystic lumen. Depending on the composition of the fluid, the cyst may produce a low, intermediate, or high signal intensity. A proteinaceous fluid, subacute blood, and fat will produce a high signal intensity on the T_1-weighted images, whereas the T_2-weighted images disclose a bright signal with fluid and subacute blood, and an intermediate signal with fat.

Such differentiation will be useful in younger patients who may have a suspected hemorrhagic bone cyst for which surgical intervention would not be necessary.[3]

TREATMENT OF CYSTS IN THE JAW BONES

The treatment of all bony cysts is removal of the cystic lesion in its entirety. The removal of the cystic fluid will relieve the pressure within the bony cavity and permit bone healing. At surgery all of the cyst lining should be removed to minimize the chance of recurrence. Regardless of the etiology or the location of the cyst, the surgical principles for removing a bony cyst are the same. The surgery may be done in a single procedure, or staged in the so-called marsupialization technique (Partsch operation).

The broad general principles guiding the approach to removing a simple bony cyst are discussed in detail in Chapter 9 on endodontic surgery. In this chapter some of the general principles may not be restated, but specific details will be outlined in relationship to location when necessary for the reader to better understand the surgery. When dealing with large radicular cysts, removal of the cyst will not be adequate treatment, and the source of the pathology must be addressed. The reader should note, however, that it is extremely important that only the nonvital tooth/teeth be treated endodontically or extracted. Just because the roots of teeth appear radiographically to be associated with the cystic cavity does not mean that they require endodontic intervention or extraction. Tooth vitality should be ascertained with an electric pulp tester.

Instrumentation

- #3 Bard Parker surgical blade handle and #15 surgical blade
- Periosteal elevator (Molt)
- Small and large double-ended Lucas type curettes
- Wieder retractor (tongue retractor) or dental mirror
- Minnesota retractor or Seldin periosteal elevator
- High and slow speed dental handpieces
- Burs: 557 square crosscut surgical bur, #6 or 8 round bur (25 mm); Pear shaped or round "non-clogging" carbide bur (acrylic bur)
- Friedman or Blumenthal type rongeurs
- Bone file
- Monoject syringe
- Sutures: 4-0 silk or Vicryl
- Needle holder
- Scissors

Procedures

The principles that must be followed in the design of the soft tissue incisions for the removal of cystic lesions are detailed in Chapter 9. Those that involve special considerations will be emphasized later in this chapter.

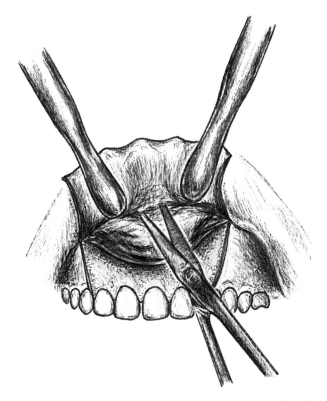

FIG. 14-1 Scissors being used to dissect the plane of fusion between the cystic lining and the adjacent soft tissue of the lip. This is done by a combination of blunt and sharp dissection.

The incision is made cleanly with a #15 Bard-Parker blade extending full thickness to the bone. The surgeon should try to avoid having to make too many attempts at the incision, as this will inadvertently lead to several cuts, tissue tags, loss of blood supply, and slow healing. The incision line should be kept away from any anticipated or actual bony defect so as to avoid wound breakdown postoperatively. The incision should be long enough to allow for proper surgical exposure and retraction without excessively traumatizing and compromising the vascularity of the flap.

A periosteal elevator is used to reflect a full thickness mucoperiosteal flap to expose the underlying anatomic site of the cyst. If the cyst has perforated the buccal cortical plate and has fused to the lateral soft tissues, the surgeon should carefully examine the area to determine a plane of demarcation between the cyst and normal soft tissue. Scissors should be used to dissect this plane using a combination of blunt and sharp dissection (Fig. 14-1). The type of scissors that are used will depend on the surgical situation. The sharpness or bluntness of the tip of the scissors should correlate with the density of the tissue being dissected. Dean or curved Metzenbaum scissors are the ones that we use most often (Fig. 14-2). The Metzenbaum scissors have a

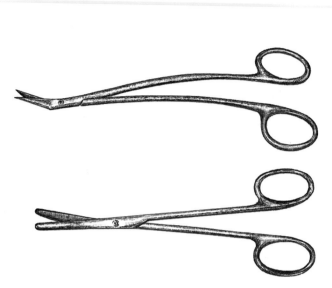

FIG. 14-2 Dean and Metzenbaum scissors which are frequently used for dissection. The Metzenbaum has a rounded tip and is used in delicate tissues whereas the Dean scissors has a pointed tip and is used in more dense tissue.

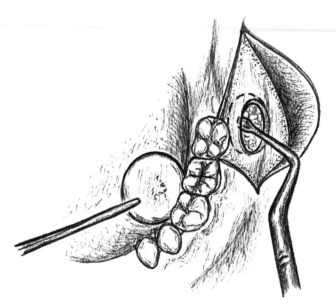

FIG. 14-3 Dissection of a cyst from its bony crypt with a curette. At the start of the peeling out of the cyst, the convex surface of the curette should be toward the membrane and the concave surface toward the bony wall.

blunted tip that can be used to separate soft tissues and to "snip" adhesions between cyst and connective tissue. When there is a history of inflammation of the area, the tissue will be more dense, thus requiring scissors with a sharper tip. The Dean scissors fulfill this role. During this step, the operator should take care not to cut into the cyst, however. Deflating it will make it more difficult to identify its borders. Careful examination, and a little experience will guide the surgeon along the plane of fusion. Retraction of the flap can be done with either a Minnesota retractor, or with the Seldin periosteal elevator.

If it is necessary to surgically create a bony window, the overlying bone can be carefully removed with a #6 or 8 surgical-length round bur in a high-speed dental handpiece. In large cysts, or in the maxilla, the bone may be so thin that access to the cyst can be attained by flaking off the bone with a curette or with the periosteal elevator. Once the window is started and the cyst wall identified, the access process is continued until solid bone is reached, and there is an adequate-sized window to remove the cyst.

The largest spoon-shaped curette that will fit into the bony cavity is used to begin the dissection of the cystic membrane from the bony wall. The reason for using a large curette is to provide a large area that will prevent tearing of the cystic wall. To start the shelling out

process, the edge of the curette is gently pushed between the epithelium-lined connective tissue capsule of the cyst and the bony crypt. At the start of the peeling out of the cyst, the convex surface of the curette should be toward the membrane and the concave surface toward the bony wall (Fig. 14-3).

As much of the periphery as can be reached from the buccal is dissected at this time, gently stripping the cyst away from its attachment to the bone by pushing it toward the center of the cystic cavity. Once more than 50% of the cyst has been liberated by this technique, the curette may then be turned so that the concave portion may be used to reach under the cyst and "spoon" out the remainder of the attachments from the bone (Fig. 14-4). The dissection may go either from one end to the other, or it could be done in increments from both ends to meet at a common point. An attempt should be made to remove the lesion intact. Following the delivery of the cyst, the bony cavity should be carefully examined to ensure complete removal of the cystic membrane and components and to ensure hemostasis. The bony edges are smoothed with a bone file, and the wound irrigated and closed.

Although the incidence of finding ameloblastic or other neoplastic changes in cyst walls is low and may not be cost-effective, we still advocate that the pathology specimen should be submitted for examination, if

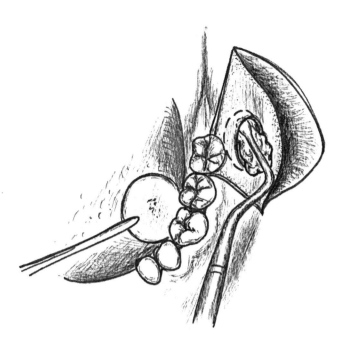

FIG. 14-4 Once 50% of the cyst has been freed the curette is turned to spoon out the remaining portion of the cyst.

only for documentation. Chaudhry rightly makes the point that it would take thousands of serial sections in a large cyst to rule out ameloblastoma or carcinoma, and that such a procedure is not practical.[4]

The use of a drain or packing of the residual bony cavity will depend on factors such as the size of the bony cavity, the control of bleeding, and the extension of the cyst into other anatomic areas (maxillary sinus, nose, palate, or floor of the mouth). The reason for placing a drain or a packing after cystectomy is to limit the formation of a hematoma or to minimize dead space. A drain is placed only to allow continuous escape from a wound of a fluid that is better outside than if left within the wound.[5] In this scenario, a latex or Penrose drain would be placed in an area from which an infected cyst was removed. Large bony defects in the jaws with continuous oozing from the marrow spaces should be packed for 24 to 48 hours to control the formation of hematoma. The packing is done with 2-inch gauze packing (Iodoform gauze) in a reversed fashion (Fig. 14-5, *A* and *B*). The gauze is placed in the superior/posterior position, held in place with a clamp, then layered inferiorly. Once the cavity is filled, the gauze is cut, and the cut end placed into the wound. The superior end is brought out of the crypt. The packing should exit the oral mucosa at a location so that when the packing is removed the hole in the mucosa will be over bone and not in direct communication with the bony defect. Failure to do so would create

a fistula between the bony defect and the oral cavity. The incision site is usually a good location to provide an exit for the packing (Fig. 14-5, *C*). After the packing is removed, the bony defect will fill with bone over a period of time.

Large bony defects in the anterior mandible and the maxilla can be managed as just described. In the posterior mandible this may not be possible with very large defects. These defects should be loosely packed with gauze impregnated with tincture of benzoin, and squeezed dry. The gauze is placed into the defect and the oral mucosa loosely approximated above it (Fig. 14-6). It will be necessary to change the packing once or twice weekly for hygiene reasons, so only a few strategic sutures, or a widely spaced continuous suture should be placed to support the mucoperiosteal flaps until they reattach. After the suture is removed the bony crypt is packed open. The gauze packing should be maintained until the entire bony defect becomes covered with granulation tissue. Once the bone is fully covered the packing may be removed, and the wound managed with irrigation. The tincture of benzoin will serve as a bacteriostatic agent and will help to control the immediate postoperative odor from the intraoral wound.

Small and medium sized defects (< 2 cm) will require no special considerations. Medium sized defects (1.5 to 3 cm) may be packed with collagen to eliminate the dead space. As cystic defects will generally fill in once the lesion is removed we do not recommend the use of hydroxyapatite or such materials in the residual cystic defect. Freeze-dried bone may be used, however, if it can be fully covered by the overlying oral mucosa. We have found no particular indication for the use of membranes (GTR) or barriers in the treatment of cystic cavities.

If a dental component (such as an impacted tooth) is present within the cyst that requires removal, it should be addressed before the cystectomy is done (see Chapter 8 on the impacted canine).

If an incisional biopsy was obtained and the lesion is a documented keratocyst (OKC), a peripheral ostectomy should be performed after the removal of the cyst. This is done by using methylene blue solution to stain the bone. The dye should be applied carefully to the cystic cavity and allowed to perforate into the marrow space for about 3 to 5 minutes. The excess dye is removed by irrigation. A large round bur is used to remove bone until all of the absorbed dye is no longer visible (Fig. 14-7). The use of methylene blue is not absolute, and even if it is not used the surgeon should still perform the peripheral ostectomy, being careful to cover the entire bony cavity.

For OKCs chemical cauterization may also be done.

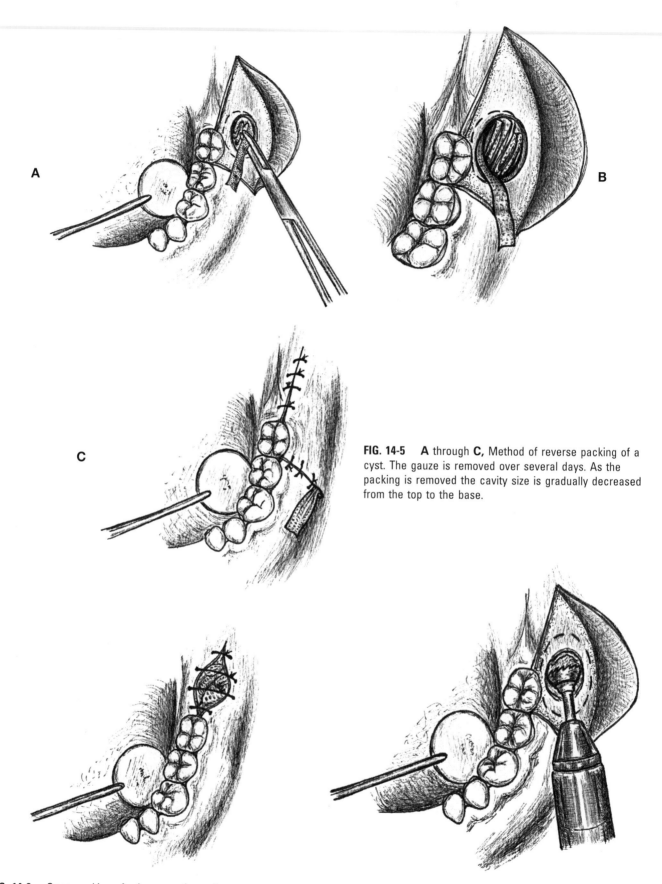

A

B

C

FIG. 14-5 **A** through **C,** Method of reverse packing of a cyst. The gauze is removed over several days. As the packing is removed the cavity size is gradually decreased from the top to the base.

FIG. 14-6 Open packing of a large cystic cavity.

FIG. 14-7 A large round bur being used to perform an ostectomy within the cyst cavity of an OKC.

Chemical Cauterization

Carnoy's Solution. This cauterizing solution is carefully placed into the bony cavity and allowed to remain there for 5 minutes. Care must be taken to prevent contact between the cauterizing solution and mucosal surfaces or with teeth. After 5 minutes, the area is irrigated copiously with physiologic saline.[6] The first irrigation should be done with high-speed evacuation so as not to spread the chemical before it is adequately diluted. Subsequent irrigations can be done more vigorously.

Composition of Carnoy's Solution

60 ml absolute alcohol

30 ml chloroform

10 ml acetic acid.

Phenol. The phenol is placed on a peanut or a cotton swab, and is used to burnish the bone. This is done for approximately 1 minute. The phenol is allowed to penetrate for 1 minute. It is then removed by rinsing lightly with 95% ethanol. This is followed by copious irrigation with physiologic saline to remove the alcohol.

The rationale of chemical cauterization is to fixate and destroy residual cells that may lead to recurrence. If the inferior alveolar nerve is exposed or is close to the surface, we do not recommend the use of chemical cauterization as it may irreversibly injure the nerve. Carnoy's solution has been shown in research studies to cause nerve injury with axonal degeneration.[7,8]

Special Considerations

Maxilla. Esthetics should be carefully taken into consideration in the design of the incision in the anterior maxilla as the results of the surgery may well be visible postoperatively. When anterior full-coverage prosthetics (crowns) are present, the incision should be kept apical sparing the marginal gingiva to minimize postoperative gingival recession and unpleasant revealing of the prosthetic margins. Where moderate to advanced periodontal defects are evident, the depth of the pockets should be measured with a periodontal probe, marking the depth of the sulcus, and placing the incision line at least 2 mm apical to the depth of the sulcus. In all other cases a sulcular incision is preferred.

In the area of the maxillary lateral incisors large cysts may become fused with the soft tissue of the palate. The anterior portion of the cyst that is attached to bone should be dissected first. Once freed the assistant then holds the specimen (Fig. 14-8) while the surgeon places one finger into the palate at the area where the cyst lining is fused with the

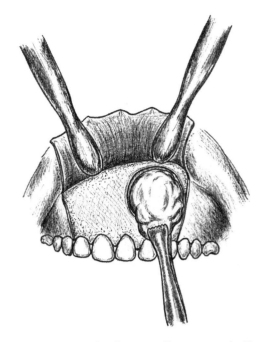

FIG. 14-8 Aspiration of a large maxillary cyst to facilitate the removal of the cystic sac.

palate. Pushing up on the palate, the surgeon carefully separates the cystic wall from the palate trying not to perforate the palate. Perforation would lead to the formation of a fistula.

Cysts in the posterior maxilla may perforate into the maxillary sinus or fuse with the palatal mucosa. These are best exposed from the buccal surface. The cyst membrane is partially dissected from its bony attachments as previously described. To facilitate the final stages of the enucleation, the cystic sac is aspirated (Fig. 14-9). The cyst lining that is fused to the palatal mucosa is dissected free from the palate (Fig. 14-10). When it perforates the maxillary sinus and fuses with the antral lining the part of the sinus mucosa that is fused with the cyst membrane is sacrificed and removed with the cyst to ensure complete removal (see Fig. 14-10). The remaining sinus membrane is not disturbed unless it is involved with polyps. To allow drainage or to pack the cavity an intranasal antrostomy is created by forcefully passing a curved rasp downward and lateral beneath the inferior turbinate into the exposed floor of the maxillary sinus. The file is used to remove irregular bony edges (Fig. 14-11). The sinus may be packed and the end of the gauze brought out through the nose.

Mandible. The anatomy of the mandible makes the surgical intervention a little more complex be-

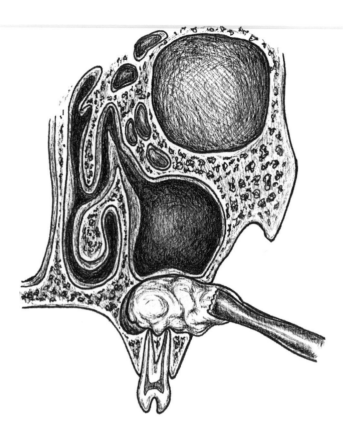

FIG. 14-9 Freeing of the collapsed cyst from its mucosal attachments.

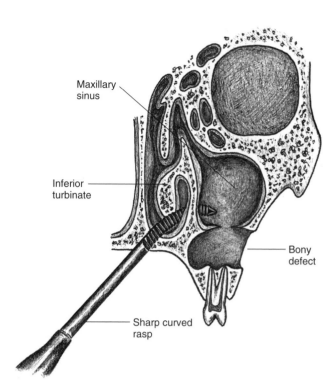

FIG. 14-11 Performance of an intranasal antrostomy to allow drainage from the maxillary sinus or to pack the cavity. The sinus is packed and the end of the gauze brought out through the nose.

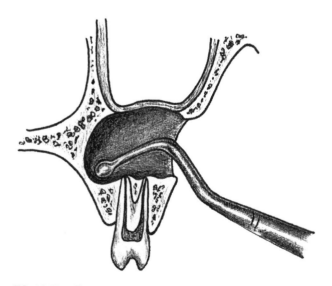

FIG. 14-10 The antral lining that is fused with the cyst membrane is sacrificed and removed with the cyst to assure complete removal.

cause of the neurovascular bundles that are associated with the mandible. The inferior alveolar neurovascular bundle runs within the mandibular canal, often in close proximity to the roots of the molars. It exits the mandible as a bundle at the mental foramen in the premolar area. The lingual nerve runs in close proximity to the lingual plate at the retromolar trigone, a common site for incisions to access cystic lesions associated with an impacted lower third molar.

If the cyst is present in the anterior mandible, a crestal incision could be safely designed without compromising cosmesis of the marginal gingiva because of its location below the smile line, even with the presence of a full coverage prosthesis. Another consideration in this location is the narrow band of attached gingiva present. For proper exposure the incision should extend two teeth beyond the radiographic margin of the cystic boundaries. Vertical release is placed to provide more relaxation of the mucosal flaps. The position of a vertical release should always be guided by the anatomic position of the mental nerve.

If the cyst is located in the posterior mandible the

incision should be kept buccal over the external oblique ridge (Fig. 14-12). This will minimize the possibility of injury to the lingual nerve and allow some of the wound to be closed over bone. The length of the incision will be guided by the size of the cyst.

In case of cystic involvement of the ascending ramus the incision is placed lateral to the mandible and extends more superiorly, about 1 cm above the occlusal plane (see Fig. 14-12). The operator should make sure that the tendonous insertions of the temporalis muscle unto the anterior portion of the coronoid process are fully sectioned. This will allow adequate elevation of the temporalis muscle to provide the necessary access. The lateral aspect of the ramal process is exposed. Dissection is then continued on the medial aspect of the ramus and carried superiorly to remove the insertions of the temporalis tendons from the anterior ramus. A V-notch retractor may be used to facilitate removal of the tendons and to position the tissue bundle superiorly (Fig. 14-13). A sharp periosteal elevator can also be

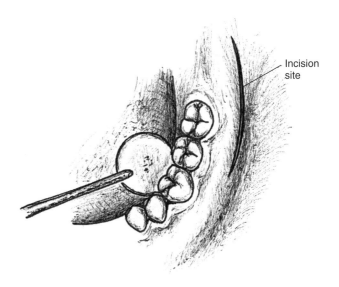

FIG. 14-12 Location of incision to approach a cyst that is located in the posterior mandible. The incision is made over the external oblique ridge. In case of cystic involvement of the ascending ramus the incision is placed to extend more superiorly, about 1 cm above the occlusal plane.

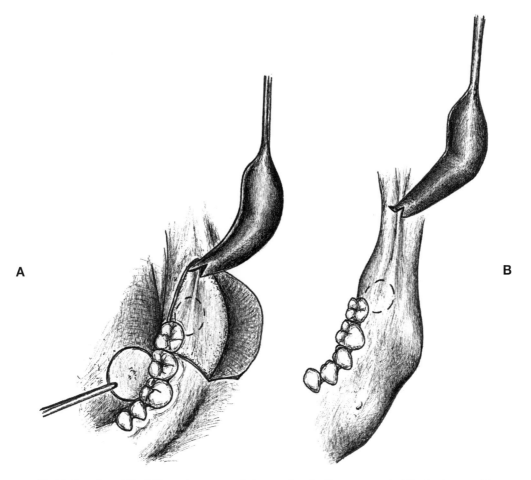

FIG. 14-13 **A** and **B,** A V-notch retractor being used to facilitate removal of the tendons and to position the tissue bundle superiorly.

used. The cyst is approached from the retromolar area, shelling out the cyst from the anterior and working backward.

Soft Tissue Cysts. Soft tissue cysts may be fissural, dermatologic, or of retention or obstructive phenomena. They are painless unless secondarily infected, and will generally be of a rubbery consistency. The diagnosis will generally be made from clinical exam, experience, and occasionally by aspiration. Although not commonly managed by the dentist, several soft tissue cysts occur in the oral/perioral region of the face that can be managed in the dental office. The removal of the intraoral dermoid cyst will be discussed here, even though this may not be an office procedure.

Dermoid Cysts. Dermoid cysts are believed to be derived from epithelial rests, which persist in the midline after fusion of the mandible and hyoid branchial arches. The cyst lumen is often filled with sebaceous material, and the wall usually contains a variety of skin appendages like hair follicles or sweat glands. This cyst usually occurs in the anterior floor of the mouth in the submental region, either above or below the geniohyoid muscle (Fig. 14-14). They are relatively uncommon in the oral cavity, and are not easily discovered unless they expand into the floor of the mouth. Although they occur in the same area as a ranula, they do not give the vesicular appearance of the ranula. CT scans are helpful in distinguishing a dermoid cyst and in locating its relative anatomic position.

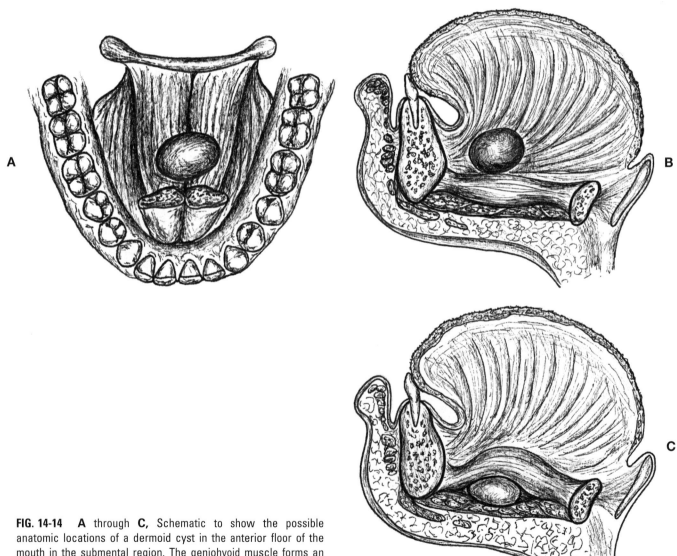

FIG. 14-14 A through **C,** Schematic to show the possible anatomic locations of a dermoid cyst in the anterior floor of the mouth in the submental region. The geniohyoid muscle forms an anatomic border that defines whether the cyst will be removed from an extraoral approach or transbuccally.

Dermoid cysts that are located above the geniohyoid muscle are removed from a transoral approach, whereas those below this muscle are removed from a transcutaneous approach. The transcutaneous approach is beyond the scope of this atlas.

Instrumentation

- #3 Parker type blade handle
- #15 surgical blade
- Curved hemostat
- Metzenbaum and Dean scissors
- 3-0 silk suture
- 3-0 Dexon and 5-0 nylon sutures
- Surgical cautery
- Holding forceps
- Allis and Bobcock forceps
- Lacrimal duct cannulas

Transoral Removal of Dermoid Cyst from Floor of Mouth

Two percent Lidocaine with Epi 1/100,000, 2 to 3 cc, are injected in the floor of the mouth around the apparent lesion. Care should be taken not to balloon the tissue excessively as this will make the dissection more difficult. Both submandibular ducts are visualized and their course is well identified to avoid severing during the procedure.

The surgical incision is made in the midline in the sagittal plane through the oral mucosa extending from the attached gingiva at the lingual aspect of the mandible to the ventrum of the tongue (Fig. 14-15). Mucosal flaps are developed superficially. 3-0 silk sutures are placed to gently retract these flaps (Fig. 14-16). Alternatively, the mucosal edges may be sutured to the lateral borders of mandible, or the sutures may be passed around the proximal dentition. Good access with good visibility should be achieved. Using blunt and sharp dissection, the capsule of the cyst is identified. This capsule will appear more white than the surrounding tissues.

Blunt dissection is then performed using curved Metzenbaum scissors with careful scissor strokes, or a fine hemostat, to separate the cystic formation from the adjacent soft tissue (see Fig. 14-16). During the time of dissection, finger pressure in the submental area extraorally will be of great value in pushing the cyst superiorly into the floor of the mouth. Once the cystic swelling is freed from the surrounding tissue it may be grasped with a Bobcock clamp, and removed. The cavity should be dry before closure. All bleeding points should be controlled with bipolar or a small cautery. Closure is done in layers carefully to avoid leaving dead spaces that

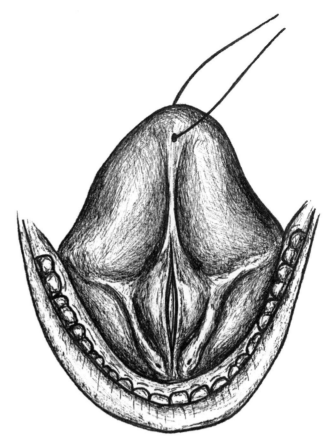

FIG. 14-15 Incision site for the transoral approach to remove a dermoid cyst from the anterior floor of the mouth.

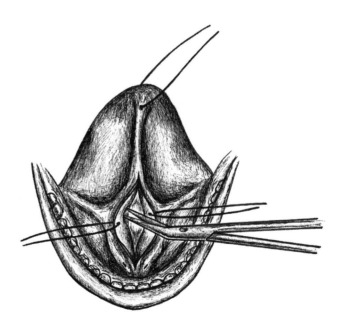

FIG. 14-16 Blunt dissection of the dermoid cyst with a curved Metzenbaum scissors. During the dissection finger pressure should be used to push the cyst into the intraoral site.

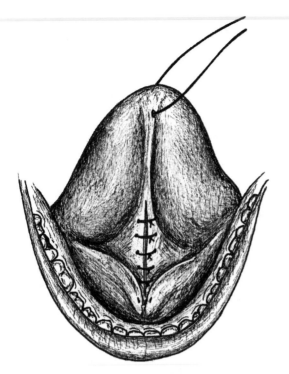

FIG. 14-17 Layered closure of the surgical site following transoral removal of a dermoid cyst from the floor of the mouth.

could be potential spaces for hematoma collection (Fig. 14-17).

Post Operation

Although the postoperative swelling is usually not extensive, some swelling and moderate pain should be expected, and the patient should be monitored for swelling in the floor of the mouth. Keeping ice cubes in the mouth after the pressure gauze is removed may be helpful. Hematoma formation in the sublingual space may be potentially serious as elevation of the floor of the mouth may cause obstruction of the airway. If the hematoma is expanding, it should be addressed immediately and managed by drainage and, if necessary, by reopening the surgical site and controlling the source of the bleeding (see Chapter 5 on control of bleeding). Intraoral sutures are removed 5 to 7 days postoperatively.

REFERENCES

1. Peterson LW: Cysts of bone and soft tissues of the oral cavity and contiguous structures. In Kruger GO, editor: *Textbook of oral surgery*, St. Louis, 1974, Mosby, pp. 223-247.
2. Lumerman H: *Essentials of oral pathology*, ed 1, Philadelphia, 1975, JB Lippincott, p. 47.
3. Weber AL: Imaging of cysts and odontogenic tumors of the jaw, *Radiol Clin North Am* 31(1):102, 1993.
4. Archer WH: Treatment of cysts of the oral cavity. In Archer WH: *Oral and maxillofacial surgery*, ed 5, Philadelphia, 1975, WB Saunders, p. 555.
5. Edgerton MT: Dressing, drains and suture removal. In Edgerton MT: *The art of surgical techniques*, Baltimore, 1988, Williams and Wilkins, p. 168.
6. Voorsmit, RA, Stoelinga PJ, van Haeist UI: The management of keratocysts, *J Maxillofac Surg* 9:228-236, 1981.
7. Frerich B, Cornelius C, Wietholter H: Critical time exposure of the rabbit inferior alveolar nerve to Carnoy's solution, *J Oral Maxillofac Surg* 52:599-606, 1994.
8. Loescher AR, Robinson PP: The effect of surgical medicaments on peripheral nerve function, *Br J Oral Maxillofac Surg* 36(5):329-332, 1998.

CHAPTER 15

Biopsy Techniques

ORRETT E. OGLE, DDS

Biopsy is the removal of tissue from a living person for microscopic examination to confirm or to establish the diagnosis of a disease. The diagnosis of most oral pathology may be made from the history, clinical appearance, and radiographic findings. On occasion, however, it will be necessary to confirm the clinical diagnosis, or to make the diagnosis itself, based on microscopy. On these occasions tissue will be needed for the pathologist to make the diagnosis, and the clinician must supply a specimen that will be of good diagnostic value.

To perform an acceptable biopsy the dentist should have a reasonable suspicion of the nature of the lesion that will be biopsied. The mental compilation of a list of possible diagnoses based on the clinical and radiographic examination is called differential diagnosis. In establishing the differential diagnosis the practitioner should use the history, clinical, and radiographic examination to first classify the lesion into one of the following groups:

- Developmental/congenital
- Inflammatory—infections, autoimmune diseases, and reactive lesions
- Neoplastic—benign and/or malignant
- Traumatic—acute or chronic
- Systemic—oral manifestations of systemic or cutaneous diseases

This list may be remembered by the mnemonic "DINTS."

After the broad category classification, the diagnosis may be further narrowed to specific disease entities. Table 15-1 gives a broad classification of oral lesions that may be biopsied based on location, and Box 15-1 gives a list of white and red lesions.

Once the differential diagnosis has been made, the need for a biopsy should be determined. The clinician should always remember that even the most expert clinical diagnosis will never be as reliable as the microscopic diagnosis made from a biopsy, and if there is ever **any** doubt of the diagnosis, a biopsy should be performed. The practitioner must also decide what type of biopsy should be done. Biopsies may be excisional, incisional, or aspirational. Box 15-2 contains a list of terms used by the pathologist on reports of biopsy, all of which the practitioner should clearly understand.

Following are some considerations that should be observed to ensure full diagnostic value of the biopsy:

1. The tissue being removed for microscopic examination should be taken from a representative area of the lesion. Examine the extent and nature of the lesion carefully, and take the biopsy from the area that best represents the pathologic entity. Do not take tissue from obviously necrotic areas. Thin, deep sections should be obtained in partial (incisional) biopsies rather than broad, shallow ones (Fig. 15-1). Both epithelium and connective tissue should be included in the biopsy specimen, because superficial tissue may simply show an inflammatory reaction.

2. When doing a partial biopsy from an ulcerative lesion or an epithelial one, always attempt to include an adequate border of normal tissue. This will allow for comparison during the microscopic examination. In some total (excisional) biopsies, a good border of normal tissue should also be included all around the lesion to be sure that the lesion has been totally removed.

3. Use extreme care with tissue forceps. Careless handling of the tissue with forceps may crush the tissue, place artificial clefts in the specimen, or otherwise mutilate it. The specimen should be carefully held at one end with a fine-tooth forceps, or a suture may be used to manipulate the specimen. The suction should be kept away from the surgical site when the tissue is ready to be removed so as to avoid sucking up the specimen.

4. Avoid drying out of the specimen. The tissue should be placed into saline or formalin immediately after removal. Drying out of the specimen may cause cellular distortion, making the microscopic diagnosis difficult or inaccurate.

5. Always accompany the specimen with a good report that will include the clinical and radiographic examination, and a listing of the differential diagnosis. Also be sure to include age, sex, and

TABLE 15-1 Commonly Occurring Oral Lesions Listed by Region

Location	Disease Entity
Face	Sebaceous cysts, fibroma, lipoma, hemangioma, neurofibroma, nasolabial cyst
Lips	Mucocele, fibroma, white lesions, herpetic lesions, salivary gland tumors, basal and squamous cell carcinoma, hemangioma
Oral mucosa	Fibroma, granulomas, reactive lesions, aphthous ulcers, papilloma, red lesions, white lesions, oral manifestations of mucocutaneous diseases, epulis, salivary gland tumors, hemangioma
Jaws	Periapical pathosis, periapical cysts, keratocyst, other jaw cysts, fibroosseous diseases, giant cell lesions, ameloblastoma, AOT, other odontogenic tumors, osteomyelitis, central hemangioma, Paget's, other primary bone pathology
Palate	Fibroma, papillomatosis, granulomas, traumatic ulcers, ulcerative diseases, white lesions, red lesions, benign and malignant salivary gland tumors, sialometaplasia
Tongue	Fibroma, traumatic ulcers, granuloma, squamous cell carcinoma, papilloma, white lesions, granular cell myeloblastoma, hemangioma
FOM (floor of mouth)	Ranula, sialolith, carcinoma in situ, squamous cell carcinoma, white and red lesions, hemangioma

BOX 15-1 White and Red Lesions of the Oral Mucosa

WHITE LESIONS	RED LESIONS
Scar tissue of mucosa	Traumatic macules and erosions
Papilloma	Reddish ulcers or ulcers with red halos
Leukoderma	
Healing chemical or thermal burns	Cellulitis
	Acute chemical or thermal burns
Hyperkeratosis (leukoplakia)	Erythroplakia
Squamous cell carcinoma	Carcinoma in situ
Verrucous carcinoma	Kaposi sarcoma
Candidiasis	Atrophic candidiasis
White hairy tongue	Denture stomatitis
Nicotine stomatitis	Nicotine stomatitis
Vesicular bullous disease	Primary herpes
Lichen planus and lichenoid reactions	Erosive lichen planus
	Erythema multiforme
White spongy nevus	Xerostomia
Smoker's lip lesion	Median rhomboid glossitis
Migratory glossitis	Pyogenic granuloma
Necrotic tissue	

race as this information will be helpful to the pathologist.

Box 15-3 lists further "Dos and Don'ts" of biopsy.

TYPES OF BIOPSIES
Excisional Biopsy

Excisional biopsy is removal of a lesion in toto. It is a combination of a diagnostic procedure and definitive therapy, and should be reserved for lesions

■ that are surgically reasonably accessible.

■ less than 2 to 2.5 cm in diameter and that are clinically benign.
■ that may be "shelled out."
■ that are small, well-defined bony lesions.

Incisional Biopsy

Incisional biopsy is the removal of a small, representative, portion of the lesion for microscopic examination. Indications for incisional biopsy are as follows:

■ Large intrabony or soft tissue lesions
■ Diffuse lesions
■ Suspected malignancies

The specimen submitted for examination should include the maximum volume of *abnormal* tissue, as this is what the pathologist needs to establish a definitive diagnosis. With this in mind, it is not necessary to always include a border of normal tissue. For ulcerative lesions, however, the specimen should consist of suspected diseased tissue and adjoining normal tissue. Such a specimen will give the pathologist a picture of "normal" and "abnormal" which will assist in producing an accurate microscopic diagnosis.

In an incisional biopsy a rectangular or pie-shaped wedge is removed from the margin of the lesion (remember, however, that the goal is to supply the largest volume of *abnormal* tissue) (Fig. 15-2). The incision should be deep enough to include normal tissue deep to the lesion because histologic changes may be very different from those in superficial tissue. Clinical judgment must be used, however, in deciding the appropriate depth of incision so as to prevent injury to vital underlying structures.

Mixed red and white lesions should be biopsied in an area from which both types of tissue can be obtained in

15-2 Glossary of Terms

Anaplasia: A regressive change in adult cells to more primitive embryonic cell types that is irreversible. These cells show differences in size, shape, chromaticity, and mitotic detail. Anaplasia is characteristic of malignant disease.

Anisocytosis: Abnormal variations in the size of cells.

Atypical: The condition of being irregular, or unusual. This should serve as a vague warning to the surgeon that the pathologist is concerned about something, but that it cannot be classified as a malignancy.

Dysplasia: A reversible change in adult cells characterized by variations in size, shape, and architectural organization. This may be thought of as a state between hyperplasia and neoplasia. Although not totally accurate, the clinician may consider dysplasia as premalignant.

Granuloma: A special type of inflammation that is characterized by the accumulation of macrophages, some of which coalesce into giant cells. It is notably characteristic as a reaction to a foreign body (i.e., calculus).

Hyperchromatic: A state in which the cell is more intensely stained than is normal. It represents a form of degeneration of the cell nucleus in which the nucleus becomes filled with particles of chromatin. It represents a de-differentiation to immature type tissues and may imply malignancy, but is not definitive.

Hyperkeratosis: An increase of the corneous layer of the oral mucosa. It may be a result of a specific disease that shows this condition as a part of its course, or it may be secondary to external factors (cigarette smoke, denture irritation, cheek biting, etc.)

Hyperplasia: A proliferation of new cells that are not neoplastic. In some cases, this is the result of the body's normal reaction to an external stimulus.

Metaplasia: A reversible change in which one adult cell type is replaced by another adult cell type that is not normal for that tissue.

Necrosis: Tissue death. It may be seen in inflammatory, traumatic, or neoplastic conditions.

Neoplastic: An area that shows new growth, comprising an abnormal aggregation of cells whose growth exceeds and is not coordinated with that of the normal surrounding tissue.

Pleomorphic: Cells of the same tissue that assume various distinct forms.

Poikilocytosis: Abnormal variations in the shape of cells.

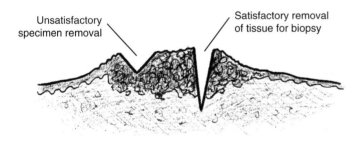

Unsatisfactory specimen removal

Satisfactory removal of tissue for biopsy

FIG. 15-1 Thin, deep sections should be obtained in partial (incisional) biopsies rather than broad, shallow ones. Both epithelium and connective tissue should be included in the biopsy specimen.

15-3 Dos and Don'ts of Biopsy

DO

1. Get a representative sample when doing an incisional biopsy.
2. Remove sufficient tissue, because the larger the sample, the greater will be the chance of getting an accurate diagnosis.
3. Always use a new sharp blade.
4. Handle the specimen carefully.
5. Biopsy all large and suspicious lesions before they are totally removed.
6. Always aspirate bony cavities before opening into them.
7. Always submit diseased tissue that is removed to the oral pathologist.

DON'T

1. Vascular lesions should never be biopsied incisionally.
2. Intrabony radiolucent lesions should not be biopsied without prior diagnostic aspiration.
3. Pigmented lesions should not be biopsied incisionally.[1]
4. Do not deposit local anesthesia closer than 1 cm from the lesion.
5. Try to avoid the use of electrocautery, as the thermal effect may result in cellular histologic distortion.

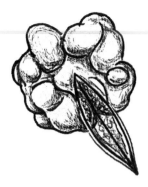

FIG. 15-2 An incisional biopsy showing the removal of a pie-shaped wedge from the margin of the lesion. Specimen will include both normal and abnormal tissue showing the area of transition.

the same specimen. If this is not possible, multiple incisional biopsies should be done in order to get the required representative sample of the lesion. If this is done, each sample should be tagged and placed in separate specimen bottles. It is more important, however, to biopsy the red areas, as these red areas represent more active and significant dysplastic changes.

Punch Biopsy. This is a form of incisional biopsy that in the oral cavity is best suited for the diagnosis of mucosal abnormalities that may require multiple biopsies.[2] Keyes biopsy punches are the type recommended for use on oral mucosal lesions.[3] These punches range in size from 1.0 to 12.0 mm., increasing in increments of 0.5 mm.

The biopsy is done by placing the punch at the intended biopsy site, and slowly rotating the punch back and forth between the thumb and index fingers, using moderate pressure, until the bevel on the head of the punch is no longer visible. The punch is removed and the surgically created core is released at its base using a fine, curved iris scissors. Multiple plugs of tissue can be taken. The cheek, lip, and accessible regions of the tongue are sites that are amenable to punch biopsies. The cheek and lip will require counterpressure from the outside. In general, for this type of biopsy sutures are not required, but on rare occasions a single suture may be necessary to control persistent bleeding.

Because these cores are very small, proper handling of the specimen is critical. The tissue should be held with Adson's forceps with serrated tips using minimal pressure. Suction should not be used. If visibility becomes a problem, then the site should be gently blotted with gauze. When the tissue has been removed from the mouth it should be placed epithelial side down on a piece of Telfa or a stiff piece of paper. Heme from the surgical incisions will act as "glue" to allow the specimen to stick to the paper, thus when the paper with the specimen is placed in fixation, the specimen will not

distort.[4] For routine histopathologic investigations, 10% neutral buffered formalin is the preferred fixative.[5] If immunofluorescence is requested, the tissue should be placed in Michel's medium for fixation and transport. Immunofluorescence studies should be considered as adjunctive in diagnosis.[6] This study is indicated to assist the diagnosis of a suspected immunologically based disease with primary oral manifestations such as pemphigus, pemphigoid, lichen planus, and lupus erythematosus.

Fine Needle Biopsy. This is another type of incisional biopsy in which a fine needle is used to remove a very small core of cells from a deep-seated lesion. Indications for fine needle biopsy in oral surgery would be a suspected tumor of the parotid gland or enlarged lymph nodes in the submandibular or submental region. The technique of fine needle aspiration biopsy (FNAB) offers the advantages of ease of performance, cost effectiveness, convenience, and at the same time accuracy.

Under local anesthesia, a 23-gauge needle attached to a 10-cc disposable syringe containing 2 cc of air is introduced into the lesion. (*This air is needed to be able to express the specimen from the needle.*) Negative pressure is applied to the syringe, and several sharp, quick, jabbing strokes are made with the needle. These passes should be made at different angles so as to sample various areas of the mass. The operator must take care not to accidentally withdraw the needle from the mass while harvesting tissue. When the surgeon is ready to remove the needle, the negative pressure on the plunger is released so as to keep the specimen in the needle as it is withdrawn from the mass. The aspirated tissue is then expressed onto a glass slide. A second slide is placed on the first and used to spread the aspirant. One of these slides is placed in 95% ethanol fixative and the other is air-dried. The glass slide that was alcohol fixed will be stained with Papanicolaou's stain, while the air-dried one may be stained with Wright's stain (Diff-Quik). The glass slide prepared with Diff-Quik is for immediate assessment.

Aspiration Biopsy. An aspirational biopsy (not to be mistaken with FNAB) is the removal of the contents of a mass for the purpose of analysis. In oral surgery, this technique is usually used to rule out and/or differentiate fluid-filled lesions. These lesions may be cysts, abscess cavities, vascular lesions, hematomas, sialoceles, or empty cavities (traumatic bone cyst). The aspirational biopsy is applicable to both intraosseous as well as soft tissue masses.

All radiolucencies in the jaws, with the exception of small areas that are obviously periapical pathosis, should be aspirated before surgical intervention. It is very important that the surgeon rule out vascular lesions before opening into bony cavities, as the unantic-

BOX 15-4 Suggested Instrumentation for Performing Oral Biopsies

SOFT TISSUE BIOPSY
- Aspirating dental syringe
- Local anesthesia
- Scalpel handle #3
- #15 scalpel blade
- Cawood-Minnesota retractor
- 3-0 silk suture for retraction
- Small curved Iris scissors
- Dean scissors
- Halsted-Mosquito hemostats, curved (2)
- Fine teeth tissue forceps
- Adson tissue forceps
- Allis soft tissue forceps
- Atraumatic Bobcock forceps
- Needle holder
- Suture scissors
- Specimen jar

ASPIRATION BIOPSY
- Aspirating dental syringe
- Local anesthesia
- 10-cc plastic syringe
- 16-gauge needle, sharp
- Scalpel handle #3
- #15 blade
- Periosteal elevator
- Cheek retractor
- Seldin elevator for retraction
- High speed dental handpiece
- Fissure bur
- Bone wax
- 3-0 silk suture
- Needle holder
- Suture scissors

BONE BIOPSY
- Aspirating dental syringe
- Local anesthesia
- Scalpel handle #3
- #15 blade
- Periosteal elevator
- Cawood-Minnesota retractor
- Seldin elevator for retraction
- Tongue retractor (dental mirror or Wieder retractor)
- Mono-bevel chisels
- Mallet
- Double ended curettes—#11 and #12 (Lorenz Surgical*)
- Molt curettes, #2 and #4
- High speed dental handpiece
- Long fissure bur
- Bone wax
- Allis tissue forceps
- Curved Kocher forceps
- Rochester-Ochsner forceps
- Rongeurs
- Adson-Brown tissue forceps
- Needle holder
- Suture scissors
- Specimen jar

* Walter Lorenz Surgical Inc., Jacksonville, Fla.

ipated opening into a vascular lesion could present a very serious surgical complication.

TECHNIQUES

The biopsy techniques will be described according to anatomic locations. Box 15-4 gives recommended lists of instrumentation for performing oral biopsies.

Lip

The specimens from the lips most frequently submitted by dentists to an oral pathology service in Brooklyn, New York were[7]:
- Lower lip—mucocele, fibroma, pyogenic granuloma, and hyperkeratosis
- Upper lip—mucocele, fibroma, and salivary gland tumor

Anatomic Considerations. Significant anatomic structures that should be considered are the superior and inferior labial arteries. These two arteries arise at a variable distance from the corner of the mouth to enter the upper and lower lips. They are found close to the vermilion/cutaneous border on the cutaneous side deep in the orbicularis oris muscle. In both lips the right and left labial arteries anastomose widely in the midline. Bleeding from these vessels is usually not very serious as they are readily apparent and easily accessible. Bidigital pressure applied to the respective lip at the commissure during the procedure will compress the vessel and permit a relatively bloodless procedure. When incised, the vessel can easily be clamped and controlled by ligation or electrocautery.

Excisional Biopsy. This is indicated for small, benign, well-circumscribed lesions of the lip. For surgical purposes, the lip should be divided into three segments: the cutaneous portion, the vermilion, and the mucosal portion. The lips contribute highly to facial esthetics and to emotional gratification, and incisions for a biopsy should be planned to avoid or minimize disfiguring of the appearance of the lip.

Cutaneous Biopsy. For lesions totally confined to the cutaneous portion of the lip the incision for the biopsy should be planned to follow the natural facial creases and should be elliptical in shape. Elliptical excisions made parallel to or along these normal creases and

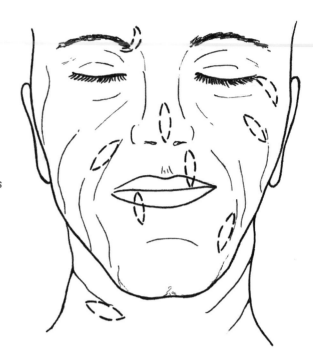

FIG. 15-3 Cutaneous biopsies should be planned to follow the natural facial creases and should be elliptical in shape. By following the natural skin creases the visualization of the scar will be minimized. Figure shows the direction of natural skin creases, and how excisions should be oriented to minimize scarring.

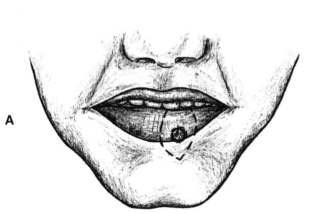

A

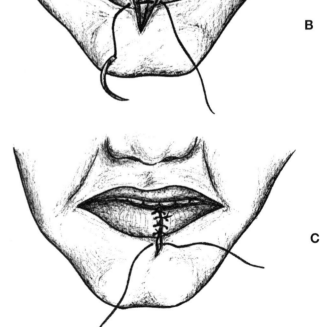

B

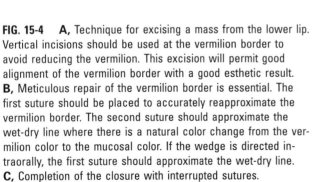

C

FIG. 15-4 **A,** Technique for excising a mass from the lower lip. Vertical incisions should be used at the vermilion border to avoid reducing the vermilion. This excision will permit good alignment of the vermilion border with a good esthetic result. **B,** Meticulous repair of the vermilion border is essential. The first suture should be placed to accurately reapproximate the vermilion border. The second suture should approximate the wet-dry line where there is a natural color change from the vermilion color to the mucosal color. If the wedge is directed intraorally, the first suture should approximate the wet-dry line. **C,** Completion of the closure with interrupted sutures.

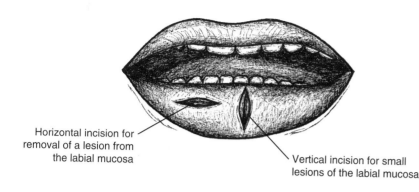

Horizontal incision for removal of a lesion from the labial mucosa

Vertical incision for small lesions of the labial mucosa

FIG. 15-5 Incision of a large lesion from the labial mucosa using a horizontally oriented incision.

folds of the lip will heal with a minimum of scar tissue (Fig. 15-3). The general rule is that the length of the incision should be three times the diameter of the lesion at its widest point to permit tension-free closure of the skin. In areas where the skin can easily be undermined, a little shorter incision may be used so as to minimize the scar. Skin should be closed with 5-0 nylon on a cutting needle.

Vermilion Border. When excising a mass from the vermilion portion of the lip every attempt should be made to avoid reducing the vermilion. To achieve this objective, vertical incisions should be used (Fig. 15-4, *A*). The wedge (shield) resection may be used to excise benign tumors from the lip. The length of the wedge should be one and one-half the width of the wedge. Up to one third of the lip may be removed with primary repair that will be esthetic. The wedge may be directed toward the skin or toward the mucosa, depending on where the mass is located.

Meticulous repair of the vermilion border is essential. When closing an excision site such as that shown in Fig. 15-4, *A,* the first suture should be placed to accurately reapproximate the vermilion border (Fig. 15-4, *B*). The second suture should approximate the wet-dry line where there is a natural color change from the vermilion color to the mucosal color. The wound closure can then be completed with interrupted sutures (Fig. 15-4, *C*). (For additional details on wound closure, see Chapter 23, "Repair of Orofacial Lacerations.") If the wedge is directed intraorally, then the first suture should approximate the wet-dry line where the color change occurs.

Labial Mucosa. Small lesions can be excised using an elliptical incision with its long axis perpendicular to the vermilion. Larger ones should be done with a horizontal incision (Fig. 15-5). The general rule of length being three times the diameter should be followed. Branches of the mental nerve are frequently encountered in this area. They can usually be seen not far below the surface of the buccal mucosa traveling within the muscle. In the excision of small fibromas, an attempt should be made to spare these nerve fibers. Their presence should not

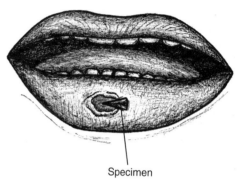

Specimen

FIG. 15-6 Incisional biopsy from the lower lip. An adequate sample of abnormal tissue should be taken, and the tissue should be large.

compromise the removal of pathology however, as these nerves will regenerate.

Incisional Biopsy. On the lips this type of biopsy is indicated for the following:
■ Large lesions that will require extensive reconstruction
■ Diffused lesions
■ Ulcerated lesions that are suspicious for malignancy

Careful examination of the lesion should be done, and a site that best represents the pathology should be selected for biopsy. An adequate sample of abnormal tissue should be taken, and the tissue should be "large" (5×5 mm) (Fig. 15-6). In suspected squamous cell carcinoma, the wound should not be closed unless sutures are needed to apply pressure to control bleeding.

Buccal Mucosa

The most frequently submitted specimens from the buccal mucosa by dentists were fibromas, hyperkeratotic lesions, ulcers, and salivary gland tumors.[7]

Anatomic Considerations. Stensen's duct will be the critical anatomic structure influencing a biopsy of the buccal mucosa. Outside of the oral cavity Stensen's duct

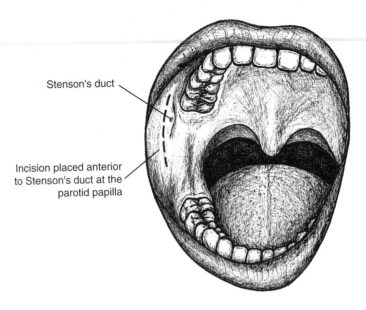

FIG. 15-7 Position of incision for a mass located anterior to the orifice and deep to the mucosa. A vertical incision is made and the mass is dissected and brought forward.

is on the facial side of the masseter muscle. It turns sharply medially around the anterior border of the masseter, often embedded in a furrow of the buccal fat pad. The anterior border of the masseter is located at about the mesial wall of the third molar. In its medial course, the duct perforates the buccinator muscle in an oblique and medial direction, to open at a papilla of the buccal mucosa opposite the midbuccal groove of the maxillary second molar tooth, or sometimes a little more anteriorly.

Excisional Biopsy. The direction of the incision will depend on whether the mass is located anteriorly to the orifice of Stensen's duct (the parotid papilla) or behind it, and on the depth and size of the mass.

For a mass located anterior to the orifice and deep to the mucosa a vertical incision is made and the mass is dissected and brought forward (Fig. 15-7). Small sessile or pedunculated masses can be removed with a vertically oriented ellipse. Horizontal incisions tend to stretch and dehisce when the mouth is opened wide, whereas vertical incisions tend to relax when the mouth is closed, and restretch to the surgical size on opening.

At or behind the parotid papilla, the ellipse should be horizontally oriented so as to avoid possible injury to the duct. In the third molar area, a vertical incision extending beyond the occlusal plane would expose the buccal fat pad, allowing it to descend into the field. This may compromise the visibility and possibly the biopsy.

Incisional Biopsy. A representative sample should be removed. The biopsy should also be deep enough to include the connective tissue layer (Fig. 15-8).

Tongue

The specimens from the tongue most frequently submitted to the oral pathology lab of SUNY Health

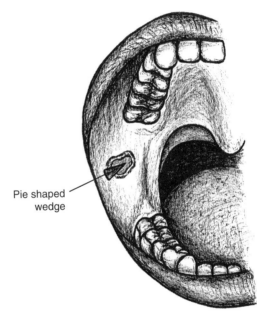

FIG. 15-8 To perform an incisional biopsy the specimen should be a representative sample of the lesion, and the biopsy should be deep enough to include the connective tissue layer.

Science Center at Brooklyn were: fibromas, granulomas, traumatic ulcers, hyperkeratoses, and squamous cell carcinomas.[7]

Anatomic Considerations. Biopsy of the lateral border and dorsum of the tongue are anatomically safe procedures. The ventral aspect of the tongue has a wide distribution of veins that may be injured during biopsy. The surgeon should be prepared to clamp, possibly ligate, and/or control bleeding from these veins.

Excisional Biopsy. This is usually achieved by elliptical incisions on both the dorsum (Fig. 15-9) and lateral borders (Fig. 15-10). (Fig. 15-10 shows a lateral border

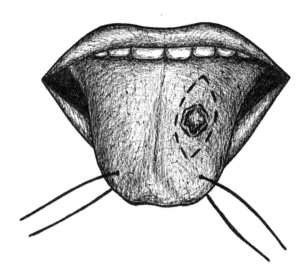

FIG. 15-9 An elliptical biopsy should be done for lesions on both the lateral border and the dorsum of the tongue. This figure shows sutures being used to control the tongue and to keep tension on it during the biopsy. The excision of the total mass is depicted.

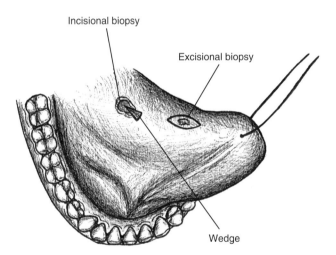

FIG. 15-10 Lateral border of the tongue showing both excisional and incisional biopsies.

with excisional and incisional biopsy.) Following local anesthesia, a #6 Martin, half circle cutting edge needle is passed through the tongue carrying a #0 silk suture. The suture is passed from the dorsal surface in the middle third halfway between the median raphe and the lateral border, through to the ventral surface, across to the opposite side of the ventral surface and back up through the tongue to the dorsal side. This type of retraction suture may be used to retract the tongue and may be tightened to control small bleeds. There is a risk, however, of impaling veins on the ventral surface of the tongue with this technique. A simpler, safer method is

to place one or two sutures in the anterior third (see Fig. 15-10).

Incisional Biopsy. This should be done for deep lesions in the tongue, and suspicious lesions (malignancies) of the lateral border (see Fig. 15-10).

Palate

As reported by personal communication with Dr. Marshal Solomon,[7] the most common lesions submitted for microscopic diagnosis from the palate were: hyperkeratoses, fibromas, pyogenic granulomas, salivary gland tumors, and squamous cell carcinomas.

Anatomic Considerations. The palate has two distinct anatomic portions. The posterior third is the movable, muscular, soft portion that terminates in the uvula; and the anterior two thirds is the nonmovable, bony, glandular hard palate. Because of the gag reflex, the possible need for a Dingman mouth prop, possible bleeding into the nasopharynx, and patient anxiety, biopsy of the soft palate may be difficult and often requires general anesthesia with intubation of the trachea. Surgery of the soft palate, therefore, should be performed by an oral and maxillofacial surgeon with cleft palate or tumor surgery experience, or by an otorhinolaryngologist, and is beyond the scope of this atlas.

Biopsy of lesions of the hard palate is a minor oral surgical procedure. Anatomic consideration of the hard palate is limited to the greater palatine vessels. Several different morphologic tissue types are found in the hard palate, and tumors and diseases may arise from any of these different structures.

Excisional Biopsy. On the palate this should be reserved for small (<2 cm in diameter) masses or ulcerations with a well-demarcated border. When this is done, the planned excision should include 1/8 of an inch (5 mm) of normal tissue around the lesion, but the three-to-one elliptical shape does not apply here. Lesions that extend to bone should include the underlying periosteum in the excised specimen. The resultant surgical defect does not require primary closure.

Microfibrillar collagen (Avitene/Helithene), a dressing of absorbable collagen (Helistat/Colatape), or Gelfoam may be used to control bleeding and left to cover the wound. The patient should avoid eating spicy foods for a week to 10 days. Hot liquids should also not be used for the first 3 to 5 days. Although these wounds are generally not very painful, the surgeon should be aware that a patient who is not in pain tends to heal better, and it is therefore prudent to minimize any postoperative discomfort that the patient may suffer. To achieve this goal topical agents should be used in addition to systemic analgesics. Some useful topical agents are the OTC preparations of benzocaine in emollient for oral lesions (Oratect Gel, Orabase-B with Benzocaine Paste),

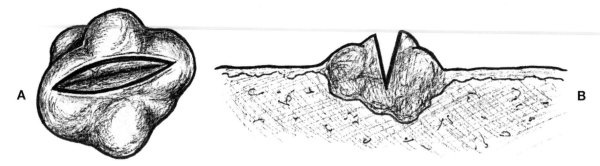

FIG. 15-11 **A,** Technique for doing a biopsy of a suspected salivary gland tumor of the palate. The wedge is taken from the center of the mass taking care not to violate the capsule and extend into normal tissue. **B,** Cross-sectional view of method of biopsy for a suspected salivary gland tumor of the palate.

topical benzocaine (Hurricane spray, Numzident), lidocaine 2% viscous solution (Xylocaine Viscous), and lidocaine transoral (DentiPatch). For larger defects a surgical splint made from a soft vacuum-forming material on a vacuum-forming machine (Sta-Vac Mini-Lab, Buffalo Dental Mfg. Co., Brooklyn, NY), or acrylic, should be fabricated preoperatively from a dental model, and used to cover the wound. This will prevent the patient from irritating the area with the tongue, and will make eating more comfortable. If the wound is covered, however, it should be examined every 3 days by the dentist. The patient should be advised to wash the splint two to three times per day, and not to sleep with it in place. Placing a surgical splint tends to trap exudates, and keep them trapped against the open wound. This may slow the healing process, cause infections, and increase scarring.

Incisional Biopsy. This is indicated for large (> 2 × 2 cm) or ominous looking lesions, diffused ones, or where the clinician is unsure of the diagnosis. (An accurate diagnosis will result in the best treatment, so the dentist should take the effort to properly identify the disease entity by a biopsy). The specimen should be taken from an area that will give the best sample of abnormal tissue. The piece removed may be rectangular or triangular in shape.

Incisional biopsy of salivary gland tumors requires special discussion. These tumors are considered *encapsulated.* Because of this, the biopsy should be done at the center of the lesion and not at the periphery (Fig. 15-11, *A* and *B*). Performing the biopsy at the periphery will violate the capsule and allow the tumor to spread into the adjacent tissue. Taking the specimen from the center will maintain the capsule, and minimize the surgical border that will be needed at the time of definitive surgery.

Bone

The tissue specimens from the jaws most frequently submitted to the oral pathology service at SUNY Health Science Center at Brooklyn[7] were: radicular and dentigerous cysts, keratocysts, fibroosseous lesions, odontomas, and ameloblastomas.

Before a bone biopsy is performed, the dentist should obtain good-quality imaging studies. If a full mouth series of periapical radiographs has been done, they should be supplemented with a panoramic radiograph of the jaws. The entire extent of the lesion must be visible along with its approximation to vital anatomic structures (teeth, nasal cavity, maxillary sinus, and inferior alveolar canal). If expansion of the buccal and/or lingual cortical plate was noted on the clinical examination, occlusal radiographs should also be taken. In rare instances CT scans or an MRI may be requested before the biopsy, but usually the panoramic radiograph will provide enough information to arrive at a working diagnosis, locate the lesion, and to plan the biopsy. A CT scan (or a DentaScan) may sometimes be necessary when planning the definitive treatment. A carefully formulated working diagnosis is important, because serious problems may be encountered by unsuspecting clinicians who may find themselves well into a surgical procedure that they were not prepared to handle. Box 15-5 provides a list that may be helpful in developing a differential diagnosis of bony lesions.

Radiolucencies. The clinician should first determine the nature of the radiolucency. Obvious periapical pathosis need not be subjected to biopsy. Other radiolucent lesions, particularly those that are not associated with teeth that are removed from the jaws must be submitted for microscopic examination. Small radiolucent lesions that have a well-demarcated border may be enucleated in toto. The procedure is similar to that used

BOX 15-5 Differential Diagnosis of Bony Lesions by Radiographic Appearance

RADIOLUCENT LESIONS	MULTILOCULATED LESIONS	MIXED LESIONS	RADIOPAQUE LESIONS
• Cysts—radicular/dentigerous • Odontogenic keratocyst • Giant cell granuloma • Unicystic ameloblastoma • Adenomatoid odontogenic tumor (AOT) • Ameloblastic fibroma • Giant cell lesion of hyperparathyroidism • Metastatic tumors	• Ameloblastoma • Central giant cell granuloma • Odontogenic myxoma • Aneurysmal bone cyst • Vascular malformations • Central hemangioma of bone • Cherubism • Burkitt's lymphoma	• Fibroosseous diseases • Florid osseous dysplasia • Chronic osteomyelitis • Osteoradionecrosis • Metastatic tumors • Osteogenic sarcoma • Odontogenic fibroma • AOT • Calcified epithelial odontogenic tumor (CEOT) • Paget's disease	• Odontoma Cementomas • Peripheral osteoma • Florid osseous dysplasia • Mature osteoblastoma • Osteogenic sarcoma • Mucosal cyst of maxillary sinus • Metastatic carcinoma of prostate • Sickle cell sclerosis

for cystectomy. (See Chapter 14, "Cysts and Their Management," for surgical details.) Central granulomatous lesions not associated with periapical pathology should be submitted for microscopic examination before definitive treatment is instituted. Large radiolucencies should first be biopsied, and a diagnosis established before they are removed.

The sequela of opening into an unsuspected vascular tumor is very serious, and will result in severe morbidity. Because the consequence of such a surgical misadventure is calamitous, it is prudent that all radiolucencies of the jaw be aspirated as the first step in developing a working diagnosis. *Vascular lesions should always be ruled out.*

Aspirational Biopsy. A 16-gauge needle attached to a 10-cc disposable syringe is used to penetrate into the radiolucency. Negative pressure is applied to the syringe, and the contents of the radiolucent lesion removed. This may be nothing (a solid mass), air (traumatic bone cyst), straw-colored or blood-tinged fluid (cyst, ameloblastoma), fluid with keratin needles (odontogenic keratocysts), or blood (a vascular lesion).

If the cortex is dense and the 16-gauge needle cannot penetrate into the underlying lesion, a sulcular incision is made, a mucoperiosteal flap reflected, and a hole is drilled through the cortex into the radiolucency. The aspirating syringe with an 18-gauge needle can now be placed into the lesion and a sample of its contents removed (Fig. 15-12).

In a high-pressure vascular lesion, the syringe will fill with blood with very little negative pressure. The blood from a vascular lesion will be obviously red. At times however, blood-tinged fluid may be aspirated from nonvascular lesions that may be mistaken for blood. This is because bleeding occurred into the lesion as a result of the trauma from the aspirating device penetrat-

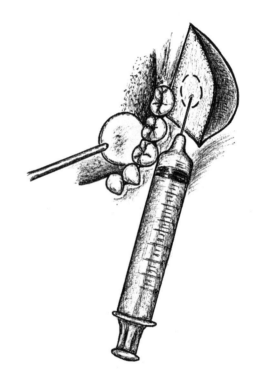

FIG. 15-12 Aspiration of a radiolucent lesion centrally located in bone. An 18-gauge needle attached to a 10-cc syringe is used to perform the aspiration.

ing the bone. Rubbing the fluid between gloved fingers is sometimes useful in determining that the fluid is not blood, but mucoid in nature. If in doubt, the lesion should be aspirated a second time. The liquid from a cystic lesion will be decreased or absent, whereas true vascular lesions would refill and give a second positive aspirant to about the same volume as the first. Any suspected vascular lesion should be aspirated twice to confirm its presence.

A negative return means that the lesion is either a solid mass or an empty cavity.

Biopsy Technique. Using a sulcular incision, reflect a mucoperiosteal flap. If the cortical plate is thin, with or without fenestration, then the periosteal elevator or a curette can be used to peel away the thinned cortex to expose the underlying pathology. If the cortical bone is intact and thick, a #6 or #8 round bur should be used to make a window through the cortex to expose the underlying pathology. The size of the window should be large enough to accomplish the goal of the biopsy. If the lesion will be enucleated in toto (an excisional biopsy), then the window should permit access to the total lesion. For an incisional biopsy, a smaller window is satisfactory. A representative sample of adequate size should be removed.

Multiloculated Lesions. These bony lesions should also be aspirated to rule out a vascular lesion. Once the surgeon has ruled out vascular lesions, a specimen may be obtained through a bony window. Try to take an adequate sample of tissue—5 × 5 mm should be smallest sample.

Radiopacities. The well-defined radiopaque lesion (an odontoma) may be removed in toto as an excisional biopsy. To do this, a round bur in a high speed handpiece is used under generous irrigation, to make a bony window to expose the pathology, which may then be enucleated.

Incisional Biopsy. An intact block of bone should be removed; this may be achieved with rotary instruments or with chisels. If a rotary instrument is used, a 5 mm dental latch type trephine (Ace Surgical, Boston, MA) may be used to remove a core (Fig. 15-13), or a fissure

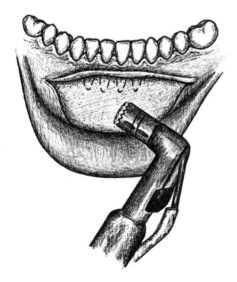

FIG. 15-13 Performing a bone biopsy with a trephine. The trephine will harvest a core of bone.

bur in combination with a chisel or bone curette may be used to remove an intact block.

The dental drill with a small fissure bur is used to outline the block. The block may then be removed by the bone curette or by a chisel. Small chisels may also be used to elegantly outline and remove the block of bone. The block that is removed should be at least 7 to 10 mm × 7 to 10 mm in size, and should go deep into the lesion.

Bony specimens will require decalcification, and the surgeon should not expect results for 10 to 14 days.

Floor of Mouth

According to the oral pathology service at SUNY Health Science Center at Brooklyn,[7] the most frequently submitted specimens from the floor of the mouth were: hyperkeratoses, ranulas, squamous cell carcinomas, and other tumors.

Anatomic Considerations. The floor of the mouth contains important anatomic structures with which the surgeon should be familiar. Excisional or incisional biopsy in the floor of the mouth should be carefully planned so as not to damage vital structures. The significant ones are the duct of the submandibular gland (Wharton's duct), the lingual nerve, and the sublingual artery.

Wharton's Duct. This structure enters the floor of the mouth in the region of the mandibular third molar medially, and close to the tongue. It first courses deep in the floor of the mouth along the upper surface of the mylohyoid muscle. Becoming more superficial, it crosses over the lingual nerve, and continues anteriorly on the undersurface of the sublingual gland. It opens into the mouth at the sublingual caruncula within a few millimeters of the lingual frenum. From the premolar forward the submandibular duct is midway between the base of the tongue and the alveolar ridge. Anteriorly, the duct widens and is superficial. The submandibular duct is a fairly large structure and is very easily identifiable below the lingual mucosa in the anterior portion of the mouth.

Behind the premolars the duct is deep and is situated below the sublingual gland, thus the chances of cutting into it during a mucosal biopsy are greatly decreased. From the premolar forward, however, the likelihood of injury during a biopsy increases as the duct is now more superficial. Mucosal biopsy done in the anterior portion of the floor of the mouth is at high risk to injure the duct. Because of this reason, the duct should be cannulated during the biopsy. This will allow the surgeon to be aware of the location of the duct during the procedure, and will also permit instant repair in case the duct is transected. If the duct is cut along its length, it need not be repaired primarily. The wound edges of the mucosa are sutured over the duct and recanalization will occur without further intervention. Transection of the duct will require an anastomosis, or a sialodochoplasty may be performed.

Cannulation of the submandibular duct is performed with lacrimal probes. The double ended, 5-inch, silver, lacrimal probes are ideal for this procedure. Sizes 3/0 to 4/0 through 1 to 2 should be available. A 2 × 2 gauze is used to dry the floor of the mouth. The operator identifies the orifice of Wharton's duct by milking the submandibular gland anteriorly and observing the flow of saliva from the duct. Starting with the 4/0 probe the operator introduces the probe into the duct (see Fig. 15-14). (Lidocaine viscous may be used to lubricate the probe to permit easy access into the orifice and to decrease sensation.) Once into the duct the surgeon gives the probe two small quarter rotations, then allows the probe to stay in the duct for 7 to 10 seconds. This will permit dilation of the duct. With the eyes of the surgeon fixed on the orifice, the probe is removed and flipped over to now introduce the 3/0 end into the duct. The same thing that was done previously is now repeated. To minimize patient discomfort, lidocaine jelly should be placed on the oral mucosa before the start of the procedure. When using lidocaine jelly, it is placed on a gauze and the end of the metallic probe placed into the blob of jelly before it is introduced into the duct.

Keeping the eyes on the duct, the operator removes the first probe and immediately introduces the 2/0 end of the next probe. For a biopsy the dilation may stop at 1/0. This probe is left in the duct during the biopsy.

Lingual Nerve. The lingual nerve descends from the pterygomandibular space to enter the oral cavity in the vicinity of the mandibular third molar teeth. Here it turns anteriorly into the floor of the mouth and is superficially located at the level of the third molar. A little further anteriorly (second/first molar area) the nerve is in close proximity to the posterior border of the sublingual gland. The nerve then turns medially, passing underneath the submandibular duct, to divide into a variable number of branches that enter the substance of the tongue.

The lingual nerve is superficial in the posterior portion of the mouth and injury is most likely to occur in the third molar area. Incisions for a biopsy at this area should be medial and close to the tongue.

Sublingual Artery. This is a branch of the lingual artery that is situated in the floor of the mouth, at the base of the tongue, medial to the sublingual gland and Wharton's duct. In the region of the first molar-premolar area the sublingual artery is of considerable volume. Injury to the artery at this location may produce hemorrhage that may be a serious incident. Local clamping of the artery should be attempted, but this is sometimes difficult. Pressure is often the most successful method to control bleeding here. Pressure is applied by packing the area with gauze and by the surgeon applying the pressure bimanually. Constant pressure should be maintained for about 3 to 5 minutes, though longer periods may be required. If attempts to stop the bleeding at the place of injury fail, the pressure should be maintained and the patient rushed to a hospital for ligation of the lingual artery.

It must be mentioned, however, that the sublingual artery is sometimes only a small insignificant branch of the lingual artery and may even be missing. In such

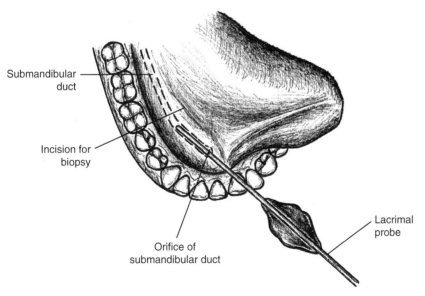

Submandibular duct

Incision for biopsy

Orifice of submandibular duct

Lacrimal probe

FIG. 15-14 Canulation of the submandibular duct with lacrimal probes and location of incision for taking a biopsy from the floor of the mouth.

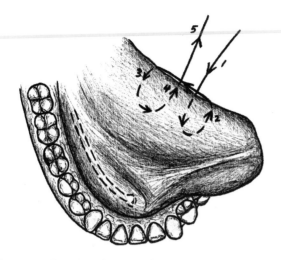

FIG. 15-15 Technique for retracting the tongue using a suture. A Wieder retractor may also be used to assist with the retraction of the tongue.

cases it is replaced by branches of the submental artery, which is a branch of the facial artery. When this is the case, ligating the lingual artery will obviously not stop the bleeding. Vessel ligation, therefore, should be attempted only after all attempts at control by pressure have been exhausted, and it should be done in the controlled environs of the operating room. Angiography should be performed to identify the bleeding vessel and its origins.

Excisional Biopsy. This should be confined to small pedunculated lesions, or to small white or red lesions in the anterior floor of the mouth. In the midline of the floor of the mouth the incision for the biopsy may be oriented vertically between the openings of Wharton's duct if they are widely separated. In all other locations the incision should be parallel to the body of the mandible (Fig. 15-14). This would avoid total transection of vital structures.

Incisional Biopsy. This is most often done for hyperkeratotic or ulcerated lesions. The direction of the incision should be oriented as depicted in Fig. 15-14. The surgeon should use experience and common sense in deciding how deep to take the biopsy. The operator should make sure that the sample that is removed is adequate to provide the pathologist with sufficient abnormal tissue to be able to make a good microscopic diagnosis.

Although tumor formation in the sublingual gland is very rare (less than 0.5% of all tumors that occur in the major salivary glands[8]), when they do occur they are almost 100% malignant.[8] Because of this, an incisional biopsy should always be performed for suspicious masses in this gland or of ulcerations of the oral mucosa that are associated with the sublingual gland.

Control of the Tongue. How the tongue is controlled is determined by where the biopsy is to be performed. For biopsy in the anterior portion of the floor of the mouth, it will be necessary to elevate the tongue. This can be achieved by passing a 0-silk suture through the tip of the tongue (Figs. 15-9, 15-10, and 15-14). In the lateral aspects of the floor of the mouth, the surgeon will need to keep the tongue steady and off to the side. This can be accomplished by using a retraction suture on the lateral tongue along with a Wieder (sweetheart) retractor (Fig. 15-15).

REFERENCES

1. Epstein E, Bragg K, Linden G: Biopsy and prognosis of malignant melanoma, *JAMA* 208: 1369, 1969.
2. Bertram U, Hjorting-Hansen E: Punch biopsy of minor salivary glands in the diagnosis of Sjogrens's syndrome, *Scand J Dent Res* 78:295-300, 1979.
3. Denis DP, Morris LF: The oral mucosal punch biopsy: indications and techniques. *JADA* 121:145-149, 1990.
4. Bernstein M: Biopsy techniques: the pathologic considerations, *JADA* 96:438-443, 1978.
5. Sheehan DC, Hrapchak BB: *Theory and practice of histotechnology*, ed 2, Battelle Pr., 1987, St. Louis.
6. Daniels TE, Quandra-White C: Direct-immunofluorescence in oral mucosal disease: a diagnostic analysis of 130 cases *Oral Surg* 51:38, 1981.
7. Solomon M: Personal communication. Oral Pathology Section, Dept. of Pathology, State University of New York, Health Science Center at Brooklyn, Brooklyn, NY, Aug. 1998.
8. Shafer WG, Hine MK, Levy BM: Tumors of the salivary gland. In: *A textbook of oral pathology*, Philadelphia, 1974, WB Saunders, Ch. 3.

PROSTHETIC SURGERY

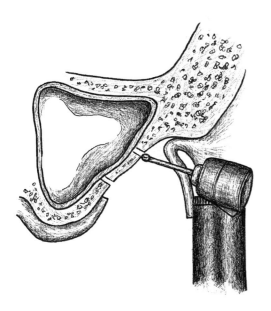

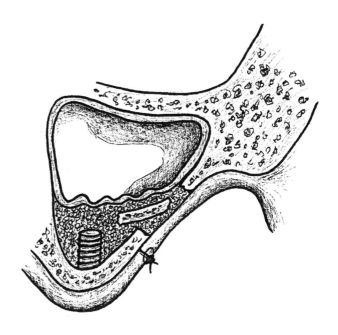

SECTION

VI

16 Minor Preprosthetic Surgery

DARSHAN J. PANCHAL, DDS
ORRETT E. OGLE, DDS

Preprosthetic surgery is concerned with the surgical modification of the alveolar process and its surrounding structures to enable the fabrication of a well-fitting, comfortable, and esthetic dental prosthesis. When the natural dentition is lost, changes will occur within the alveolus and the surrounding soft tissue. Some of these changes may interfere with the satisfactory fabrication of a denture. There may be edentulous bone loss (EBL), irregularities, undercuts, scarring, and changes in insertions of the perioral muscles. A careful and systematic evaluation of the intraoral denture-supporting tissues should therefore be performed before attempting masticatory rehabilitation with dentures.

An alveolar ridge with irregular bony projections and undercuts may pose a problem with adaptation and/or insertion of the prosthesis. Maxillary and mandibular tori may be areas that will be constantly irritated by a removable prosthesis. The maxillary tuberosity is also a well-known problem area in full denture construction. It is often an area of undercut that interferes with insertion; it may be enlarged, resulting in decreased interarch space, or it may be close to the mandibular ramus, allowing the denture to become unstable during opening. Inflammatory hyperplasia and epulis fissuratum can cause chronic irritation and infection such as candidiasis. Shallow vestibular depth adversely affects denture stability because it will result in denture displacement as a result of muscle function. In short, a number of anatomic factors affects dental prosthetic rehabilitation. Successful prosthetic treatment, therefore, involves recognition of these factors and their surgical management before final impressions are done. The goal of this chapter will be to provide basic techniques for the surgical management of some of these problems.

The following areas will be addressed:
1. Immediate dentures
2. Basic alveoplasty
3. Maxillary tori
4. Mandibular tori
5. Maxillary tuberosity
6. Epulis fissuratum
7. Papillary hyperplasia
8. Vestibuloplasty
9. Palatal grafts

GENERAL ARMAMENTARIUM

The following instruments will form the basic surgical tray for performing preprosthetic surgery:
- #15 surgical blade
- Bard Parker scalpel handle #3
- Molt periosteal elevator
- University of Minnesota cheek retractor
- Seldin elevator
- Blumenthal bone rongeurs
- Monobevel chisel and small mallet
- Straight fissure bur (surgical length)
- Large round or oval nongouging bur
- Tissue forceps
- Curved mosquito hemostat
- Metzenbaum scissors
- Bone file
- Needle holder
- Silk suture (3-0 on a cutting needle)
- Suture scissors

IMMEDIATE DENTURES

At times, because of periodontal disease, and sometimes rampant caries, it may be necessary to remove the teeth and go immediately to the prosthesis so that the patient will not face the embarrassment of having to go without teeth. The technique for immediate dentures requires specific planning and timing. In general, extraction of all remaining teeth at one sitting and insertion of immediate dentures is indicated only when the teeth can be extracted without complications and with minimal or no alveoplasty. When this is not the case, complicated extractions should be done before taking impressions because considerable changes of bony contour can occur. Complicated extractions consist of grossly carious teeth, teeth with large restorations, endodontically treated teeth, teeth with widely separated or curved roots, and impacted teeth. Patients with a history of difficult extractions should also be added to this menu. In addition, tori, if present, should be removed before taking impressions for immediate dentures.

When sequencing extractions for immediate dentures the mandibular molars should be removed first. The premolars should be spared for assessment of vertical dimension. The maxillary posterior teeth are removed at the second visit and the upper and lower anterior teeth are removed at the final visit of immediate denture insertion. The immediate dentures, as the name implies, are placed at the time of the final extractions.

Technique

After the posterior extraction sites are allowed to heal (approximately 6 weeks) the final impressions are taken. The impression technique for full dentures should be used. A custom tray is used, and border molding should be accurately performed. Accurate vertical dimension and centric occlusion are recorded. A wax set-up of the posterior teeth is done to verify the occlusion and the vertical dimension. Minimal occlusal adjustment should be done at the time of surgery. Special attention should be given to the tuberosity area as well as to the post-dam region.

Model surgery is performed by the dentist on the master cast to remove the remaining teeth, irregularities, and/or undercuts. When planning the model surgery, bone loss evident on the radiograph from periodontal disease, without a comparable recession of soft tissue, should be reflected in the shaping of the cast. Table 16-1 presents detailed steps for trimming of the cast for the immediate denture. Following the model surgery a clear surgical stent is fabricated on the altered master cast. The stent will aid the surgeon by acting as a guide during the procedure for alveolar contouring. The stent, when placed into the mouth at surgery, will

TABLE 16-1 Steps for Trimming the Cast for Immediate Dentures

Steps	Laboratory Procedure	Rationale
Step 1	Remove those parts of the crowns of the teeth that are visible above the free gingival margin.	This step will remove the major portion of the clinical crown, but not the portion that lies beneath the gingiva.
Step 2	Trim the cast at the previously removed crowns so that each site is recessed another 1 mm.	This represents the removal of the entire crown of each tooth.
Step 3	The third step is a beveled cut across the buccal surface of the ridge. Draw a line at the junction of the gingival and middle third of the buccal aspect of the alveolar ridge. Start removing stone at the labial depth of the recess made in the cast during step two. Stone is removed from this point in a continually diminishing amount to the line mentioned above.	The removal of this amount of stone represents the collapse of the labial gingiva toward the alveolus.
Step 4	Trim the labio/lingual aspect of the cast. This step involves contouring of the cast from the irregularities created from steps 2 and 3.	This step is to round out the occlusal and buccal aspects of the cast. This trim should be conservative.
Step 5	Completely remove all stone that represents the gingival cuff on the lingual/palatal aspect.	Most casts represent a reproduction of the continuous roll of gingival tissue that normally lies against the lingual aspect of the teeth. This roll of tissue will collapse into the alveolus after the teeth have been extracted and nothing is there to physically support it.
Step 6	Contour the cast further, if anatomic considerations dictate.	When mechanical, biologic, or aesthetic requirements dictate an alveoplasty, additional stone must be removed from the cast in an amount equal to the planned reduction of the bony process.
Step 7	Shape and smooth the surface of the cast. A Buffalo bench knife is used to remove sharp angles. Fine sandpaper is used to finish the master cast. (The laboratory technician can finish this step.) The vestibular third of the cast is never trimmed.	A smooth cast will give a better surgical stent with less irregularities.

Modified from Jerbi FC: Trimming the cast in the construction of immediate dentures. *J Prosth Dent* 16(6):1047-1054, 1966.

contact the soft tissue at various points. This will be seen as a blanching or flattening of the gingival tissue through the clear stent. These areas will require alveoplasty to prevent sore spots below the immediate denture. Sequential adjustments in this manner will lead to the final result of the stent seating intraorally in a similar fashion as it did on the model. This will now make the oral denture-bearing area similar to the altered cast. (The stent is constructed with a heat-cured clear acrylic.) The final cast (the trimmed cast) is used by the lab to complete the denture set-up and processing.

Surgery

The remaining teeth are extracted as atraumatically as possible. A buccal flap is then reflected. The extent of the flap is dependent on which areas of the alveolus will require modification. This is determined from prior knowledge of the model surgery. After each plastic recontouring of the ridge, the gingiva is repositioned, the stent inserted and examined by the surgeon. When the clear stent fits the ridge adequately, without rocking and without pressure points, the area is irrigated and closed with continuous sutures. Care must be taken not to pull the sutures too tight, to the point where they will place undue tension on the height of the buccal vestibule, or overlapping of the margins of the gingiva. The denture is inserted and the occlusion checked. The occlusion must be adjusted before the patient is discharged.

Analgesics and antibiotics are prescribed. The patient is advised not to remove the denture for 24 hours. The following day the patient is seen by the surgeon who will remove and clean the denture with water. Oral hygiene is performed daily by the patient, and sutures are removed in 7 days. A reline may be done in 6 months.

ALVEOPLASTY

Alveoplasty is defined as the contouring of the alveolar process. It is performed to smooth out bony irregularities, eliminate undercuts, and prepare the residual ridge for prosthesis. The goals are to create a firm and stable base for a dental prosthesis while preserving as much alveolar tissue and bone as possible. Conservatism should be the preeminent guide. Alveoplasty should never be used to correct jaw discrepancy problems (such as overjet). Jaw size discrepancy should be corrected by orthognathic surgery and not radical removal of the buccal cortical plate. Biologically sound techniques such as maxillary segmental surgery have been described and give good results without sacrificing the anterior alveolar bone or invading the cortical plate.[1]

Technique

Adequate local anesthesia is obtained. A few milliliters of the local anesthesia is injected subperiosteally to facilitate elevation of the mucoperiosteal flap from the irregular ridge without tearing of the mucosa. Using a #15 blade, a crestal incision is made over the target area and extended in both directions to allow for adequate access to permit the surgical objective (Fig. 16-1). Minimal raising of the gingiva is recommended so that only a minimum of the alveolar bone is exposed. Large flaps will increase bone resorption and will cause further obliteration of the sulcus as it will be displaced by the sutures. Infrequently vertical releasing incisions may be used for additional access. A full-thickness mucoperiosteal flap is reflected using the periosteal elevator and retained with a Seldin elevator or the Minnesota retractor (Fig. 16-2).

Bony contouring is accomplished with a bone file, rongeurs, and/or a large nongouging round bur mounted atop a slow speed handpiece (see Fig. 16-2). A bone file should be the final instrument used to smooth out any sharp irregularities. As a rule, the ridge need not be perfectly smooth, but sharp edges, large prominences, and deep undercuts should be eliminated. Digital palpation is used to determine uniformity and smoothness. This is done through the gingiva which is repositioned and not directly on the bone. When the surgeon is satisfied with the plastic remodeling of the bone, the underside of the flap is irrigated to remove all loose pieces of bone and bone dust. The flap is replaced to its original position and the wound closed using interrupted or continuous sutures to obtain a watertight seal (Fig. 16-3). The sutures should not strangle the soft tissues, however, neither should they displace the sulci

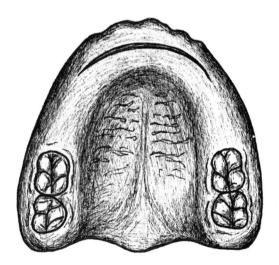

FIG. 16-1 Site of crestal incision for performing alveoplasty of the maxillary anterior. The same incision may be used for alveoplasty at any other location.

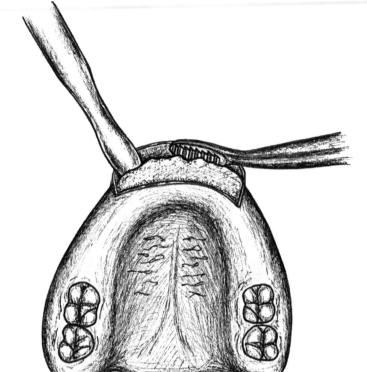

FIG. 16-2 Reflection of a full thickness mucoperiosteal flap to expose the buccal aspect of the alveolar crest for alveoplasty. The tissue is reflected and gently retracted with a Seldin elevator.

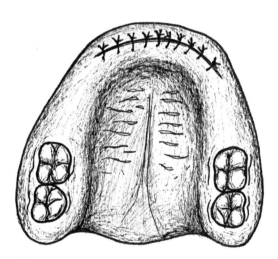

FIG. 16-3 Closure of incision following alveoplasty.

significantly. The sutures are left in place for 5 to 7 days. An antibiotic is recommended, but is not absolutely necessary. Adequate analgesics should be prescribed.

In the age of dental implants, compression alveoplasty (squeezing of the cortical walls of the socket following removal of teeth and interseptal bone) is not recommended so that buccolingual width may be preserved for future implant placement. Secondary alveoplasty should also not decrease the width of the alveolar crest significantly.

MAXILLARY TORUS

A maxillary torus is a sessile mass of dense, cortical bone in the midline of the palate. Not all tori need removal. The following are indications to remove a palatal torus:

- Constant trauma to the overlying mucosa during mastication
- When the torus interferes with denture construction by preventing a good post dam seal or has large undercuts that interfere with impression techniques
- Very large lobulated tori
- Speech impediment
- Psychological phobia (malignancy paranoia)

A maxillary torus should be studied by a true lateral radiograph to rule out the possibility of pneumatization of the torus. It has been reported that on occasion the nasal floor dips downward in the area of the palatal torus.[2] Removal of such a torus could lead to a traumatic cleft palate (oronasal communication). This phenomenon, however, seems to be rare as we have never seen a case in over 25 years.

Technique

A maxillary impression is taken and a cast poured. The torus is removed on this cast and a clear acrylic stent is made. The stent will aid to support the flap, prevent

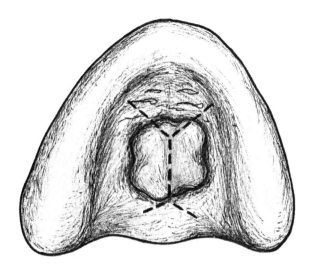

FIG. 16-4   Outline of the soft tissue incision used to expose the maxillary torus. An inverted Y incision is used, but in a large torus a double Y incision is used. This will permit easier retraction of the palatal tissue.

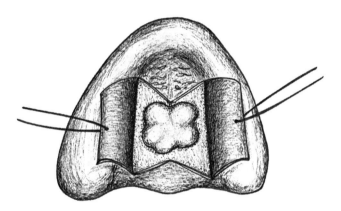

FIG. 16-5   A periosteal elevator is used to reflect a full thickness mucoperiosteal flap, which is then retained with 3-0 silk retraction sutures. The palatal tissue over the torus is very delicate and care must be taken not to tear this extremely thin and friable mucosa of the flap by pulling excessively on the retraction sutures.

hematoma formation, wound protection from food intake, and in postoperative patient comfort. (Some surgeons, however, opt not to use a stent, but it is our opinion that the patient will be more comfortable with the stent.)

Local anesthesia with a vasoconstrictor is given around and also into the torus to facilitate elevation of the thin mucoperiosteal tissue that usually covers the torus. (This technique is referred to as hydrodissection.) The operator should wait for at least 7 minutes to ensure the full hemostatic effects of the vasoconstrictor.

An inverted Y incision is used to expose the torus (Fig. 16-4). Using the periosteal elevator, a full thickness mucoperiosteal flap is elevated and retained

with 3-0 silk retraction sutures (Fig. 16-5). Care is taken not to tear the extremely thin and friable mucosa of the flap by pulling excessively on these sutures, however.

After the entire torus is fully exposed, it is scored to the desired depth in a crisscross pattern with a fissure bur using copious irrigation (Fig. 16-6). The depth should be to about 1.0 to 2.0 mm above the level of the horizontal palatal shelf. The creation of these multiple segments will allow removal of the torus with little risk of fracturing of the palate and inadvertent perforation into the nasal cavity. A chisel and mallet are used to remove the individual segments (Fig. 16-7, *A*). The final smoothing is done with a large, oval, nongouging bur (Fig. 16-7, *B*) under copious irrigation, taking care not to perforate into the nasal cavity. (The entire torus may be removed by a large acrylic bur without the use of chisels. This is, however, more prone to complications as the bur may traumatize the tongue, lip, or palatal mucosa. Perforation and gouging is also more common). It is better to leave a small elevation rather than risking perforation into the nasal passageway. The area is thoroughly irrigated, the flap trimmed and loosely sutured with 3-0 silk or Vicryl using interrupted sutures. The stent is inserted and secured. In the edentulous patient the stent may be made from thermoplastic material used in the Vacu-Form as this will be easily retained. Alternatively, an acrylic splint may be fabricated with the flanges made short of the vestibule, which is relined with a soft relining material at the time of surgery.

The splint is retained in place for 48 hours, after which time it is removed by the surgeon to clean and to inspect the wound. The stent is worn over the operative site until healing is satisfactory (usually about 2 weeks). The splint is removed after each meal and in the mornings and at bedtime for cleansing.

Complications

Because of the thin nature of the palatal bone, the patient must be informed of the possibility of an oral-nasal fistula.

Postoperative sloughing of the mucosal flap is common and not a problem because granulation tissue will eventually cover the defect. Denuded palatal bone is not excessively painful and it heals very well without significant scarring within about 1 month. Sloughing can be minimized by trimming away any dusky, friable, and macerated tissue during closure.

MANDIBULAR TORI

The mandibular torus is usually located on the lingual surface of the mandible in the region of the premolars

FIG. 16-6 After the entire torus is fully exposed, it is scored to the desired depth in a crisscross pattern with a fissure bur using copious irrigation. The depth should be to about 1.0 to 2.0 mm above the level of the horizontal palatal shelf. The creation of these multiple segments will allow removal of the torus with little risk of fracturing of the palate and inadvertent perforation into the nasal cavity.

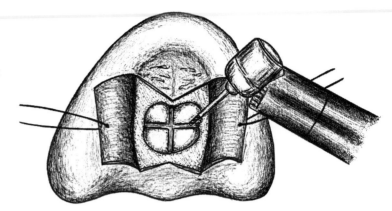

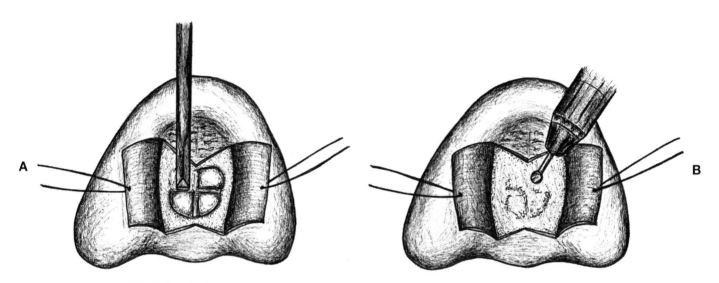

FIG. 16-7 **A,** A chisel and mallet are used to remove the individual segments. When a monobevel chisel is used the bevel is placed against the palatal shelf. A bibevel chisel may be used as shown in this figure. **B,** Following removal of the gross segments, the final smoothing is done with a large oval nongouging bur under copious irrigation, taking care not to perforate into the nasal cavity. It is better to leave a small elevation rather than risk perforation into the nasal passageway. *(The entire torus may be removed by a large acrylic bur without the use of chisels.)*

and the first molar. They are commonly bilateral and may be single or multiple. They almost always will require removal if a mandibular removable prosthesis is being considered. On occasion, a dentate patient will want removal secondary to chronic irritation or malignancy phobia.

Technique

Local anesthesia consisting of an inferior alveolar block, lingual nerve block, and local infiltration onto the torus is performed (hydrodissection).

In an edentulous patient, the incision is made crestally of sufficient length to expose the entire torus (usually 2 teeth's width in both directions beyond the torus). In dentate patients, the incision is placed in the lingual gingival sulcus (Fig. 16-8).

An envelope flap is reflected with the periosteal elevator to about 1 cm below the torus, and long enough to expose the entire torus. A 2×2 gauze sponge may be placed below the torus, or a wide elevator (Seldin) placed below the segment of bone to be removed. This is to prevent the loss of the excised bone into the soft tissues of the floor of the mouth (Fig. 16-9). Vertical releases are never done.

Next, a 2-mm deep groove is placed with a fissure bur

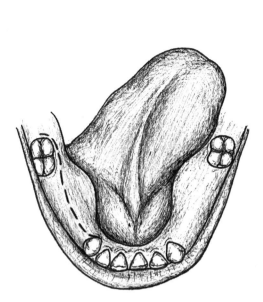

FIG. 16-8 Placement of an incision on the lingual aspect of the gingiva for the removal of a mandibular torus. In an edentulous patient, the incision is made on the crest of sufficient length to expose the entire torus (usually two teeth's' length in both directions beyond the torus). In dentate patients, the incision is placed in the lingual gingival sulcus.

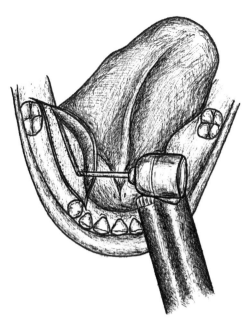

FIG. 16-10 A 2-mm deep groove is placed with a fissure bur onto the superior margin of the torus at the junction of where the exostosis of the torus meets the lingual body of the mandible.

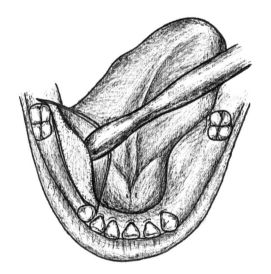

FIG. 16-9 An envelope flap is reflected with the periosteal elevator to about 1 cm below the torus, and long enough to expose the entire torus. A 2×2 gauge sponge may be placed below the torus, or a wide elevator (Seldin) placed below the segment of bone to be removed. This is to prevent the loss of the excised bone into the soft tissues of the floor of the mouth.

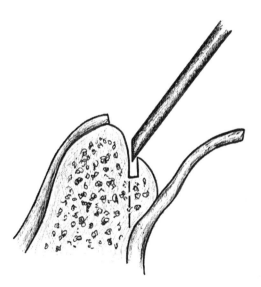

FIG. 16-11 A monobevel chisel being used to remove the mandibular torus. The chisel is introduced into the crestal groove with the angled bevel facing the body of the mandible, and is tapped with a mallet while the jaw is being supported by the patient or by an assistant.

onto the superior margin of the torus at the junction of where the exostosis of the torus meets the lingual body of the mandible (Fig. 16-10). If the torus is long, then vertical cuts should be carefully placed in the torus to create multiple segments. A monobevel chisel is intro-

duced into the crestal groove with the angled bevel facing the body of the mandible (Fig. 16-11). The chisel is then tapped with a mallet while the chin is supported manually. After the bony mass is dislodged, the rough bony surface may be smoothed with a bone file or a large round nongouging bur. The flap is irrigated and closed with either interrupted or continuous suturing technique using 3-0 silk or Vicryl sutures. If edges of the soft tissue overlap, the excess tissue should be trimmed with a curved Metzenbaum scissors so that the edges will approximate each other. A gauze pack is placed beneath the tongue to facilitate readaptation of the lingual flap as well as to prevent hematoma formation.

Complications

When removing bilateral tori, it is important to keep the midline between the two flaps intact. This prevents the formation of a bilateral sublingual hematoma, which can potentially pose a threat to the airway.

Displacement of bone chips and other debris can also lead to a late infection in the sublingual space. This can be minimized by limiting the depth of the flap dissection and by placing a protective Seldin retractor at the inferior portion of the flap, and by thorough irrigation after the procedure.

MAXILLARY TUBEROSITY

Hypertrophy of the maxillary tuberosity may be either fibrous or bony in nature. The enlargement may either be in the vertical or horizontal planes (or both). A lateral bulbous tuberosity can be tolerated if it is unilateral and adequate space exists for the buccal flange of the denture base. This can be determined clinically by seeing if there is sufficient space for a dental mirror to fit between the tuberosity and the ascending ramus of the mandible without difficulty in opening and closing. Bilateral tuberosity enlargement on the lateral aspects, however, will require reduction.

Vertically enlarged tuberosities will need reduction if the interarch space is less than 1 cm at the vertical dimension of occlusion (to provide space for the denture bases). In general, the intermaxillary distance measured from the crest of the tuberosity to the retromolar area of the mandible should equal at least a centimeter when the mandible is placed in a position corresponding to the correct vertical dimension of occlusion.[3] Before the attempted reduction of the tuberosity, adequate radiographs should be obtained (a good quality panographic radiograph). This will determine if the enlargement is fibrous or bony in nature, and to make sure that the maxillary sinus has not dipped down into the tuberosity itself.

General Technique

Reduction of Fibrous Tuberosity. The objective of this procedure is to reduce the fibrous enlargement of the tuberosity to a size and shape that will change its contour to conform with the rest of the alveolar ridge. Wedge resection is the preferred technique. As a rule, one third of the bulbous mass will be removed from the center and the remaining two sides undermined submucosally, compressed, and then sutured. However, the larger the tuberosity, the greater the wedge will have to be. Using a #15 blade, an elliptical incision is made over the crest of the tuberosity down to bone (Fig. 16-12). The wedge-shaped cuts should start on the crest of the ridge at the junction of normal ridge and the area of fibrous hypertrophy, and end at the most posterior part of the tuberosity close to the pterygomaxillary fissure. The wedge is grasped with an Allis forceps, and lifted while it is freed from the cortical bone at the base. This may be achieved by a combination of sharp and blunt dissection until the resulting wedge is removed (see Fig. 16-12).

A periosteal elevator is used to reflect a buccal flap. A Minnesota retractor is used to hold the flap (Fig. 16-13). Submucous resection is then accomplished through both buccal and palatal flaps using the #15 blade. These cuts are made parallel to the bony surface. The submucous wedges are then excised (Fig. 16-14, *A* and *B*). The surgeon removes the submucosa fibromatous tissue until by trial both flaps will meet in the midline without being under tension.

Reduction of Bony Tuberosity. A crestal incision is made starting from behind the tuberosity to approximately 10 mm beyond the intended area of bony reduction. To incise behind the tuberosity a #12 blade should be used. At the end of the crestal incision a vertical releasing incision is placed. This incision should angle 135° to the crestal incision to provide a wide-based flap. This incision should be down to bone. A periosteal elevator is used to raise a buccal flap to expose the entire aspect of the bony tuberosity. If there is an undercut area, care should be taken not to perforate or lacerate the mucosa at the depth of

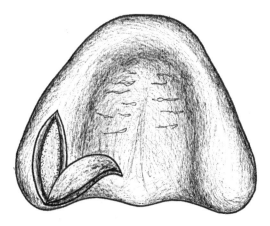

FIG. 16-12 An elliptical incision made over the crest of the tuberosity down to bone.

the undercut as this may compromise the blood supply to the flap and cause subsequent sloughing of the mucosa. Bone may now be removed using a side cutting rongeur or a large oval acrylic bur if rotary instruments are preferred. After the buccal contouring is completed, free the palatal mucosa, and make whatever plastic contouring that will be necessary. (See Chapter 2, "Regional Surgical Anatomy," for anatomy of the palatine artery.)

The area is smoothed with a bone file and irrigated. Replace the soft tissues over the bony tuberosity and note the overlap. With the Metzenbaum scissors cut away the excess soft tissue so that the flaps may be closed without tissue overlap or undue tension. It is better to have a little excess tissue than not to have enough. Closure is made by a running continuous 3-0 suture.

Complications

The major complication will be accidental perforation into the maxillary sinus. If the maxillary sinus is exposed, good soft tissue closure will usually avoid fistulation.

EPULIS FISSURATUM

Arising from chronic denture irritation, epulis fissuratum can interfere with denture stability and comfort. Epulides fissurata are histologically submucosal fibroses. They are usually inflamed, and will benefit from some treatment before surgical removal. This may be done by discontinuation of the denture for 2 weeks prior to surgical treatment, or by relieving the denture in the area of irritation and lining it with tissue conditioner. This method may require several weeks for maximal resolution. The patient should be followed weekly and the remaining epulis removed when the surgeon determines that maximal spontaneous resolution has occurred.

General Technique

Following the administration of local anesthesia with a vasoconstrictor the base of the tumor-like growths are carefully grasped with as many Allis forceps as are necessary to outline the base so that an incision line is well demarcated. When the Allis forceps are in place they are held by the surgeon. The assistant should retract the upper lip to ensure that the lip muscles are

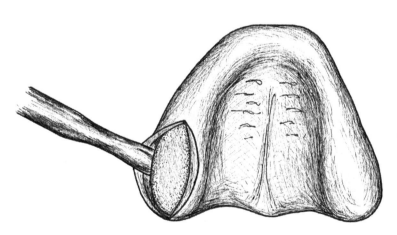

FIG. 16-13 Reflection of a buccal flap to expose the bony tuberosity. A Minnesota retractor is used to hold the flap.

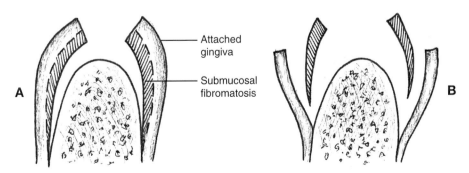

Attached gingiva

Submucosal fibromatosis

FIG. 16-14 **A** and **B,** Excision of submucosal fibrous tissue for the reduction of a fibrously enlarged tuberosity.

not excised with the epulides. The superior line of the epulis is incised first, staying parallel to the bone and not violating the periosteum. The mass is raised by the Allis forceps and the inferior cut is made to remove the entire growth. In placing the inferior mucosal incision, it is preferable to retain as much attached mucosa as possible. This is done by making certain that there is a clearly defined line of separation between the epulides and the crestal gingiva. In this way the fibrotic tissue can be fully excised and the attached mucosa may be spared. The incisions may be done with a scalpel blade, but our preference is to use an electrosurgery unit (Bovie). Excess tissue tabs are trimmed with a Dean scissors. Bleeding points are controlled with electrocautery.

We do not try to get primary closure of the wound as we have found that this tends to roll the lip inward and decrease the amount of vermilion show. This makes the lip look short, bulky, and unaesthetic. Instead we prefer to trim the overextended, ill-fitting denture and re-line it with soft reline at surgery. This dressing is removed at 48 hours and cleaned. The patient wears this prosthesis until adequate healing has occurred. At about 6 weeks new prosthetic rehabilitation may be started. If alveolar height is not adequate for a suitable removable denture then some form of implant restoration should be considered (see Section VII, Chapters 19 and 20 on implants). The excised tissue should be sent for histopathologic examination.

PAPILLARY HYPERPLASIA

Papillary hyperplasia (denture stomatitis) generally occurs in edentulous patients wearing ill-fitting dentures. Around-the-clock denture use is associated with increased incidence but the condition has been known to occur in denture-free patients. Treatment is initially conservative, entailing a denture reline and decreased use. Existing candidiasis should be treated with the appropriate fungicides. The practitioner should keep in mind that when candidiasis is present, both the oral cavity and the denture should be treated. Digital massage therapy has also been shown to be of benefit. If conservative therapy is not sufficient, then surgical therapy must be considered.

General Technique

A biopsy is initially performed to confirm the diagnosis. A small elliptical wedge is taken from the anomaly avoiding the greater palatine vessels. Radical excision of this lesion is unjustified. The lesions can adequately be removed with the use of an antral curette. The small pedunculated masses are removed by scraping with the

curette until the corium (the dense white tissue below the epithelium) is reached (Fig. 16-15).

Mucoabrasion with a large, slow-moving, nongouging round bur is another option. Irrigation should be used for this technique. Electrocautery can also be used if it is available and preferred. If electrocautery is used, the patient should be grounded. Care should be taken not to burn the perioral tissues. A looped electrode is very effective for this procedure. The loop is used to slowly remove the papillomatosis in a paintbrush fashion. Total removal may require several procedures.

Following excision, the relined denture or prefabricated acrylic stent with soft reline (e.g., Coe-Comfort) may be used for hemostasis and wound protection. Healing by secondary epithelialization is usually complete within 3 to 5 weeks.

VESTIBULOPLASTY
General Considerations

Traditionally, the goal of preprosthetic surgery has been to provide for a large and comfortable tissue foundation (denture-bearing area) to support the prosthesis. Vestibuloplasty and ridge augmentation are the most commonly used techniques. More currently, the success of osseointegrated implants has revolutionized the treatment of edentulism. Appropriate selection between vestibuloplasty, ridge augmentation, and implants is a multifactorial decision based on anatomic, medical, social, and financial considerations. In general, vestibuloplasty is used when adequate alveolar bone exists but the surrounding soft tissue impedes denture flange construction. Specific indications are discussed with the individual procedures. Ridge augmentation is necessary when severe resorption has occurred, rendering the bony anatomy as unusable or at risk for jaw fracture.

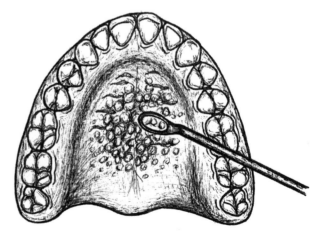

FIG. 16-15 The small pedunculated masses of papillary hyperplasia are removed by scraping with an antral curette until the corium (the dense white tissue below the epithelium) is reached.

Ridge augmentation is also used to provide a substrate for implant placement. Ridge augmentation for implants is discussed elsewhere in this text. This section will discuss the various forms of vestibuloplasty and their related procedures.

In vestibuloplasty the soft tissue and insertions of the muscles of facial expression are detached surgically and allowed to heal in a more apical position thus exposing more of the basal bone. The incision is placed at the junction of the attached and unattached mucosa (Fig. 16-16, A). This incision should only be through the superficial mucosa and should not violate the periosteum. A supraperiosteal dissection is done (Fig. 16-16, B). It is easier to do this dissection with a blade. This is done by filleting the muscular attachments from the periosteum. The dissection is then completed by further displacing the remaining soft tissues from the periosteum. An attempt should be made to be as close to the periosteum as possible. Small perforations through the periosteum will not cause major problems, but they should be avoided.

The purpose of the vestibuloplasty is to expose more bone preventing dislodgment of the denture by the abnormal muscle insertions into the remaining alveolar ridge. The denuded area that is surgically created may be handled in several ways. The simplest method is to let the area heal by secondary intention (Fig. 16-16, C). This method, however, has up to a 50% relapse rate. Another more successful method is to graft the defect with palatal mucosa, commercially available collagen membranes, or cadaveric mucosal membranes.

Lipswitch Vestibuloplasty[4,5]

Also known as the crestally pedicled mucosal graft, the lipswitch procedure is designed to increase a shallow mandibular labial sulcus anterior to the mental foramina. At least 15 mm of vertical ridge height is essential in the anterior mandible for a successful result. Local anesthesia is given in the form of bilateral inferior alveolar blocks and local infiltrations along the ridge and lower lip for hemostasis. The desired vestibular depth is visualized. This incision is started 1.5 times this desired depth away from the attached mucosa on the lower lip (Fig. 16-17). A mucosal flap is elevated and pedicled at the crestal attached gingiva (Fig. 16-18). This is done with the use of a Metzenbaum scissors. An incision is placed through submucosa and periosteum at below the pedicle near the crest and a subperiosteal flap is elevated inferiorly to the desired vestibular depth (Fig. 16-19). This periosteal flap is then sutured to the incised lip margin with interrupted resorbable suture. The free mucosal flap is then sutured to the base of the dissection inferiorly with a 4-0 resorbable suture (Fig. 16-20).

A pressure dressing is placed over the chin to provide close adaptation of the mucosal flap to bone. This is performed using 0.5 inch medical tape running from cheek to cheek crossing over the chin. The dressing is worn for 48 hours. Denture construction can begin in 3 months.

Complications. The mental nerves may be traumatized during the procedure and a temporary and/or permanent paresthesia may develop. The patient must

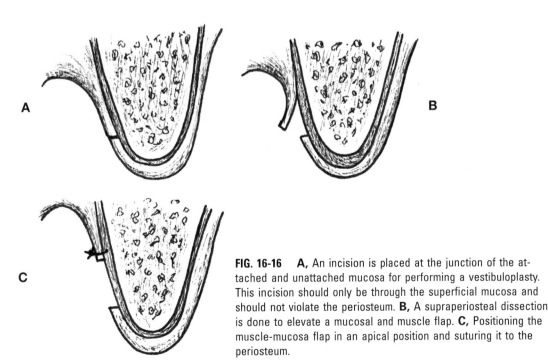

FIG. 16-16 **A,** An incision is placed at the junction of the attached and unattached mucosa for performing a vestibuloplasty. This incision should only be through the superficial mucosa and should not violate the periosteum. **B,** A supraperiosteal dissection is done to elevate a mucosal and muscle flap. **C,** Positioning the muscle-mucosa flap in an apical position and suturing it to the periosteum.

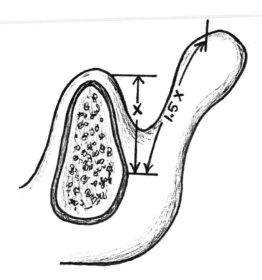

FIG. 16-17 The incision for the lipswitch vestibuloplasty is started 1.5 times this desired depth away from the attached mucosa on the lower lip.

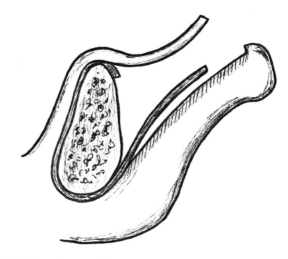

FIG. 16-19 A second incision is placed through submucosa and periosteum below the pedicle near the crest, and a subperiosteal flap is elevated inferiorly to the desired vestibular depth. This periosteal flap is scored at the intended vestibular depth to permit the placement of sutures.

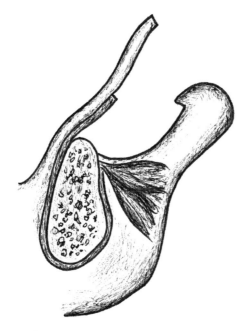

FIG. 16-18 Development of the crestal pedicled mucosal flap.

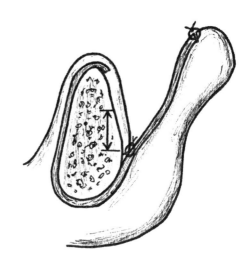

FIG. 16-20 The superior portion of the periosteal flap is sutured to the incised lip margin with an interrupted resorbable suture. The free mucosal flap is then sutured to the base of the dissection inferiorly with a 4-0 resorbable suture.

be fully informed of this possibility before the procedure.

Submucous Vestibuloplasty

The submucous vestibuloplasty, or Obwegeser vestibuloplasty, is primarily advocated for the anterior maxilla. It has been used for the mandible but with generally poor results (as shown by Obwegeser in 1959[6]). This vestibuloplasty is commonly indicated in patients who have low mucosal and muscle attachments but have adequate bone structure in the maxilla.

To test if this procedure can be done a dental mirror is placed into the depth of the mucobuccal fold and is pushed up about 1.0 cm to simulate the increase in vestibular depth. The surgeon pays attention to the vermilion of the upper lip. If the upward push in the vestibule has no effect on the vermilion

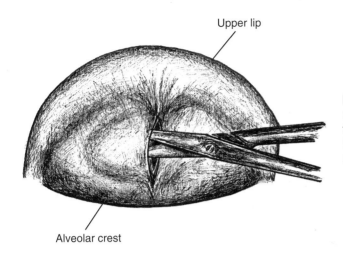

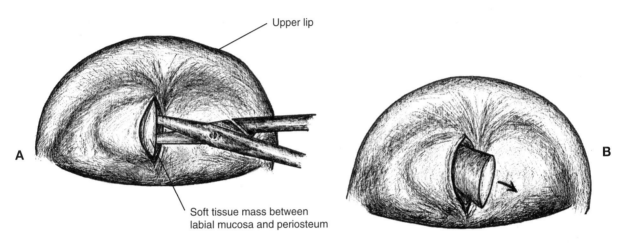

FIG. 16-21 A midline incision made just through the mucosa of the upper lip and through the gingiva to the periosteum, but not through the periosteum itself. Using a Metzenbaum scissors, a flap consisting entirely of labial mucosa is raised from the inner aspect of the upper lip.

FIG. 16-22 **A** and **B,** Using a combination of blunt and sharp dissection, the underlying submucosal tissues are removed from between the mucosal flap and the periosteum.

then the procedure can be done. If the vermilion of the lip rolls inward, however, then the procedure should not be done, as it would compromise the esthetic of the face.

General Technique. In essence, the submucous vestibuloplasty uses mucosa of the upper lip to increase the vestibular depth. The lip is raised and held taut. A midline incision is made just through the mucosa of the upper lip and through the gingiva to the periosteum, but not through the periosteum itself (Fig. 16-21). Using a Metzenbaum scissors, a flap consisting entirely of mucous membrane is raised from the inner aspect of the upper lip (see Fig. 16-21). This is done by using blunt dissection with the scissors to separate the mucosa from the submucosa. From this midline pocket, the dissection is taken to about the first premolar area, or to an area where the depth is already adequate. Using a combination of blunt and sharp dissection the underlying submucosal tissues are removed from between the mucosal flap and the periosteum (Fig. 16-22, *A* and *B*).

This supraperiosteal dissection is done to a distance superiorly that would correspond to the envisioned height of the new vestibule.

Using horizontal mattress sutures the labial mucosal flap is adapted directly to the periosteum and repositioned superiorly to increase the vestibular depth (Fig. 16-23). This tacking of the labial mucosa to the periosteum is done with 3-0 Vicryl on a large tapered needle. The needle is passed down to the bone, slides along the bone for 7 to 10 mm and then exits the mucosa, and is tied to keep the labial mucosa firmly adherent to the periosteum. Sutures are placed at several points. The space between each suture should be about 5 mm. Placing these sutures may be tedious and not being able to engage the periosteum is sometimes problematic. The choice of needle size is important, and the surgeon should have access to needles of at least two sizes. A prefabricated stent is used to maintain the new vestibular depth and ensure close adaptation of the mucosa. It is left in place for 1 week. The denture may be con-

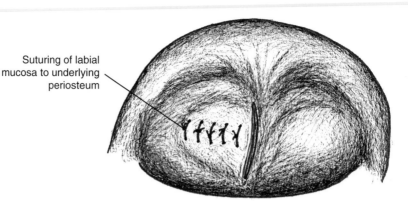

FIG. 16-23 Using horizontal mattress sutures, the labial mucosal flap is adapted directly to the periosteum and repositioned superiorly to increase the vestibular depth. This tacking of the labial mucosa to the periosteum is done with 3-0 Vicryl on a large tapered needle.

Suturing of labial mucosa to underlying periosteum

structed soon after the patient is comfortable enough to tolerate the impressions for full denture prostheses.

Complications

If enough labial mucosa is not present in the vestibule, the upper lip may roll inward, resulting in a thinning effect of the upper lip. This can usually be tested for preoperatively with a dental mirror pushed up into the labial fold to evaluate the degree of roll in. In any case, the patient should be well aware and informed of this possibility.

PALATAL GRAFT

The hard palate is a very versatile and useful donor site for grafting relatively small defects in the dental area of the oral cavity. The palatal graft can provide keratinized gingival tissue for coverage, supplementation, and reconstruction of oral soft tissue defects. It is conveniently harvested and affords minimal donor site morbidity. It can be used to restore defects for gingival recession, provide keratinized tissue for an implant collar, or even supply depth for various vestibuloplasty procedures.

General Technique

Local anesthesia is given to the donor site. A vasoconstrictor is preferable for hemostasis and the local should be allowed to sit for at least 7 minutes before the harvest. The required area of graft is determined and outlined. To judge the depth of the incision we have found that using a #10 blade, and sinking it to the depth of the bevel on the blade will provide an adequate thickness of palatal tissue for grafting. Going too deep into the palatal mucosa runs the risk of injuring the greater palatine artery, which can be a source of brisk bleeding. The palatine vessels usually run very intimately with the periosteum.

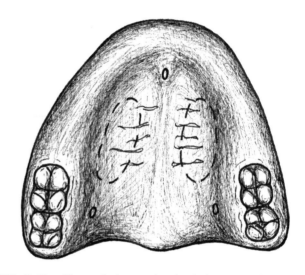

FIG. 16-24 Site and shape of palatal tissue which may be harvested for soft tissue grafting procedures.

Once the incision is outlined it can sometimes be difficult to start the removal of the graft. One trick is to take the anterior 1 mm deeper after the outline has been made, then start the harvesting at this point with a #15 blade. Lifting the edge with a mouse tooth forceps, and using a combination of a blade and a Metzenbaum scissors, the wedge of palatal tissue is carefully dissected supraperiosteally and removed (Fig. 16-24). Bleeding points are controlled with cautery. Collagen may be placed to further control bleeding.

After removal, the graft is inspected for the presence of fatty and glandular tissue on its undersurface. All excessive fatty tissue is removed so that adequate diffusion of nutrients can occur between host bed and the free graft. The graft may then be adapted to the host site. Critical to the success of any free graft is its stability and close adaptation. Thus, it should be sutured to a snug fit to the host bed. Angiogenesis into the graft occurs within 48 hours and complete healing may take up to 5 weeks.

SECONDARY EPITHELIALIZATION PROCEDURE

This technique has been mentioned previously but has very little use today. The only time that we use this procedure is in the treatment of maxillary epulis fissuratum. It is named as such because the additional vestibular depth is gained from tissue healing by secondary intention (granulation). The effectiveness of this procedure is limited because of the commonly observed relapse of the muscle and soft tissue attachments back to their existing levels. The lipswitch procedure and a palatal graft will give better and more stable results. In severe cases the use of endosseous implants should be considered.

Although the results are poor, we still will present the technique for this procedure.

General Technique

In order to increase the labial sulcus of the maxilla, an incision is made at the junction of the free and attached gingiva from tuberosity to tuberosity or as needed.[7]

An oblique releasing incision may be placed posteriorly on both sides if desired. A submucosal flap is elevated, leaving only the periosteum (see Fig. 16-16, A and B). This flap is elevated superiorly to the floor of the nose in the anterior and to the buttress of the zygoma in the posterior. The edge of this repositioned flap is sutured as far apically as possible with 3-0 Vicryl suture in an interrupted fashion (see Fig. 16-16, C). A stent fabricated with its flange extended to the projected new vestibular depth is inserted, and is kept in for 1 to 2 weeks. On the mandible, these stents were traditionally held to the mandible with circumferential wiring. (circummandibular wiring). Where retention is more on the maxilla the stent may be retained with a bone screw. If the bone is not exposed, a pseudomembrane will form which will then be replaced by granulation tissue. Dentures should not contact this membrane until epithelialization is complete (4 to 6 weeks). The operator can expect a 50% loss of the attained increase in vestibular depth within the first year. This occurs despite the patient wearing a prosthesis.

REFERENCES

1. West RA, Burke JL: Maxillary osteotomies for preprosthetic surgery, *J Oral Surg* 32:13, 1974.
2. Goodsell J, Morin GE: Abnormalities of the mouth. In Kruger GO: *Textbook of oral surgery*, St. Louis, 1974, Mosby, ch. 6.
3. Scott RF, Olson RAJ: Minor preprosthetic procedures. In Fonseca RJ, Davis WH, editors: *Reconstructive preprosthetic oral and maxillofacial surgery*, ed 2, Philadelphia, 1995, WB Saunders, ch. 4.
4. Godwin JG: Submucous surgery for better denture service. *JADA* 34:678-686, 1947.
5. Kethly JL, Gamble JW: The lipswitch: a modification of Kazanjian's labial vestibuloplasty, *J Oral Surg* 36:701-705, 1978.
6. Obwegesser HL: Die submukose Vestibulumplastik, *Dtsch Zahnarztl Z* 14:629-649, 1959.
7. Clark HB: Deepening of the labial sulcus by mucosal flap advancement. Report of a case, *J Oral Surg* 11:165, 1953.

The goal of modern dentistry is to prevent the loss of teeth, and to restore the human dentition when teeth have been lost. Today many great technological advances are at our disposal. We have used fluoride in the fight against dental caries. The mechanisms of periodontal disease have been researched extensively, which has allowed us, in many cases, to arrest the progression of bone loss allowing many people to maintain their dentition for a lifetime. Severely carious teeth can be restored with durable, esthetic materials, which will last for longer periods of time than those previously available. Yet with these great advances in knowledge and in restorative materials some teeth will not be salvageable and must be removed. With the advent of dental implants in the early 1980s we are now able to restore the dentition to a more natural state, and with better function. However, obstacles may be encountered with bony morphology when implants are considered. The major obstacle is lack of supportive bone to allow proper positioning of the dental implant in the alveolus and ultimately a functional prosthesis. This leads us to the topic of this chapter, which is dedicated to bone grafting of the alveolar ridge in preparation for the placement of dental implants. We will discuss the approach to the initial evaluation of the edentulous ridge, the types of bone grafts available with their respective harvesting techniques, the basic healing process that takes place, and finally techniques for the placement of the bone graft. A step-by-step guide to bone grafting will be presented in an easy-to-follow manner.

DIAGNOSIS AND TREATMENT PLANNING FOR BONE AUGMENTATION

After the decision is made to place implants for the replacement of lost teeth a complete oral exam must be performed paying particular attention to the edentulous ridge. The following are prerequisite for a proper implant work-up:

- A complete intraoral examination
- Radiographs, and in select cases a CT scan (Denta Scan). This may be necessary in cases in which neurovascular bundles must be avoided or paranasal sinus must be clearly identified.
- Study models

Clinical Examination

The attached gingiva must be examined to ensure that there will be enough keratinized mucosa for emergence of the implant. The minimal amount of attached gingiva is controversial, but in my opinion there should be 1 to 2 mm of attached gingiva to create a biologic seal around the implant abutment.

Another parameter that must be carefully examined is bone height. The amount of bone necessary to support an implant may vary with its location in the oral cavity. For example, if it is to be placed in the anterior mandible 10 mm is likely to be adequate whereas in the posterior maxilla at least 13 mm would be required. Although bone height is most often the first aspect of the examination, bone morphology is also important. The bone height may be adequate but if the ridge width is narrow or a concavity exists on the buccal, implant placement is not advised unless a bone graft is used in conjunction. At this point a technique known as "sounding the bone" is used to determine bone width. After local anesthesia is administered, a periodontal probe is used to measure gingival thickness at five different points around the ridge as depicted in Fig. 17-1, A and B. The areas that are "sounded" should be noted. After these measurements are recorded they will be transferred to a study model. This is accomplished by cutting the study model in the exact vertical location where the planned implant will be placed and transferring the probe measurements to the study model in the same manner in which they were recorded on the patient. Using a pencil the dots recorded are connected simulating the approximate bone width. This is a simple method that takes a few extra minutes but is cost effective when compared with a CT scan and gives the

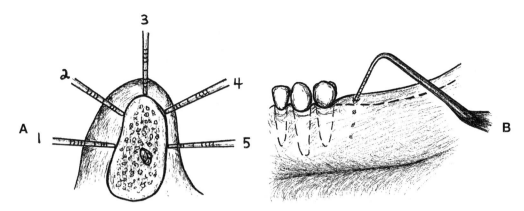

FIG. 17-1 A, Cross section of the alveolus depicting periodontal probe placement for "sounding the bone." **B,** Lateral view of the ridge showing probe placement.

necessary information to carefully place a dental implant. It must be noted here that placement of implants is a team effort including the implant surgeon, prosthodontist/restorative dentist. It must be a carefully orchestrated process to ensure a functional final prosthesis, which the patient finds esthetically pleasing. If it is determined after examination that bone height or width is insufficient, the process of bone augmentation must be considered.

Radiographic Examination

A basic radiographic examination should include a panoramic radiograph for evaluation of the edentulous areas and contiguous anatomic structures. If the panographic film is to be used for measurements it must be kept in mind that there is a 20% to 30% distortion/magnification of the anatomic structures when viewed in a panoramic radiograph (consult the owner's manual of your particular machine). If a single tooth replacement is the treatment planned, individual periapical radiographs will give reasonable information on alveolar bone height, adjacent teeth, and anatomic structures. However, buccal to lingual width will not be appreciated. In few cases an occlusal radiograph may be useful, but will be affected by angulation of the central beam.

Study Models

Maxillary and mandibular study models are an integral part of the initial work-up. They can be used to fabricate a surgical stent, which can guide the surgeon to the exact site of implant placement. Diagnostic wax-ups are used to simulate the final restoration. The original casts can be duplicated to preserve their integrity. If removable full dentures are to be the final prosthesis a surgical stent can be made by simply duplicating the denture tooth wax-up. Arch form, tooth spacing, and bony contour can all be evaluated in the lab, thus reducing chair time.

TYPES OF BONE GRAFTS

Before discussion of the possible bone grafting techniques, a brief description of the types of bone grafts, and in the case of autografts, the techniques used for harvesting will be presented. Four major types of grafts are available to the surgeon (Table 17-1). They include:

- Autografts
- Allografts
- Alloplasts
- Xenografts

THE BIOLOGY OF BONE GRAFTS

It is essential that the implant surgeon performing augmentation grafts be familiar with the basics of bone healing as it pertains to bone grafting. Here we will discuss the two types or phases, as they are commonly called, of bone healing.

The two basic types of bone healing are simply referred to as Phase I and Phase II.[1,2] Phase I bone healing is strictly osteogenesis. This is an immediate proliferation of transplanted osteocytes and subsequent formation of osteoid (immature bone). When an autogenous bone graft is taken from the hip for example, the cells, which survive the transplant process, will start to form new bone immediately upon placement in the recipient site. This type of bone healing is the most favorable type and results in the formation of normal physiologic bone. Phase II bone healing consists of two processes: osteoinduction and osteoconduction. The process of Phase II

TABLE
17-1 Types of Grafts

Type	Description
Autograft	A graft taken from one anatomic location and placed in another location in the same individual (e.g., iliac crest to maxillary sinus)
Allograft	A graft taken from a cadaver treated with certain sterilization and antiantigenic procedures and placed into a living host
Alloplast	A chemically derived nonanimal material for medical implantation
Xenograft	A graft taken from a nonhuman host for implantation into a human host

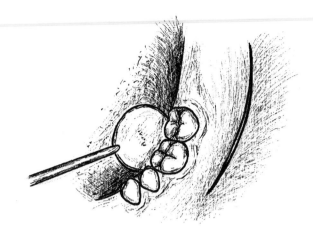

FIG. 17-2 Mandibular left showing incision for access to the ramus for bone harvesting.

bone healing takes a greater period of time than Phase I bone healing. Osteoinduction is defined as the inducement of mesenchymal cells to produce bone. This occurs when bone morphogenic protein (BMP) acts on nondifferentiated mesenchymal cells causing their differentiation into osteoblasts and an "induction" into bone forming cells. Osteoconduction is defined as a framework or scaffold for the formation of new bone tissue and it begins with a period of osteoclastic activity. What takes place is the removal of osteoid and unorganized bone matrix, and its replacement by new, more organized bone. Autogenous grafts heal by both phases of bone healing making them the grafts with the most favorable prognosis for healthy bone formation.

TECHNIQUES USED TO HARVEST MANDIBULAR RAMUS, CHIN, AND MANDIBULAR TORI

As bone grafting becomes more common in the practice of implant dentistry more and more techniques are being developed. The techniques most commonly being used today will be discussed.[3]

Mandibular Ramus

This site of harvest is indicated when small bone grafts are needed. Local anesthesia is administered in the normal manner used to extract mandibular teeth with the addition of local infiltrations in the area of the proposed surgery. This local infiltration will induce hemostasis and allow the surgeon greater visibility. The

local anesthetic of choice is 2% lidocaine with 1:100,000 epinephrine.

1. A #15 scalpel blade on a standard #3 scalpel handle is used to create an incision starting on the lateral border of the ramus approximately 1.5 cm above the mandibular occlusal plane and ending at the mandibular second molar region (Fig. 17-2). To facilitate closure at the completion of the case the incision should not be directly in the buccal vestibule. It should be about 1 cm lateral to the vestibule. The scalpel is used to create a full thickness incision to bone at the level of the external oblique ridge.

2. Using a #9 Molt periosteal elevator a full-thickness mucoperiosteal flap is developed lateral to the mandibular ramus. Once the area exposed is large enough to allow harvesting of the properly sized bone graft a Minnesota retractor may be used to retract the buccal flap while the dental assistant retracts the tongue with a Wieder retractor.

3. Using a rear exhaust high speed handpiece with a #557 surgical length bur the bone is scored in the pattern necessary for the bone graft specimen. It is good practice to maintain the crest of the external oblique ridge of the mandible (Fig. 17-3). Using copious amounts of irrigation while performing the osteotomies will prevent burning the bone and facilitate cutting by removing debris from the bur. After the osteotomies are through cortical bone a small monoplane chisel is placed with the bevel directed medially (toward the cancellous bone). Several taps with a mallet are then used to

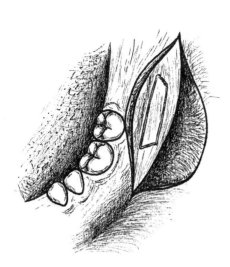

FIG. 17-3 Mucoperiosteal flap reflected showing osteotomy for graft harvesting.

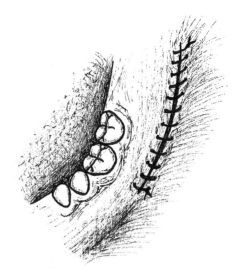

FIG. 17-5 Closure of incision with continuous suture technique.

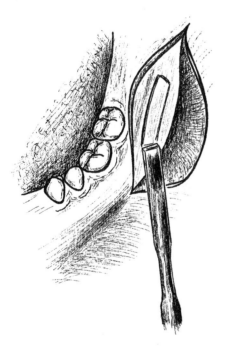

FIG. 17-4 Monoplane chisel being used to separate buccal cortex to complete the harvesting process.

separate the cortex from the underlying medullary bone (Fig. 17-4).

4. The harvested bone is immediately placed in room temperature 0.9% sodium chloride solution. Irrigate the wound thoroughly with sterile water or normal saline using a 60 ml syringe with an 18-gauge IV catheter. The wound is closed primarily using 3-0 Vicryl (Ethicon, Somer-

ville, NJ) or silk suture on a tapered needle. A continuous suture may be used to close this incision (Fig. 17-5).

5. The bone harvested may be crushed into small particles or used as a block.

Mandibular Chin Graft Harvesting

The procedure is described later in this chapter.

Mandibular Tori as a Donor Site

In most instances the mandibular tori are used only as a supplement, not the sole donor site.[4] However, moderate amounts of bone may be harvested. This can be used when, during the placement of an implant, a dehiscence occurs and a minimal amount of bone is needed. The following is a brief description of the procedure to remove mandibular tori.

1. An inferior alveolar nerve block is administered after anesthesia is obtained. Infiltration directly over the tori is performed to produce hemostasis and also dissect the mucosa away from the bone.

2. Next, using a #15 blade on a #3 scalpel handle a sulcular incision is made on the lingual of the existing mandibular teeth or in the case of edentulism a crestal incision is made (Fig. 17-6, *A*).

3. Using a #9 Molt periosteal elevator a full-thickness mucoperiosteal flap is raised on the lingual side of the mandible (Fig. 17-6, *B*). It is important to note that if the tori are to be removed bilaterally the dissection should not proceed across the midline. This will help to minimize the possibility of a

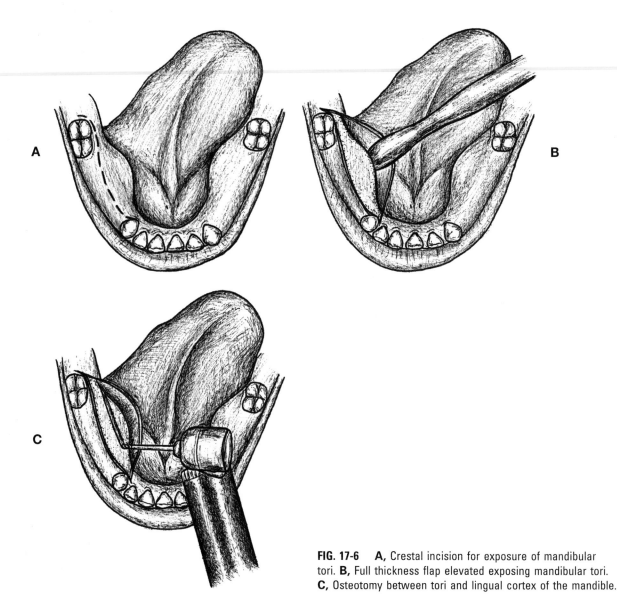

FIG. 17-6   A, Crestal incision for exposure of mandibular tori. **B,** Full thickness flap elevated exposing mandibular tori. **C,** Osteotomy between tori and lingual cortex of the mandible.

hematoma developing and crossing the midline. If this were to occur airway embarrassment may occur. Careful dissection is necessary to prevent tearing of the flap.

4. Once the tori are visualized a high speed hand-piece is used to create a trough between the tori and the lingual cortical plate of the mandible. The depth of this trough should extend approximately three-quarters the width of the tori (Fig. 17-6, C).

5. Next, a monobevel chisel is used to complete the harvesting. With the bevel positioned facing the lingual cortex the tori can be removed with a few taps with a mallet.

6. Immediately the bone is placed into room temperature 0.9% sodium chloride until it is to be placed into the recipient site.

7. Finally, the wound is thoroughly irrigated with normal saline and the flap is reapproximated using 3-0 Vicryl or silk in an interrupted fashion.

PLACEMENT OF A PARTICULATE CORTICOCANCELLOUS BONE GRAFT

If after a complete work-up it is noted that adequate bone remains at the crest but narrows apically, a particulate corticocancellous bone graft should be adequate to allow proper implant placement. This graft is also convenient because it can be placed at the same time as the implant so long as primary stability of the implant can be obtained at the time of surgery. Assuming the implant has been placed securely the following procedure can be followed

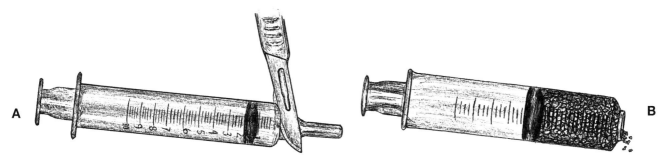

FIG. 17-7 **A,** A #10 blade being used to modify a 10 cc syringe for graft compression. **B,** Modified 10 cc syringe with corticocancellous in place.

for the placement of a particulate corticocancellous bone graft:

1. After obtaining graft material from a donor site it is minced into a fine particulate coagulum. This may be accomplished with the use of a Rongeur or a bone mill. This coagulum is compressed into a modified hypodermic syringe as depicted in Fig. 17-7, *A* and *B.*
2. The graft is now packed around the apical perforation of the implant. After sufficient bone graft is placed to cover the perforation 3-0 Vicryl is used to reapproximate the soft tissue. It is important to maintain strict sterile conditions during the procedure, obtain watertight closure, and protect the surgical site from trauma during the healing period.

GRAFTING OF THE EXTRACTION SOCKET

Edentulous bone loss begins shortly after tooth removal. The majority of alveolar bone that is lost occurs within a year of tooth extraction. Because of this fact some surgeons advocate immediate bone grafting at the time of tooth extraction in the hope of preventing excessive loss of bone height and width. Immediately after tooth extraction a bone graft material is placed in the socket, usually DFDBA (demineralized freeze-dried bone allograft) followed by placement of a membrane barrier (Gore) and 3-0 silk suture in a figure-8 configuration.[5,6] This will allow bone healing to occur with the exclusion of soft tissue ingrowth.

If multiple teeth are to be removed in consecutive order a full thickness mucoperiosteal flap should be used to facilitate closure after the bone graft is placed.

1. First, using a #15 blade a sulcular incision is made approximately 2 teeth beyond the proposed extraction sites.
2. Using a #9 Molt periosteal elevator a full thickness mucoperiosteal flap is raised on the buccal being careful not to tear the tissue. The teeth are ex-

tracted atraumatically preserving the buccal bone.
3. Once the teeth are removed all granulation tissue is excised with the use of a surgical curette or a Rongeur.
4. Next, the bone graft material is packed into the extraction sockets, the flap repositioned and held in place using 3-0 silk sutures. When repositioning the flap near primary closure can be accomplished if the interdental papillae are interdigitated as demonstrated in Fig. 17-8, *A* and *B.*

If success of the graft is to be expected the patient must be instructed to keep the operative site clean. This will help to prevent wound infection and ultimately graft failure. I have found chlorhexidine mouth rinse to be beneficial in preventing postoperative infections.

CORTICAL ONLAY BONE GRAFT

For edentulous areas with inadequate buccal to lingual/palatal width there are several choices for the graft material:

1. Autogenous bone: donor sites may be the mandibular symphysis, mandibular ramus, calvarium, or iliac crest.
2. Allografts: demineralized freeze dried bone allograft (DFDBA) blocks, freeze-dried blocks, and/or particles.

The following procedure can be performed in the office setting under local anesthesia and IV sedation for placement of small onlay bone grafts.

Bone Harvesting from the Chin

1. After local anesthesia is achieved a #15 blade is used to make an incision in the buccal sulcus starting proximally and moving distally, but going slightly toward the lingual aspect of the crest in the edentulous area. This design will permit adequate mobility of the buccal flap to accommodate the increased bulk of the graft and allow the suture line to be away from the graft itself (Fig. 17-9, *A* and *B).*

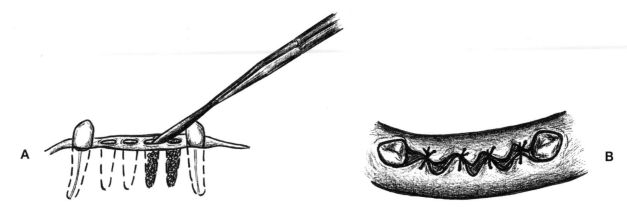

FIG. 17-8 **A,** Extraction socket with particulate graft in place. **B,** Closure of extraction site with interdigitating papillae.

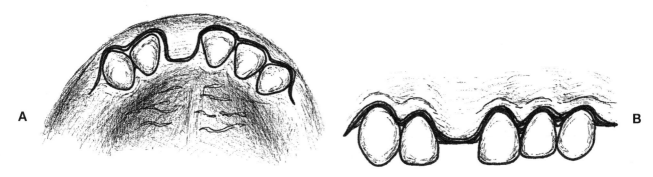

FIG. 17-9 **A,** Sulcular incision with extension onto the palatal aspect of the edentulous ridge. **B,** Buccal view of the sulcular incision.

2. A full-thickness mucoperiosteal flap is raised using a #9 Molt elevator being careful not to tear the tissue. Once the flap is raised the edentulous ridge is examined to estimate the approximate amount of bone that will be necessary. Once an estimate of the approximate amount of bone that will be needed is established a second surgical site must be developed.

3. Harvesting from the mandibular symphysis: Using a #15 scalpel blade on a #3 Bard-Parker scalpel handle a mucosal incision is made 1 cm labial to the depth of the vestibule in the anterior mandibular from canine to canine (Fig. 17-10 *A*).

4. Using blunt dissection with a small curved hemostat a mucosal flap is developed to the approximate level of the vestibule (Fig. 17-10, *B*), being careful to avoid the mental nerves as they exit the mandible into the soft tissue. Once the flap is well developed bilaterally down to the periosteum a scalpel is used to expose the bone with an incision carried from canine to canine at the level approximately 5 mm below the apices of the mandibular anterior teeth.

5. Now using a #9 Molt periosteal elevator, the periosteum is reflected down to the inferior border of the mandible (Fig. 17-10, *C*). Using a #8 surgical length round bur on a straight handpiece two bur holes are placed a minimum of 5 mm inferior to the apices of the mandibular anterior teeth.

6. Next two additional bur holes are placed to form a rectangle approximately the size of the bone graft needed. To complete the osteotomy a #557 surgical length bur (25 mm friction grip, W. Lorenz, Jacksonville, FL) is used with copious amounts of irrigation to connect the four bur holes creating a cortical osteotomy (Fig. 17-11). To finalize the harvesting of the graft a small curved monoplane osteotome is used with a mallet to separate the cortical bone from the underlying marrow (Fig. 17-12). Hemostasis can be achieved by placing Avitene (MedChem Products Inc., Woburn, MA) in the osteotomy site. (See Chapter 5, Perioperative Hemorrhage.)

7. Once hemostasis is achieved the flap is closed in two layers using 3-0 Vicryl suture on a tapered needle. First approximate the periosteum with multiple interrupted sutures being careful to maintain the mentalis muscle in its proper position. The mucosa is then closed using a continuous suture.

8. Immediately after harvesting the graft it should be placed in room temperature 0.9% sodium chloride.

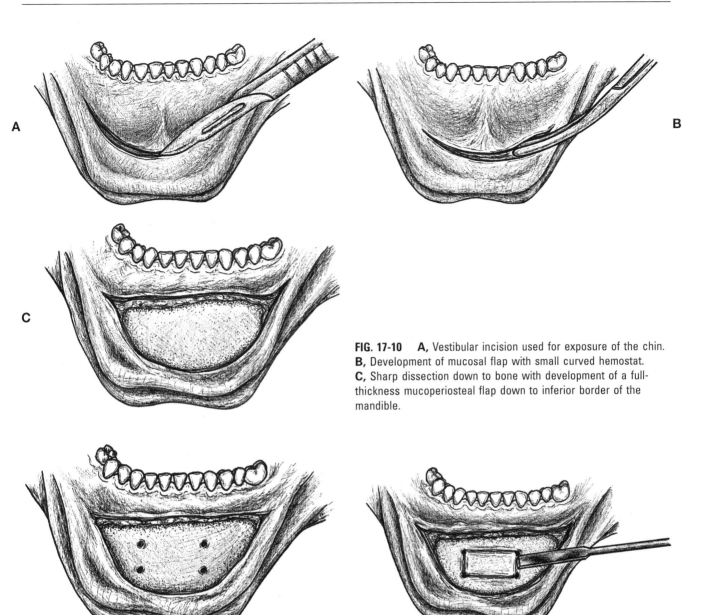

FIG. 17-10   A, Vestibular incision used for exposure of the chin. **B,** Development of mucosal flap with small curved hemostat. **C,** Sharp dissection down to bone with development of a full-thickness mucoperiosteal flap down to inferior border of the mandible.

FIG. 17-11 Exposed chin showing 4 bur holes indicating the four corners of the proposed graft.

FIG. 17-12 Monoplane chisel being used to separate graft.

In order for an onlay graft to succeed it must be stabilized to allow phase II bone healing to occur.

Fixation of the Cortical Bone Graft

1. Before fixation of the bone graft to the recipient site multiple small perforations in the cortex should be placed with a #6 surgical length round bur under copious irrigation. This will allow additional blood supply to the marrow cells (Fig. 17-13).
2. Finally, using a mini fixation system (Osteomed, Irving, TX) the cortical bone graft is secured into place with one or two screws (Fig. 17-14).

3. Once the graft is secured into position all sharp edges are smoothed with a large round bur.
4. The flap can now be repositioned using 3-0 Vicryl or silk under minimal tension. The bone graft is allowed to heal for 3 to 12 months depending on the size and type of graft. At the time of implant placement the fixation screws are removed to prevent interference with implant placement.

INTERPOSITIONAL RIDGE GRAFT

On rare occasions the height of the bone may allow the properly sized implant to be placed, however, the width

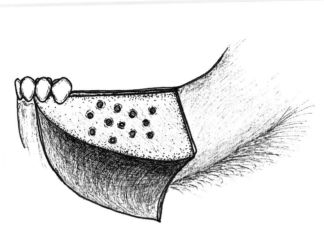

FIG. 17-13 Multiple small bur holes in buccal cortex.

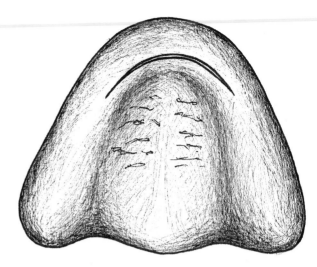

FIG. 17-15 Crestal incision of maxilla for graft placement.

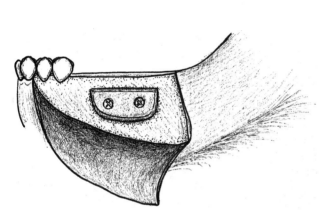

FIG. 17-14 Block graft fixated to the buccal cortex using two fixation screws.

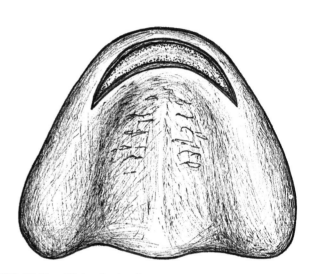

FIG. 17-16 Minimally developed buccal flap in preparation for split ridge technique.

may be inadequate. One technique for resolving this problem is the interpositional bone graft.[7]

1. First, as with all procedures, adequate local anesthesia must be obtained. The ideal local anesthetic for this procedure would be 2% lidocaine with 1:100,000 epinephrine, which will allow enough time to perform the procedure and also provide a hemostatic operative site. The procedure will be described for the anterior maxilla but it may be used in other areas of the oral cavity.

2. Using a #15 scalpel blade on a standard #3 scalpel handle an incision is made from the maxillary right first molar area to the contralateral first molar area along the crest of the ridge. The incision is a full-thickness incision (Fig. 17-15).

3. Using a #9 Molt periosteal elevator a buccal flap is elevated minimally to maintain maximal perios-

teal attachment necessary to ensure adequate blood supply to the buccal bone (Fig. 17-16).

4. The osteotomy is now performed using a 45-degree rear exhaust high speed handpiece with a #557 surgical length bur and copious amounts of irrigation. The osteotomy is started midcrest in the area of the maxillary second premolar and advanced to the contralateral second premolar area. The depth of the osteotomy is very important so as to prevent inadvertent horizontal fractures of the buccal plate. An adequate width of buccal bone is required to permit a well-vascularized outfractured portion of bone and an adequate periosteal pedicle. The approximate depth of the osteotomy should be 1 cm. A bibevel chisel is used to gently outfracture the buccal plate and allow enough width for the proposed implant (Fig. 17-17).

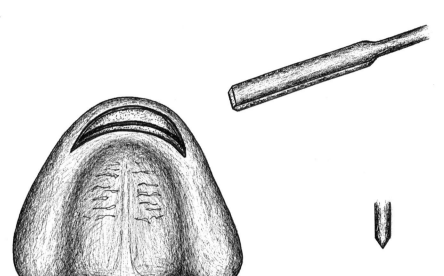

FIG. 17-17 Maxilla depicting crestal osteotomy and bibevel chisel.

TABLE 17-2 Examples of Bone Fill Materials

Category	Examples	Particle Size
Autografts	Chin, maxillary tuberosity, mandibular tori, mandibular ramus	Variable
Allografts	DFDBA (demineralized freeze-dried bone allograft) FDBA (freeze-dried bone allograft)	250-500 Micron
Alloplast	Resorbable HA: Osteograf LD, OsteoGen Tricalcium phosphate: Augmin Bioactive glass: Biogran, Perioglas Resin material: HTR (hard tissue replacement)	Various particle size and texture
Xenograft	Osteograf-N 300, Bio-Oss	

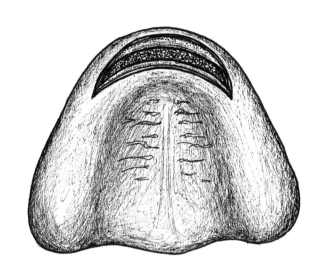

FIG. 17-18 Buccal cortex out fractured with corticocancellous graft in place.

5. At this time the bone graft can be placed either as a particulate corticocancellous graft or as a block graft. The particulate bone may be harvested from the tuberosities and mixed with DFDBA to increase the volume and eliminate the need for another operative site. The harvesting of tuberosity is performed simply using a side cutting Rongeur and scraping bone from the ridge.

If the split ridge technique is used in the mandible the particulate bone graft may be taken from tori if they are available. Other donor sites may be the tuberosity or ileum. Harvested bone may be augmented with allografts or alloplasts depending on the clinical situation and what is available to increase the volume in a 1:1 ratio (Table 17-2). Using a surgical curette, the graft is placed in the recipient site and compressed vertically with a moist 4 × 4 gauze (Fig. 17-18). The incision is closed in one layer using 3-0 Vicryl suture in a continuous manner. The wound must be watertight to prevent the loss of the bone graft and reduce the incidence of infection. This is allowed to heal for a minimum of 3 months and possibly up to 9 months.

CONCLUSION

These are only a few of the techniques at the disposal of the oral and maxillofacial surgeon to augment the alveolar ridge in preparation for the placement of dental implants. Other techniques are available and some will be discussed in other chapters; others are beyond the scope of this book. The clinician performing these operations must always pay particular attention to the case selection and institute strict surgical protocol in order to ensure the most favorable environment for the success of the bone graft.

REFERENCES

1. Marx R: Biology of bone graft. Oral & Maxillofacial Surgery Knowledge Update, Vol I Part I, RCN 3-62, *AAOMS*, 1995.
2. Rissolo A, Bennett J: Bone grafting and its essential role in implant dentistry, *Dent Clin North Am* 42:91-116, 1998.
3. Triplett R, Schow S: Osseous regeneration with bone harvested from the anterior mandible. In Nevins M, Wellonig J: *Implant Therapy Clinical Approaches & Evidence of Success*, Chicago, Quintessence, 1998, Ch. 15.
4. Ganz S: Mandibular tori as a source for onlay bone graft augmentation: a surgical procedure, *Practical Periodont Aesth Dent* 9:973-982, 1997.
5. Koerner K, Tilt L: Alveolar ridge aesthetics: Extraction site bone grafting for the general dentist, *Dentistry Today* 82-87, 1999.
6. Kois J: Esthetic extraction site development: The biologic variables. *Contemp Esths Restorative Practice*, March/April 1998.
7. Lustmann J, Lewinstein I: Interpositional bone grafting technique to widen the narrow maxillary ridge, *Int J Oral Maxillofac Implant* 10:568-577, 1995.

18 The Sinus-Lift Procedure

HARRY DYM, DDS

It is a well-established clinical finding that alveolar bone will undergo resorption following tooth extraction in both vertical and horizontal directions. If the underlying crestal bone is subjected to the constant traumatic occlusal forces of a denture, more rapid resorption will occur.

The posterior maxilla represents a problematic area regarding crestal bone loss and atrophy. In addition to having an alveolar crest that is more cancellous[1] than cortical in nature (thus less likely to resist resorption as a result of masticatory forces) its volume can be further reduced by pneumatization of the maxillary sinus. Misch[2] has described how the antrum expands in both inferior and lateral directions after maxillary posterior teeth are lost.

All these factors are responsible for decreasing available posterior maxillary bone for the placement of implants. Various techniques have been developed to augment this compromised region of the oral cavity prior to implant placement. The following surgical procedures have been described:

1. Iliac crest cancellous grafts
2. Rib grafts
3. Allograft alveolar augmentation
4. Le Fort I osteotomy with interpositional bone grafts
5. Alloplastic augmentation

All these procedures are indicated in case of severe maxillary atrophy in which the interarch distance is extremely increased. In most cases, however, the interarch distance is normal or reduced and another approach, such as the grafting of the maxillary sinus, is indicated. In 1977 Tatum introduced a crestal approach to the sinus membrane and in 1986[3] changed to a modified Caldwell-Luc lateral window. The graft material is inserted between the antral floor and the Schneiderian membrane (the lining of the maxillary sinus floor) and the technique is referred to as the *sinus-lift procedure*.

EVALUATION OF THE POSTERIOR MAXILLA

In addition to the usual clinical evaluation performed, radiographic examination should include periapical and panoramic radiographs. These films may sometimes fail to give the operator the adequate information needed for determining the amount of bone available for implant placement because the images are only two-dimensional.

If the operator has any doubt concerning the amount of available bone for implant placement, a reformatted CT scan (such as a DentaScan program) is a most helpful tool. This particular format gives cross-sectional views at 2-mm intervals and thus permits evaluation of the exact amount of bone present.

Because of the cancellous noncortical quality of bone present in the posterior maxilla, a high failure rate for implants of 8-mm height has been noted. When 10 mm to 13 mm of bone is available in the area, the usual maxillary implant installation techniques are appropriate. However, one should be careful not to penetrate the sinus (in a nongrafted case) with any implant fixture for more than 1 to 3 mm.[4,5] It is thought that fixture failure will result because of the downgrowth of antral epithelium around the fixture rather than by the superior growth of oral epithelium.

AUGMENTING MATERIALS (Box 18-1)

In 1980, Boyne and James[6] reported on subantral sinus grafting with a combination of autogenous bone and hydroxyapatite. Autogenous cancellous bone is the ideal grafting material because it is osteoinductive, osteoconductive, and contains osteoblasts that can produce bone.

Bone donor sites include: (1) chin, (2) tuberosity, (3) hip, (4) calvaria, (5) ramus, and (6) tibia. Other grafting materials currently used include allografts such as freeze-dried bone, and demineralized freeze-dried

BOX 18-1 Graft Materials for Sinus Lift

AUTOGENOUS BONE
1. Hip
2. Tibia
3. Symphysis
4. Ramus
5. Maxillary tuberosity

ALLOGRAFT
(Obtained from Human Cadavers)
1. Freeze-dried bone
2. Demineralized freeze-dried bone

XENOGRAFTS
(Bone from Nonhuman Species)
1. Bovine bone (Bio-Oss)

ALLOPLASTIC
(Natural and Synthetic Bone Substitute)
1. Hydroxyapatite
2. Tricalcium phosphate (TCP)
3. Bioactive glass ceramics

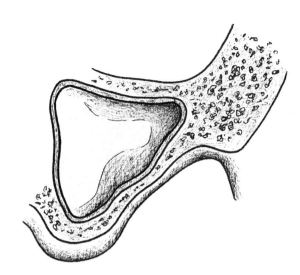

FIG. 18-1 Sagittal view of maxillary sinus showing relationship of sinus membrane, antrum, and maxillary bone.

bone. Demineralizing bone is the process by which the inorganic matrix is removed, releasing bone morphogenic proteins. BMP is felt to be an osteoinductive agent helpful in the bone forming process.

Increasingly alloplastic materials like hydroxyapatite (HA) mixed with allograft material are becoming the augmentation materials of choice. HA is felt to be an osteoconductive agent that acts as a bridge to facilitate new bone formation.

Most clinicians prefer to use autologous blood as a mixing solution, which gives the mixture a thicker cohesive form and facilitates handling of the graft material.

PATIENT SELECTION AND TIME TABLES

The relative contraindications for this procedure include uncontrolled diabetes, ongoing radiation therapy, active sinus infections, and any unstable medical condition. Excessive smoking is a contraindication for grafting and implant placement and patients should be counseled to stop smoking before surgical treatment. Patients who have received radiation treatment to the maxilla may require hyperbaric oxygen therapy prior to grafting and implant placement.

Current protocols call for waiting between 4 and 9 months after grafting for implant placement and an additional 4 to 6 months before placing final restorations.

SURGICAL PROTOCOL
(Figs. 18-1 through 18-4)

1. Obtain appropriate consent.
2. Have all implant/surgical equipment prepared and checked.

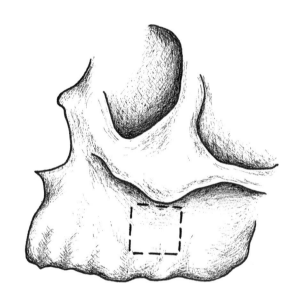

FIG. 18-2 Direct view of posterior maxilla, showing outline of bony cuts for creation of lateral window.

3. Local anesthesia is achieved with buccal and palatal infiltration along with a division II block through the anterior palatal foramen at the posterior palate.
4. Make a 3-mm incision on the palatal side of the alveolar crest of the edge with two vertical releasing incisions. Make certain that vertical releasing incisions are over solid bone and not over planned antral opening.
5. Using a sharp periosteal elevator, raise a full

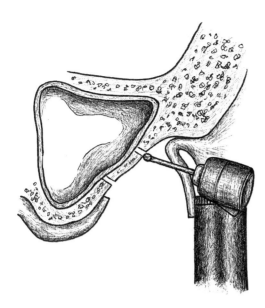

FIG. 18-3 Mucosal flap elevated and slow round bur being used to create bony window.

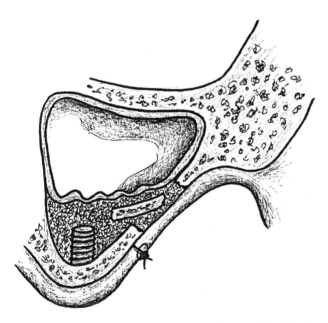

FIG. 18-4 Antral membrane shown tented upwards with implant placed and bone filling sinus.

thickness flap to gain access to the underlying bone. Care should be taken to *not* tear the periosteum.

6. Use a fiberoptic light to transilluminate the maxillary sinus to help outline the antrum and carefully plan bony cuts.

7. Place an inferior horizontal bony cut no more than 2 to 4 mm above floor of sinus.

8. Use a round diamond #6 burr, held at a 45-degree angle to the surface of the bone, to outline a rectangular bony window. Be careful to use a high torque low velocity handpiece to better control the osteotomy. Using a round bur will also avoid any sharp edges that may cause perforation of the antral lining.

9. Under copious irrigation bone should be feathered until the gray hue of the antral membrane becomes apparent.

10. At this point, a surgical curette is placed in the edges of the inferior osteotomy between the bone and the antrum and gently used to peel away the membrane from the inside wall of the sinus. This gentle sliding motion is continued all around and then the bony window is gently pushed in.

11. If a perforation of the membrane should occur, it can be repaired by placing a small piece of resorbable collagen (CollaTape, Calcitek Corp., Carlsbad, CA) barrier material against the tear, where it should easily adhere.

12. Begin grafting the floor of the sinus at the far wall. If enough inferior alveolar bone exists (4 mm or more) to stabilize endosseous implants, place the implants at this time.

13. Continue to pack and condense graft material against the hinged window of bone, which will become the new superior wall of the sinus. The grafted lateral defect can be covered with a resorbable membrane or left uncovered.

14. The flap, with its periosteum intact, is approximated over the bone graft and closed with interrupted sutures. Leave sutures in place for 7 to 10 days.

15. Place patient on appropriate antibiotic coverage (Amoxil or Zithromax for penicillin-allergic patients) and analgesics and instruct the patient to take a decongestant and not to blow his/her nose for at least 1 week after surgery.

Patients should not wear a removable appliance for the first 2 postoperative weeks. If this is not possible the denture should be adjusted so that it does not rest on the surgical site.

The most common postoperative complication is infection at the surgical site. If this should occur the surgical site should be irrigated daily until resolution occurs.

REFERENCES

1. Pietrokovski J: The bony residual ridge in man. *J Prosth Dent* 34:456-462, 1975.
2. Misch C: Treatment planning for edentulous maxillary posterior region. In Misch CE, editor: *Contemporary implant dentistry*, ed 2, St. Louis, Mosby, 1998.

3. Tatum OH: Maxillary and sinus implant reconstruction, *Dent Clin North Am* 30:207-229, 1986.

4. Jensen OT: Treatment planning for sinus grafts. In Jensen OT (ed): *The sinus bone graft*, Chicago, Quintessence, 1999, p. 49.

5. Branemark PI, Adell R, Albrektsson T: An experimental and clinical study of osseointegrated implants penetrating the nasal cavity and maxillary sinus, *J Oral Maxillofa Surg* 42:497, 1984.

6. Boyne PJ, James RA: Grafting of the maxillary sinus floor with autogenous marrow and bone, *Oral Surg Oral Med Oral Pathol* 28:613, 1980.

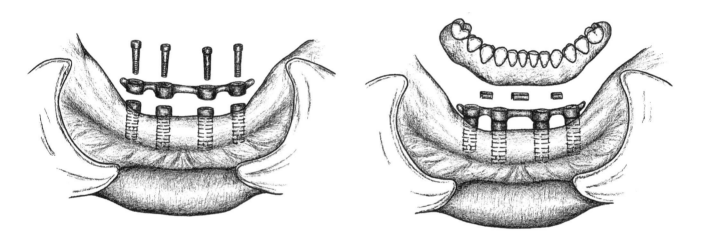

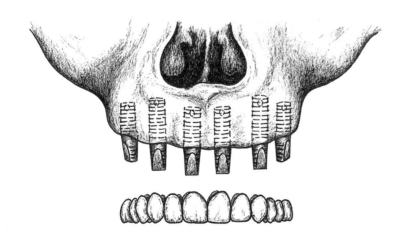

MICHAEL KLEIN, DDS

The phrase dental implants strikes fear, disinterest, or apathy in many restorative dentists. This is a result of misunderstanding the function of the dental implant, where to use it appropriately, and how to use it. This chapter will unravel the mystery of implant dentistry to make it a user-friendly discipline.

Dental implants are adjuncts to restorative dentistry. Implants are used to support and/or retain prostheses. The restoration must, therefore, drive the treatment plan. It is imperative for the restorative doctor to understand the entire implant process from the patient's diagnosis and prosthesis selection through the surgical and restorative treatment steps, so that appropriate treatment decisions can be made.

IMPLANT PROSTHESES

The four groups of implant prostheses are: the overdenture, single tooth replacement, fixed prosthesis for the partially edentulous arch, and fixed prosthesis for the completely edentulous arch.

Overdenture

The overdenture is a removable prosthesis. It can be used for both the mandible and the maxilla. The overall prosthetic design for the mandibular overdenture is similar to a mandibular complete denture. The maxillary overdenture design is usually a palateless/horseshoe shape denture design.

The two types of overdentures are implant-retained overdentures and implant-retained and supported overdentures. Implant-retained overdentures are held in place by implants but their support comes from the soft tissue and underlying bone. They use individual attachments on the implant.

The implant-retained and supported overdentures are overdentures that are held in place by implants and get some or all of their support from the implants. This overdenture uses a connecting bar with attachments for

overdenture retention. A removable partial denture may also use implants for retention. Individual attachments would be used on the implants for the removable partial denture.

Single Tooth Replacement

The single tooth replacement is used to replace missing single teeth. Prosthesis support and retention come from the implant. Retention may be achieved through screws or cement.

Fixed Prosthesis for the Partially Edentulous Arch

The fixed restoration for the partially edentulous arch is a porcelain to metal restoration. It gains both its support and retention completely from the implants. The retention may be in the form of screw retention or cement.

Fixed Prosthesis for the Completely Edentulous Arch

The three types of fixed prosthesis for the completely edentulous arch are: porcelain to metal fixed prosthesis, hybrid bridge prosthesis, and the spark erosion prosthesis.

The porcelain to metal fixed prosthesis is a restoration made in a style similar to conventional crown and bridge. It gains its support and retention from the implants. Retention may be gained through the screws or cement.

The hybrid bridge is a fixed prosthesis made of denture teeth processed to a metal framework. The support and retention for this prosthesis comes from the implants. Retention to the implants is achieved through screws.

The spark erosion prosthesis is a cross between a hybrid bridge and an overdenture. Denture teeth are processed to a metal overcasting which fits intimately to an underlying precision milled bar. This overcasting usually locks to the bar. It is removable by the patient, but because of its rigidity is it considered a fixed prosthesis. Its support and retention come from the implants. The bar is retained by screws to the implants and attachments lock the prosthesis to the bar.

INDICATIONS AND IMPLANT REQUIREMENTS

The single tooth replacement is a treatment option for the following scenarios.

1. The teeth on either side of the edentulous space are nonrestored or minimally restored and would not benefit from a conventional fixed bridge.
2. The teeth on either side of the edentulous span have been recently restored and it is undesirable to replace the restorations.
3. The teeth on either side of the edentulous span are restoratively or periodontally compromised and placement of a fixed prosthesis on them would have a poor prognosis.

Implant Requirements

One implant will support one tooth. However, in a molar replacement, consideration of placement of two implants for one molar is given if the space between the bordering teeth is 14 mm or greater.

OVERDENTURE

The overdenture is indicated for patients who need retention for their denture or psychologically want the retention for their denture. The maxillary palateless overdenture is also a useful prosthesis for patients who cannot tolerate coverage of their maxillary palate by the denture base because of gagging or intolerance to it.

Maxillary Palateless Overdenture

Individual attachments are generally not used in the maxilla. Splinting the implants with a bar is usually the treatment of choice. A minimum of four implants is recommended.

Mandibular Implant Retained Overdenture

The implant retained overdenture is indicated when prosthesis retention is required, but the patient will tolerate slight movement of the denture caused by soft tissue resiliency. Two implants are required for retention. This prosthesis is usually not used into the maxilla.

Mandibular Implant Retained and Supported Overdenture

This prosthesis is indicated when prosthesis retention and stability is required. A minimum of two implants are required, and they are splinted with a bar. As more implants are added, more support can be placed on the bar and the implants, making the overdenture more rigid as a result of less tissue support.

Removable Partial Denture Retained By Implants

Implants may be used to retain removable partial dentures. This is a useful technique when one does not want to clasp teeth, these teeth may be poor abutments, the clasps present an esthetic problem, or tooth abutments for retention may not be in the necessary position within the dental arch. Individual attachments on the implants are generally used in this application.

FIXED PROSTHESIS FOR THE PARTIALLY EDENTULOUS PATIENT

Implants are indicated for the partially edentulous patient when existing support is inadequate for a fixed prosthesis. This may be because of a long edentulous span; potential abutment teeth for a fixed prosthesis have a poor prognosis and are, therefore, unreliable as bridge abutments; or tooth abutments are nonexistent, as in a free-end saddle scenario.

An implant per tooth to be restored is usually indicated unless inadequate space for that number of implants exists or that number of implants cannot be restored because of implant and/or abutment positioning and proximity. Molars may also be replaced with more than one implant.

FIXED PROSTHESIS FOR THE COMPLETELY EDENTULOUS ARCH

A fixed prosthesis is indicated when the patient wants teeth that are nonremovable, when the patient does not want to have to think about their teeth, or when the patient wants teeth as close to natural teeth as possible.

Porcelain to Gold Bridgework

The porcelain to metal prosthesis is indicated when the tooth form emerging from the tissue is to be as natural as possible. A porcelain to metal implant prosthesis should also be considered if the opposing arch is a porcelain to metal restoration

Hybrid Bridge

The hybrid bridge is indicated when a fixed prosthesis is required and the opposing arch is a denture prosthesis or another hybrid bridge. The hybrid bridge has a lower laboratory cost than a porcelain to metal prosthesis and is technically easier to fabricate when severe bone atrophy exists and additional lip support is required. The hybrid bridge may provide a more esthetic restoration than a porcelain to metal restoration.

The Spark Erosion Prosthesis

The spark erosion prosthesis is used when the prosthesis design is such that it does not allow for proper home care of the implants by the patient. Removal of this style of prosthesis allows access for hygiene but the patient still has a fixed-type prosthesis that is very rigid, stable, and retentive with no tissue support. Such a patient is one with significant alveolar atrophy (usually in the maxilla) who requires a lot of lip support in the form of a denture phalange from the prosthesis.

All these fixed prostheses for the completely edentulous arch require some implant support. Maxillary restorations should have eight to ten implants with no cantilever on the prosthesis. Mandibular fixed prostheses should have a minimum of five implants. Cantilevers of 10 to 15 mm are allowed depending upon the positioning of the implants (anterior to posterior spread).

DATA COLLECTION

An initial interview should be conducted to ascertain what it is that the patient really would like to have when treatment is complete. Patient expectations of treatment time, provisional prosthesis requirements, and esthetic demands should be discussed. This information can help in the thought process of developing the treatment plan as you examine the patient.[1]

The medical history should be reviewed with all dental patients. Conditions that should raise red flags are: diabetes, smoking, extensive steroid usage, or any other medical condition that may affect bone and/or soft tissue healing. These conditions are not contraindications to treatment, but require consultation with the patient's physician and a carefully developed and thoughtful treatment plan. The patient should also be advised of the possible limitations of treatment.[2]

The clinical exam must be complete, including chart-ing of the hard and soft tissue, taking note of the following:

- Status of the remaining teeth
- Mobility
- Furcations
- Probing depth
- Keratinized tissue
- Interarch space
- Interteeth distance
- Ridge width
- Supereruption
- Tilting of adjacent teeth
- Occlusal/incisal plane
- Smile line
- Does soft tissue appear in the smile?
- How many teeth appear in a wide smile?
- Do the present teeth appear esthetic?
- Is the current removable prosthesis stable and retentive?
- Can the current denture be used as a provisional prosthesis?
- Are any acute infections present?

Various radiographs may be taken. The panoramic radiograph is useful in almost all situations. Periapical radiographs are needed in single tooth sites or when placing implants adjacent to tooth roots. Cephalometric radiographs are only useful in determining the maxillary/mandibular relationship but should not be used for evaluating available bone for implantation. Occlusal radiographs only show the greatest dimension of bone but do not demonstrate the narrowest dimension and are, therefore, not useful in implantology.[3,4]

CT scans give us a three-dimensional view of bone and are therefore an invaluable aid in treatment planning and placement of implants. Three-dimensional surgical simulations on CT scans may also be done. These simulations serve both a surgical and prosthetic role. Blueprints for treatment can be created and with the recent advent of computer-generated surgical templates, easily carried out. All patients do not require CT scans. However, as cases become more complex, CT scans become mandatory.

Diagnostic casts allow a second look at the patient. Although not a mandatory item to develop in every treatment plan, they should be considered for every potential implant patient. The more complex the treatment, the more necessary the diagnostic casts become. The less experienced clinician in implant treatment may not be aware of how complex a case may be and it, therefore, may be advisable to make diagnostic casts on all patients.

Photographs of the existing dentition and patient smile line are a very helpful adjunct to written clinical data, radiographs, and study casts when developing the treatment plan.

Once all the data is collected, the patient should be sent home and a thoughtful treatment plan may be developed using all collected data. This treatment plan should be developed with discussions between the implant surgeon and restorative doctor. Consideration to final prosthesis design and provisional prosthesis design and management, timing, costs, implants, CT scans, CT scan appliances, bone grafts, root canals, periodontal treatment, or any other adjunctive treatment should be put into the treatment plan. Any possible contingencies should also be listed.[5,6,7]

CT SCAN APPLIANCE

If the patient is to have a CT scan taken, then a CT scan appliance should be fabricated. The critical factor in the CT scan appliance is the placement of radiopaque markers to demonstrate the tooth position and orientation on the CT scan. Available bone may then be evaluated relative to tooth positions. Without anterior radiopaque markers, only bone may be seen but not its relevance to where the prosthesis will be. Several different styles of CT scan appliances can be fabricated including duplicating an existing prosthesis or using an Omnivac form of tooth position. Radiopaque material such as barium sulfate and die hardener, gutta percha on amalgam, and acrylic may be applied to show tooth position.

The exact final tooth position and shape must be known before the surgical placement of any implant. This may be accomplished through a diagnostic wax-up, the setting of denture teeth, or by impressioning the existing prosthesis/teeth if their shape and position are to be replicated. This information will then be used to develop the CT scan appliance and/or a surgical template.[8]

SURGICAL TEMPLATE

A surgical template should be used to direct appropriate implant positioning during surgical placement of a dental implant. The surgical template must demonstrate final prosthesis shape and position. The surgical template may be a duplication of an existing prosthesis or diagnostic set-up/wax-up. Alternatively, an Omnivac form may be used if the adjacent teeth are available for the Omnivac to seat on.

PROVISIONAL PROSTHESIS

A provisional prosthesis may be worn during implant healing, but should be designed so that pressure is not placed on the healing implant. A removable prosthesis should be broad based and stable. The removable prosthesis should be relieved and soft relined over the healing implants. A fixed provisional[9] supported by adjacent teeth, healed implants, or provisional implants is ideal but must also be relieved over the healing implants so that no pressure is placed during the implant healing. Healing periods vary depending upon implant systems. These periods usually vary between 4 and 6 months for the maxilla and 3 to 4 months for the mandible. Quality of bone and new implant surfaces may lengthen or shorten these healing times.

Provisional restorations placed onto dental implants should be considered when design of the final prosthesis should be tested out or when provisional loading of the implants is a consideration. Design considerations include overall esthetics and functional contours, design of the emergence of the restoration from the soft tissue, and support of the soft tissues by the prosthesis. Provisional restorations may be fabricated on temporary or final components supplied by the implant manufacturers.[10]

PROSTHESIS DESIGN

Implants are restored with abutments, superstructures, and an occasional mesostructure. An abutment is that portion of the prosthesis that connects directly to the implant. The superstructure is that portion of the prosthesis that is seen in the patient's mouth. A crown, fixed bridge, or overdenture is a superstructure. On occasion the crown or fixed bridge and abutment are made as one piece. A mesostructure is the portion of the prosthesis that may sit between the superstructure and abutment, usually in the form of a bar. This is mostly found in overdenture or spark erosion prostheses.[11]

ABUTMENTS

Abutments may be screwed, cemented or friction-fit onto the implant. The mesostructure or superstructure in turn may be screwed or cemented onto the abutment. The abutments come as prefabricated components or may be custom cast. The abutments come in a variety of shapes, sizes, angles, and materials to individually fit each circumstance.[12]

SINGLE TEETH

Design considerations for single teeth include the incorporation of an antirotational device in the abutment to prevent rotation and loosening of the crown. Occlusion should include light centric contact and elimination of excursive contact if possible.

MULTIPLE UNITS OF CROWN AND BRIDGE

Design considerations include splinting of multiple implant units to aid implants under shear forces. The limitation to splinting is dependent upon the amount of porcelain that may be baked while maintaining a passively seating restoration. If splinting is required beyond this number of units, then post soldering and the use of rigid interlocks should be considered.

In the fully edentulous arch, cross-arch stabilization is to be considered. Flexure of mandible must be taken into account when designing full arch fixed mandible restorations. If implants are to be placed far posteriorly (first or second molar area) and anteriorly, then making the prosthesis in two sections is a design consideration. Splinting of natural teeth to implants is to be avoided when possible. When teeth must be connected to implants, the use of gold copings on natural tooth abutments or interlocks placed between the natural tooth and abutment are planned. The steps for crown and bridge restorations include abutment selection and insertion, impression making, provisionalization where appropriate, centric record and vertical dimension records, casting try-in and solder index, framework try-in and pick-up, porcelain try-in, and insertion.

If the restoration is to be cemented, a temporary cement should be used to allow removal of the bridge if necessary. Abutment screws should be tightened to the manufacturer's recommended torque before cementation of the restorations. Screw-retained restorations should also be tightened to the manufacturer's recommended torque.

OVERDENTURES AND HYBRID BRIDGES

Overdentures and hybrid bridges follow similar prosthetic steps as in conventional removable dentures. Abutments are initially chosen and inserted, then preliminary and final impressions are made, centric record and vertical dimension taken, and teeth are selected. The position of the abutments within the master cast are verified. A trial denture set-up tried in with esthetics, centric record, and vertical dimension is confirmed for the overdenture. A cast metal framework within the denture base should be fabricated, the teeth reset, and the bar fabricated (if a bar is to be used). A second denture try-in and try-in of the bar should now be done. The denture is now processed and the bar, attachments, and denture are inserted.[13]

The hybrid bridge metal framework is cast after the initial trial denture stage. The framework may be tried in with denture teeth if an accurate master cast was confirmed before this step. When verification of the master cast was not obtained, the metal frame is re-turned in segments for a solder index and then soldered and returned with teeth reset for a final confirmation of a passively seating restoration, correct esthetics, centric record, and vertical dimension. The hybrid bridge may then be processed and inserted in the patient's mouth.[14-17]

PASSIVE SEATING

All implant restorations must seat passively. Passive seating means that the implant prosthetic components including superstructure and mesostructures (and abutments if they are part of the mesostructure) or superstructure must seat completely on the implant head or abutment head without being torqued down to place with multiple screws. This is evaluated by placing one screw into one end of the prosthesis and tightening it. All the other interfaces between implant, abutment, mesostructure, and/or superstructure are then evaluated by direct and/or radiographic examinations. If complete seating is not seen, the restoration is sectioned appropriately. All segments are secured with screws and a solder index made. Once the framework is resoldered, it is then rechecked for passive seating.

ORAL HYGIENE

Patients are taught oral hygiene regimens that effectively maintain their restorations. Oral hygiene implements routinely used include proxibrush, rubber tip, Superfloss, electric toothbrushes, and Water Pik. Implant patients are placed on 3- to 6-month recalls to be determined by the doctor.

MAINTENANCE

Periodontal probing, evaluation for gingival inflammation, bleeding, suppuration, mobility, and bone loss are to be considered. Implants, abutments, and superstructures are cleaned and maintained using instruments that will not mar their surfaces such as plastic curettes, gold plated scalers, and prophy cups. Subgingival irrigation should be employed to flush out the gingival crevice or pocket. Yearly radiographs are taken of the implants to evaluate for bone loss. Exposed screws are checked for tightness. Fixed bridges are evaluated for tightness and are recemented if required. Overdentures are evaluated for stability and retention. The overdentures are relined if unstable and the attachments are replaced if nonretentive.

REFERENCES

1. Chiche GJ, Pinault A: *Esthetics of anterior fixed prosthodontics*, Chicago, Quintessence, 1994, pp 2:33-51.

2. Cranin AN, Klein M, Simons A: *Atlas of oral implantology*, ed 2, St. Louis, Mosby, 1999.

3. Rufenacht CR: *Fundamentals of esthetics*, Chicago, Quintessence, 1990, pp 4:67-133.

4. Carr AB, Laney WR: Maximum occlusal forces in patients with osseointegrated oral implant prostheses and patients with complete dentures, *Int J Oral Maxillofac Implants* 2:101-108, 1987.

5. Misch CE: *Contemporary implant dentistry*, ed 2, St. Louis, Mosby, 1998.

6. Eckert SE, Laney WR: Patient evaluation and treatment planning for osseointegrated implants, *Dent Clin North Am* 33:599, 1989.

7. Lindh C, Peterson A: Radiologic examination for location of the mandibular canal: A comparison between panoramic radiography and conventional tomography, *Int J Oral Maxillofac Implants* 4:249, 1989.

8. Klein M, Cranin AN, Sirakian A: A computerized tomography (CT) appliance for optimal presurgical and preprosthetic planning of the implant patient, *Practical Periodont Aesth Dentistry* 5:6, August 1993.

9. Laney WR: Critical aspects of removable partial denture service. In Goldman HM, et al, editors: *Current therapy in dentistry*, St. Louis, Mosby, 1968, pp 3:287-304.

10. Klein M, Smith R: Tough-temps. Esthetics and implants, *Isr J Practical Esth Implant Dentistry* 1:15-18, May-August 1995.

11. Hobo S, Ichida E, Garcia L: *Osseointegration and occlusal rehabilitation*, Tokyo, Quintessence, 1990, p 60.

12. Branemark, PI, Zarb GA, Albrektsson T: *Tissue-integrated prostheses*, Chicago, Quintessence, 1985.

13. Naert I, Quirynen M, et al: prosthetic aspects of osseointegrated fixtures supporting overdentures, a 4-year report, *J Prosth Denture* 65:671, 1991.

14. Adell R, Lekholm U, Rockler B, Branemark PI: A 15-year study of osseointegrated implants in the treatment of the edentulous jaw, *Int J Oral Surg* 10:387-416, 1981.

15. Blombeg S: Psychological response. In Branemark PI, Zarb GA, Albrektsson T, editors: *Tissue integrated prosthesis*, Chicago, Quintessence, 1985.

16. Lekholm U, Zarb GA: Patient selection and preparation. In Branemark, PI, Zarb GA, Albrektsson T, editors: *Tissue integrated prosthesis*, Chicago: Quintessence, 1985.

17. Zarb GA, Schmitt A: The longitudinal clinical effectiveness of osseointegrated implants. The Toronto study part II: The prosthetic results, *J Prosthet Dent* 64:53, 1990.

20 Principles of Implant Surgery

HARRY DYM, DDS

It is only within the past 20 years that the surgical placement of dental implants has become a predictable procedure with a sound basis of underlying scientific knowledge.

Prior to the groundbreaking innovative work by Professor P.I. Branemark and his group at Gothenburg University in the late 60s and 70s in Sweden,[1] the majority of practitioners and academic centers shunned dental implants because of their poor success rate and the poor scientific studies associated with the field of implant dentistry and surgery.

Before Professor Branemark's work and the current use and development of the endosseous implant, the implants used most often were the subperiosteal and blade-type implant. These implant systems were almost always plagued by the presence of a peri-implant fibrous capsule, which eventually led to implant failure as a result of infection and bone loss.

Branemark innovated the current use of titanium as the implant material of choice and coined the term "osseointegration" when describing the implant/bone interface of endosseous implants. Early reports claimed the possibility of a direct implant-to-bone contact without intervening soft tissue layers.[2]

The essential critical factors that Branemark elucidated that have significantly contributed to dental implant placement success and predictability include:

1. Minimal trauma should be applied to the recipient bone site during implant surgery.
2. The use of a biocompatible material, titanium, which would allow maximal bone integration.
3. Leaving implant buried and untouched for 3 to 4 months before prosthetic loading to allow for osseointegration to occur.
4. The use of sequentially larger drill bits with copious internal or external irrigation to minimize thermal bone damage at time of implant placement.
5. The prosthesis would have to be attached to the underlying implants by means of screws.
6. The critical importance of evaluating biomechanics before implant placement.

Branemark's original work was with an external hex screw-type implant but currently a multitude of implant types is available for use. Whether the implant is tapered, wide body, narrow, internal hex, external hex, fluted, basket shaped, pure titanium or hydroxyapatite-coated, all are placed under similar surgical protocols and principles.

This chapter will discuss the perioperative management and surgical principles involved in implant placement.

PRESURGICAL PLANNING

Before implant placement a thorough visual inspection of the oral cavity must be performed. The examiner must evaluate the periodontal status of the remaining dentition, as well as the soft tissue in the area of the planned implant with regard to presence or absence of keratinized mucosa.

Taut, pale, and pink attached mucosa over the planned implant site is a good clinical precondition, whereas red, edematous, non-keratinized mobile mucosa does not offer as good a prognosis and ideally should be treated before any implant placement.

As with any other surgical procedure, a thorough review of the patient's medical history is required. Advanced age is absolutely no contraindication to implant placement as long as the patient's medical state is stable and optimized. There are relatively few absolute contraindications to implant placement (Box 20-1).

Analysis of Bone

Manual palpation of the edentulous ridge should be performed to assess the width, height, and orientation of the buccal and lingual cortical plates underneath the overlying mucosa. Calipers or probes applied directly through the mucosa may be helpful in obtaining a better impression of bone width in the planned surgical site, after local anesthesia infiltration.

In evaluating the planned implant site, minimal

1. Uncontrolled diabetic patient
2. Significant smoking history
3. Jawbone irradiation less than 1 year before implant placement
4. Acute psychotic disorders
5. Severe bone resorption in patient who refuses bone grafting

1. Appropriate x-rays
   a. Panoramic film
   b. Periapical x-rays
   c. CAT scan (if deemed necessary)
   d. Lateral cephalogram (when indicated in edentulous lower arch)
2. Models of upper/lower arches
3. Mock wax-up of missing teeth on mounted upper/lower casts
4. Fabrication of plastic stent to transfer appropriate planned implant position to patient at time of surgery
5. Do paper tracing of planned surgical site and determine position of sinus and inferior alveolar nerve
6. Manual and instrument palpation of planned surgical site to detect thickness and concavities
7. Thorough evaluation of existing periodontal condition and optimize periodontium before surgery
8. Provide thorough patient education as to nature of surgery and possible risks and complications

dimensional parameters must be kept in mind to decrease and avoid complications (Box 20-2).

1. At least 1 mm of excess bone should be present on both the lingual and buccal or labial side after taking the width of the planned implant type into consideration.
2. Ideally, at least 2 mm of bone should be present on either mesial or distal side of the implant and any adjacent tooth or implant.
3. Vertical ridge height must ideally provide a 1- or 2-mm margin of safety from the inferior alveolar mandibular canal, maxillary sinus, and other adjacent vital structures.
4. Make certain that adequate vertical space exists between the crest of the residual ridge and the occlusal surface of the opposing dentition to accommodate the implant, implant abutment, and crown. As a general rule, a minimum of 8 mm of vertical height is required.[3]

Radiographic examination must be performed to allow the practitioner the information to assess the patient's available bone stock and determine the patient's ability to accommodate implants. Conventional radiographs used include orthopantomograms, lateral cephalometric views, and occlusal and periapical x-rays.

However, after a panoramic view and clinical assessment, if one is still unable to accurately determine the osseous morphology, a reformatted computerized tomogram (CT scan) should be considered.

Specialized computed tomography programs, such as DentaScan, allow the practitioner to evaluate in good detail all adjacent vital structures and their relationship to the existing bone as well as offering a three-dimensional view of both the mandible and maxillary alveolar ridge in cross-section. This view will allow for exact evaluation and measurement of available bone in those cases where uncertainty exists.

As a general rule, the widest and longest implant that can be *safely* used based on available information should be the one selected.

Treatment Planning (Box 20-3)

Diagnostic study models should be taken on all planned implant patients and mounted on an articulator. This will help demonstrate important and vital information regarding implant position and placement and help to determine if adequate vertical space exists between the crest of the residual ridge and the opposing dentition.

Waxed teeth should be placed to determine exact tooth position and in consultation with the restorative dentist, implant position is determined. A surgical template is then fabricated to be used as a guide for fixture placement.

IMPLANT SURGERY: PHASE I

1. Local anesthesia is administered, typically 2% lidocaine with 1:100,000 epinephrine for vasoconstriction. For patients who are anxious and apprehensive, intravenous sedation may be used. Injection of corticosteroids (dexamethasone 4 to 8 mgs) either intravenously or intraorally into the lateral muscle mass is helpful in reducing postsurgical edema.
2. An incision is made slightly buccal on the mandible or palatal to the maxillary crest (with or without a vertical releasing incision) and a periosteal elevator is used to raise a full thickness flap.
3. After adequate exposure and retraction, evaluate the surface contour of the ridge. Remove any irregularity with a Rongeur or round bur but keep in mind that for every millimeter of vertical bone

BOX 20-3 Diagnostic and Surgical Implant Placement Protocol

INITIAL DENTAL CONSULTATION (dentist and patient)
- Patient's reason and motivation for dental consultation
- Etiology of edentulous or partially edentulous state
- General medical history
- Indications and contraindications
- Specific dental/oral complaints
- Oral examination
- Psychosocial evaluation
- Preliminary diagnosis
- Treatment objectives and goals

PROPHYLACTIC CARE (dentist and dental hygienist)
- Prophylaxis of teeth
- Oral hygiene instruction

CLINICAL EVALUATION AND DIAGNOSIS (restorative dentist and dental surgeon)
- Review of indications and contraindications
- Oral examination
- Evaluation of existing dentition
- Periodontal evaluation
- Occlusal analysis
- Analysis of models in a semiadjustable articulator
- Radiographic findings
- Full mount Panorex radiograph
- Specific periapical and/or lateral jaw radiographs
- Photographic documentation
- Final diagnosis

THERAPEUTIC PLAN (dental implant team)
- Plan for implant position and sizes (restorative dentist and dental surgeon)
- Plan for prosthetic restoration (restorative dentist)

PATIENT COUNSELING (dentist and patient)
- Explanation of treatment plan
- Evaluation of patient's understanding of planned therapy, willingness and ability to cooperate

PATIENT COUNSELING—cont'd
- Establishment of treatment sequence and schedule
- Establishment of financial arrangements

PRESURGICAL MOUTH PREPARATION (restorative dentist and/or other dental specialists)
- Extractions
- Necessary restorative dental procedures
- Periodontal therapy
- Endodontal therapy
- Orthodontic therapy
- Prophylactic splinting
- Fabrication of the surgical template
- Presurgical measurement radiograph with surgical template in place
- Measurement of potential implant sites on radiograph

SURGICAL IMPLANTATION (dental surgeon)
- Positioning of the surgical template
- Surgical insertion of implant (Stage 1)
- Reopening of the implant sites (Stage 2)
- Removal of the first phase healing screw

PROSTHETIC MANAGEMENT (restorative dentist)
- Preparation of adjacent natural teeth
- Removal of second phase healing screw
- Making impression
- Fabrication of the master model
- Try-in and adjustment of prosthesis
- Delivery of prosthesis

FOLLOW-UP CARE AND MAINTENANCE (restorative dentist and dental hygienist)
- Oral prophylaxis
- Periodontal evaluation
- Oral hygiene reeducation and remotivation

---

reduction the implant will be driven 1 millimeter closer to a predetermined vital structure.

4. Transfer prepared surgical stent to mouth for implant placement direction (Fig. 20-1).
5. All drilling will be done with a slow-speed, latch-type contra-angle drill at 1500 rpm with copious amounts of irrigation. Bone temperature must not exceed 47° during drilling operations[4] (Fig. 20-2, *A* and *B*).
6. A pilot drill (2 mm) is used first, making certain to use the appropriate angulation (see Fig. 20-2).
7. The implant site is then enlarged to the predetermined width using special burs in sequence depending on the implant system used (see Fig. 20-2).

8. If multiple implants are being placed, special parallel pins should be inserted into the implant sites to aid in placement.
9. Avoid any contamination of the implant before its insertion into the prepared site.
10. When all fixtures are in place the cover screws are then secured.
11. The operative site is then thoroughly irrigated and all sharp bony edges smoothed.
12. The mucosal flap is replaced and closed primarily with some mattress sutures and simple interrupted sutures using 3-0 or 4-0 silk or Vicryl material.
13. Ideally, no prosthesis should be placed over the incision site for 7 to 10 days[5] (Box 20-4). Surgical

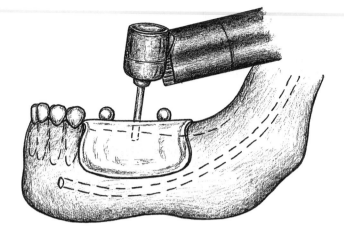

FIG. 20-1   Diagram indicating use of preoperative prepared surgical stent to aid in proper implant drill positioning.

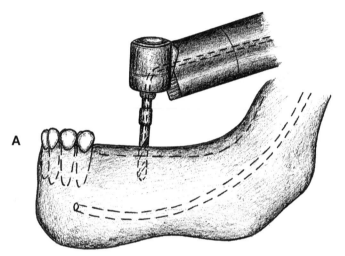

A

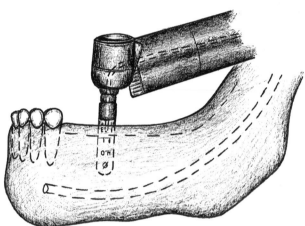

B

FIG. 20-2   **A** and **B,** Internally irrigated handpiece and drill bits in increasing dimensions used to prepare bone for the implant.

BOX
20-4   Surgical Protocol for Endosseous Implant Placement

1. Have appropriate consent form signed.
2. Have all x-rays mounted and readily available.
3. Surgical template should be available.
4. Implants and sterilized implant kit fully stocked and ready.
5. Place maxillary crestal incision more to palatal aspect.
6. Avoid leaning on handpiece and increasing drilling pressure even if bone seems quite dense and sclerotic.
7. Always place gauze curtain in oral cavity when screwing in implant cover screws to avoid inadvertent aspiration.
8. Always use parallel pins when placing multiple implants.
9. Run handpiece between 1200 and 1500 rpm during drilling.
10. Use opposing dental arch as reference guide for handpiece angulation during implant placement.
11. Always use constant irrigation during surgical preparation of bone for implant sites (external or internal or both when bone is very dense). Consider using chilled water for very dense lower mandibular bone.
12. Initial implant stability should be present at time of placement. If implant is extremely mobile and a bone/implant gap greater than 1 mm exists, immediate simultaneous bone graft should be performed.
13. Postoperative analgesics and antibiotics should be prescribed.
14. Postoperative x-rays should be taken for documentation.

stents should be used when placing multiple implants to provide for optimal biomechanics.[6]

When a precision stent is not used and when implants are placed out of alignment to the point that no prosthesis can be attached to them, the implant becomes a "sleeper" (it remains buried in the bone) and is not used.

Surgical Incision Design

Much discussion has taken place in the literature regarding incision placement design during implant surgery. Listed below are some of the different surgical incision types currently in use.

Midcrestal (Fig. 20-3, *A* and *B*). This is the easiest type of incision and perhaps the one most commonly used. It is a midcrestal incision placed directly over the alveolar bone. Its main drawback is that it leaves you with a suture line directly over the healing screw.

Palatal Based (Maxillary Implant Procedure). A technique often used during maxillary implant placement is an incision placed significantly on the palatal aspect. Its advantage is that the suture line is removed from the cover screw and allows for a complete biologic periosteal seal over the labial bone if an implant should perforate labially.

Buccally Based (Fig. 20-4). This technique places the incision closer to the buccal aspect of the alveolar crest. It allows the suture line to not sit directly over the cover screw.

Lip Incision (Fig. 20-5, *A-C*). This technique was made popular by Professor Branemark and advocated when placing implants in the lower anterior mandible in edentulous patients (especially those with shallow vestibular depths). The incision is placed out on the lip and a careful submucosal flap is raised, making certain to avoid damaging any branches of mental nerve as they travel to the lower lip. The advantage of this incision is that it allows one to reposition the mentalis muscle and decrease any postimplant muscle pull that may lead to peri-implant problems.

Implant Placement

All implant systems currently in use in the United States package their implants in sterile containers. Though all implant systems have different transfer techniques they all share a common bond in that they should be inserted into the prepared bony site under sterile technique.

Once the implant is firmly placed and seated, cover

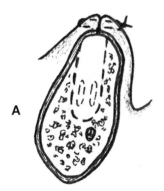
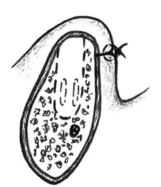
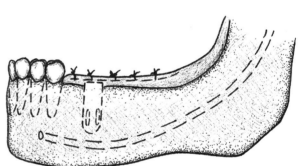

FIG. 20-3 **A,** Basic soft tissue incision design for implant surgery: *left,* midcrestal. *right,* buccally placed. **B,** Midcrestal flap closed with interrupted sutures. Note how suture line lies directly over screw and how implant sits above neurovascular canal.

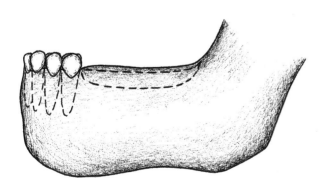

FIG. 20-4 Posterior mandible with stippled lines indicating the outline for both a midcrestal and buccal soft tissue incision.

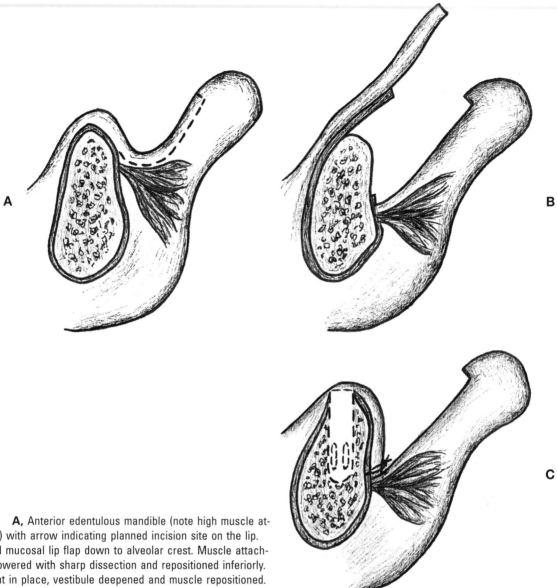

FIG. 20-5   A, Anterior edentulous mandible (note high muscle attachment) with arrow indicating planned incision site on the lip. **B,** Raised mucosal lip flap down to alveolar crest. Muscle attachment is lowered with sharp dissection and repositioned inferiorly. **C,** Implant in place, vestibule deepened and muscle repositioned. Note the one drawback to this incision; the denuded lip.

screws are then placed into the implant body. The surgical site is irrigated and the mucosal flap sutured closed with 3-0 black silk sutures. It is better for the patient not to place any prosthesis over the surgical site and to wait until after the sutures are removed (7 to 10 days later) before inserting any type of prosthesis. If this is not possible, the patient's existing prosthesis should be relieved and relined with a soft tissue-conditioning material before immediate postimplant placement.

Following implant surgery, the patient should be given prescriptions for both pain medication and antibiotic coverage. Penicillin 500 mg every 6 hours for 5 days is indicated, with erythromycin (or one of the newer forms of macrolide antibiotics for those unable

to tolerate erythromycin) a good secondary choice for the penicillin-allergic patient.

Most patients do well with Tylenol and codeine and experience only mild to moderate discomfort. Of course the patient should be advised of the usual post–oral surgery precautions, including swelling, ecchymosis, and how to contact the treating dentist in case of emergency.

IMPLANT SURGERY: PHASE II

After 3 or 4 months of undisturbed healing, the osseointegrated implant is ready for exposure and the placement of healing caps. The surgical template that was used for marking the original surgical sites can be

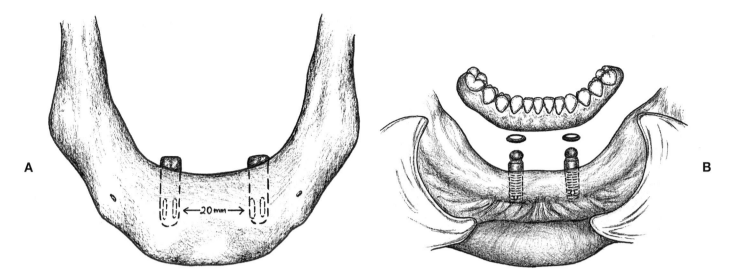

FIG. 20-6 **A,** Two lower mandibular implants placed approximately 20 mm apart in the lower anterior jaw. **B,** An overdenture can also be fabricated over two or three implants to be retained with a ball and cap attachment or an O-ring.

used to locate the osteointegrated implants. This is often not necessary as the implants can be palpated beneath the overlying mucosa.

Under local anesthesia the mucosa overlying the implant can be removed either with a scalpel, or a biopsy punch cutter device. Depending on the thickness of the overlying gingivae, the proper width and length of the transitional titanium healing collar is selected and screwed into place.

It is interesting to note that it is not uncommon for excessive bone growth to have occurred during the healing phase resulting in a layer of bone that occludes the cover screw. It can easily be removed with a Rongeur.

The prosthetic restoration can begin about 2 weeks following implant exposure.

Immediate Implantation Following Extraction

The degree of resorption of the alveolar process depends on the period of time that has passed after tooth loss. In the maxillary anterior region, severe horizontal bone resorption may be observed within a few months after extraction. In the entire mandible, the greatest reduction of bone volume (up to 30%) occurs during the first 2 years after tooth loss. It has been shown that early implantation may preserve the alveolar ridge.

With guided tissue regeneration and bone grafting techniques, even large spaces between the extraction bony socket crypt and implant are not now regarded as contraindications to implant placement.

However, some clinical studies[7] have shown that

implants placed 8 weeks postextraction, often referred to as secondary immediate implantation, have better results than primary implant placement.

Number of Implants

The number of implants to be placed will obviously be determined by the clinical findings and the patient's needs, both esthetic and financial. However, close communication is essential among everyone involved in the patient's treatment: patient, restorative dentist, and surgeon.

In cases of partial edentulism where fixed prosthetic work is planned, it is helpful to follow a guideline called Antes' law, that the total surface area of the abutments should equal the total surface area of the missing teeth. Implants can be thought of as replacing a tooth root and it is felt that in the posterior jaw area, where the quality of bone is the poorest, one implant should be placed to replace each missing tooth.[4]

When fixed bridgework is desired and indicated in totally edentulous patients, multiple implants will be necessary. If all the implants are positioned between the mental foramina, it is recommended that six implants be incorporated into the treatment plan and the superstructure be cantilevered no more than 10 mm distal to the last implant abutment.

If a removable implant-supported denture is planned as the restorative mandibular procedure, two implants can be placed in the anterior lower jaw, 20 mm apart (Fig. 20-6) to allow for adequate space for a prefabricated bar to be placed in certain cases. However, patients who present with narrow arch-shaped mandibles are better suited to four implants and a retentive connector bar (Fig. 20-7, *A* and *B*).

Finally, it is important to always remember when treatment planning for a totally implant-supported prosthetic restoration that the placement of too few implants with improper distribution will lead to excessive forces being distributed upon insufficient support. This overloading of implants may induce bone loss, increasing the risk of implant failure.

Implant Placement in the Atrophic Mandible

Mandibular resorption is a common finding in edentulous mandibular patients seeking implant therapy. The severely resorbed mandible (8 mm and less) presents a reconstructive surgical challenge to the surgical team. Though some claim success in reconstructing patients with 7-mm implants,[8] many clinicians feel that bone grafting to augment the atrophic mandible is required.

Intraoral onlay grafting to superiorly increase vertical height with simultaneous implant placement has been advocated by some,[9] however, many feel this procedure carries a higher risk of sensory impairment, infection, and greater subsequent resorption. The alternative approach is to graft the lower border of the atrophic mandible using an extraoral approach.

The Bosker implant has become a popular alternative for the treatment of the severely atrophic mandible. It is a transosteal implant system that allows for an implant-supported overdenture prosthesis. It has been reported to actually increase bone apposition over time in certain patients.

The partially edentulous posteriorly atrophic mandible presents special problems for implant placement because of the limiting factor of the neurovascular canal. A surgical technique of temporary nerve displacement does offer a practical solution but it is often

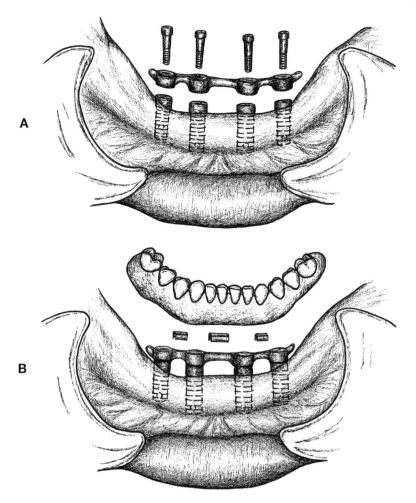

FIG. 20-7   **A,** The special bar is fabricated and attached to the four implants with screws. **B,** Newly fabricated denture snaps over retentive bar; now most stable.

accompanied by a sensory change and patients should be informed of this possible sequela.

Onlay grafting and recently reported alveolar osteogenesis distraction are alternate treatment solutions.

Implant Placement in the Edentulous Maxilla

For a maxillary removable implant-supported prosthesis, the placement of two or three implants on each side of the maxilla in the canine to the first molar area provides the most predictable esthetic and functional result.

For a maxillary fixed implant-supported prosthesis, precise placement of the implants is critical. Implants are usually placed in the central incisor, canine, premolar, and molar areas (Fig. 20-8), with the exact location determined by the surgical tray fabricated from a diagnostic wax-up and information obtained from the radiographic work-up. Care must be taken to not place an implant too far posteriorly as it may be difficult to obtain clearance to work with the prosthetic components. Ideally four implants should be placed on each side of the arch.

BONE GRAFTING FOR IMPLANT SURGERY

Patients who present for implant treatment often lack the necessary quantity of bone in either the vertical or horizontal dimension required for implant placement. This bone loss is usually secondary to the natural atrophy that occurs in both the maxilla and mandible after early tooth loss but can be secondary to traumatic jaw injuries.

Bone atrophy is no longer an absolute contraindication to implant therapy and current bone grafting techniques exist that will allow most patients to ultimately receive endosseous implants.

Types of Bone Grafting

Bone graft materials available for use are of three basic types and the clinician will determine which to use based on:

1. Quantity of bone needed
2. Health status of patient
3. Type of defect to be grafted

Allogeneic Bone

Allogeneic bone is bone harvested from human cadavers that have been thoroughly screened for any transmissible disease. It is properly sterilized and is available from certified bone banks. Both cortical strips as well as cancellous bone are available along with bone chips, powder, or granules.

Autogenous Bone

This bone material is the most biologic in that it is harvested directly from the patient. Of course, this will require an additional surgical procedure and will add cost, time, and discomfort to the planned implant procedure; however, it is often the only surgical reconstructive solution for the rehabilitation of the severely atrophic maxilla or mandible in need of implant placement. The amount and type of bone needed will also determine the donor site required for harvesting (Figs. 20-9 and 20-10).

When significant amounts of both cancellous and cortical bone are needed, the preferred bone site is the patient's ileum or hip. The anterior hip is easily harvested if one is in need of 40 cc's of cancellous bone or

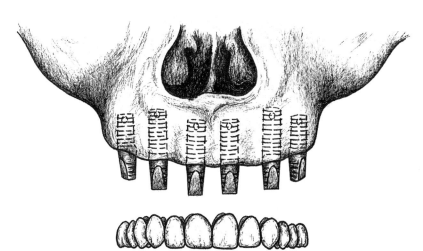

FIG. 20-8 A twelve unit fixed bridge can be placed over the implants and cemented directly to the posts.

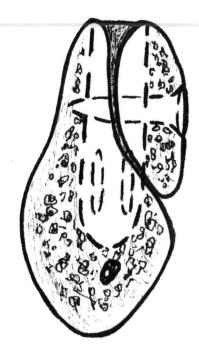

FIG. 20-9 Cortical onlay graft to augment narrow ridge with simultaneous implant placement.

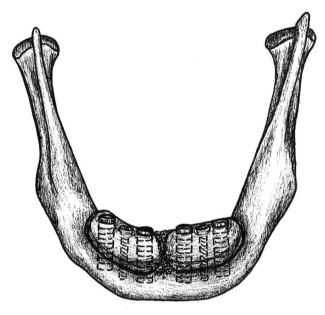

FIG. 20-10 Vertical onlay grafts to augment atrophic mandible.

less; the posterior ileum can be used if significantly more bone is required. If smaller amounts of bone are needed the following intraoral donor sites are available and can be accessed easily with the patient in an ambulatory dental setting.

1. The chin is easily approached either through a sulcular or vestibular incision after the administration of local anesthesia. One should be certain to be clear of the roots of the anterior teeth by 2 mm before starting the bony cuts. The harvest should be limited to the outer cortical plate as perforation of the lingual plate will result in more bleeding and postoperative complication. Special care must be taken to avoid injury to the mental nerve. The donor site itself, if large, can be filled with allogeneic bone mixed with collagen fibers to aid in hemostasis and to prevent any intraoral dimpling before closure.

2. The maxillary tuberosity is an easier available source for some limited amount of bone. It is easily accessed but care should be taken to avoid any significant oral antral communication.

3. Posterior lateral ramus in the area of the third molar region is a possible donor site. Little cancellous bone is available but it is a good source of cortical plate for onlay grafting.

4. Calvaria and ribs are both possible sites but require operating room conditions and offer little cancellous bone.

HOME CARE MAINTENANCE

Like the natural dentition, good oral hygiene is one of the most important and critical factors associated with long-term success and health of implants. Poor hygiene resulting in heavy plaque and calculus build-up around implants will lead to peri-implant mucositis (inflammation limited to the soft tissue) and peri-implantitis (loss of supporting bone secondary to inflammation).

The periodontal pathogens that affect the natural dentition can be equally damaging to the supporting structure of the implant and one should strive to eradicate preexisting inflammatory periodontal disease before actual implant placement.

Plaque control procedures can begin immediately following implant placement; especially if a mucosal dehiscence occurs and exposes the implant cover screw, the patient can be placed on chlorhexidine mouth rinses and taught to clean the exposed implant components by using a cotton applicator dipped in chlorhexidine. After stage two surgery the patient should rinse with chlorhexidine twice a day for 14 days and then begin mechanically cleaning the abutment above and below the tissue margin. Metal hand instruments and ultrasonic tips should be avoided when debriding around implants because they alter the titanium surface, fostering plaque retention and maturation.[10] Plastic instruments recently introduced with similar designs to traditional periodontal scalers should be used.

After delivery of the prosthesis to the patient, the patient should be placed on a recall system for routine evaluation.

The implant patient must be thoroughly instructed in

the use of various periodontal cleansing aids available to adequately maintain peri-implant health.

REFERENCES

1. Branemark PI, Hansson BD, Adell R, et al: Osseointegrated implants in the treatment of the edentulous jaw. Experiences from a 10 year period, *Scand J Plast Reconstr Surg* 16(Suppl):1, 1977.
2. Branemark PI, Adell R, Breine U, et al.: Intra-osseous anchorage of dental protheses. I. Experimental studies, *Scand J Plast Reconstr Surg* 3: 81-100, 1969.
3. Sheperd NJ: A general dentist's guide to proper dental implant placement from an oral surgeon's perspective, *Compendium* 22: 118-130, 1996.
4. Eriksson AR: Heat induced bone tissue injury. Thesis, University of Gothenburg, Sweden, 1984.
5. Collins TA: Branemark-Basic and Beyond. In Bell WH (ed.): *Modern practice in orthognathic and reconstructive surgery*, Philadelphia: WB Saunders, 1992.
6. Brose MU, Michney R, Rieger G: A precision alignment frame for endosseous post dental implants, *J Prosth Dent* 60:591, 1988.
7. Mensdorff-Pouilly N, Watzek J, Solar P, et al: Immediate implantation for rehabilitation of the jaw after extraction of all residual teeth. In Lill W, Spiekermann H, Watzeh J, editors: *Abstracts of the 5th International Congress on Preprosthetic Surgery*, Vienna, April, 1993.
8. Triplett RG, Mason ME, Alfonso WF: Endosseous cylinder implant in severely atrophic mandible, *Int J Oral Maxillofac Implant* 6:264-269, 1991.
9. Astrand P: Onlay bone grafts to the mandible. In Worthington P, Branemark PI, editors: *Advanced osseointegration surgery: Application in the maxillofacial region*, Chicago, Quintessence, 1992, pp 123-128.
10. Rapely JW, Swan RH, Hallman WW, et al: The surface characteristics produced by various oral hygiene instruments and materials on titanium implant abutments, *Int J Oral Maxillofac Implant* 5(1):47-52, 1990.

TRAUMA

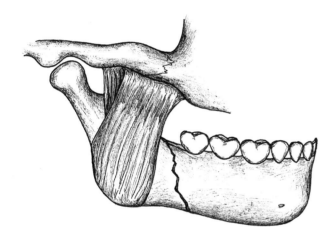

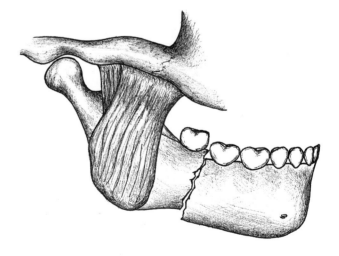

21

Evaluation and Treatment of Dentoalveolar Injuries

WAYNE MAURER, DDS
RYAZ ANSARI, DDS
HARRY DYM, DDS

INITIAL ASSESSMENT

Severe or life-threatening injuries to the mouth, jaws, and facial regions should be treated in a hospital setting, whereas isolated mild trauma to the oral cavity in which life-threatening or severe injury have been ruled out can be treated on an outpatient basis.

MEDICAL HISTORY

A thorough medical history should be taken for all patients seen with facial and dental trauma. The medical history should include the place and time as well as any other circumstances surrounding the trauma. It is important to ascertain whether the patient can respond to specific details so as to evaluate the neurologic status of the patient at the time of the incident. If the patient's recollection is cloudy or the patient is unable to recall, a full neurological work-up is necessary. With injuries to the dentition it is extremely important to ascertain the length of time that has elapsed between the trauma and the initial therapy. If teeth have been completely luxated from the mouth, the length of time they have been outside the mouth and the transport medium used are critical for the prognosis of any attempted reimplantation.

EXTRAORAL EXAMINATION

A complete and thorough facial examination should be carried out. Special attention should be given to tissue contours, point tenderness, step defects, ecchymosis, occlusion, and tooth mobility. A left and right comparison should be made throughout the examination in order to interpret correctly any abnormalities. Any significant inconsistencies between clinical observations and the description of the trauma by the patient should be noted. It is also of importance to note whether the observed injuries coincide with the time of the trauma. Clinical signs of previous surgery or trauma should be noted and entered in the patient's clinical records.

SOFT-TISSUE INJURIES

It is vital to establish that no foreign bodies have lodged within the adjacent soft tissues in patients who have experienced dentoalveolar trauma. This is true particularly in cases in which the patient has bitten the soft tissues and when fractured teeth are evident; fragments of enamel may have become embedded in the soft tissues. In any wound involving a danger of infection the patient should be assessed for a tetanus booster. Debridement of soft tissue wounds should be limited and the wound margin should be excised. Primary closure should be obtained in all cases if possible. The need for antibiotic prophylaxis should be evaluated on a case to case basis, although in the authors' opinion antibiotics should be used in all extensive trauma involving the oral cavity, as infection caused by oral bacterial contamination is a significant possibility.

The wound should be carefully cleaned using normal saline or peroxide-soaked gauze squares and then disinfected using an alcohol/povidone-iodine mixture. Coagulated blood and tissue fragments should be removed and the wound should be thoroughly inspected. Visual inspection and probing with a blunt probe will provide information on the depth and involvement of the underlying bony structures. Muscle and connective tissues are best approximated using resorbable sutures (3-0 or 4-0 Dexon), and the mucosa and skin can then be closed using monofilament sutures (5-0 or 6-0 Nylon).[1]

INTRAORAL EXAMINATION

Examination of the teeth and supporting tissues should be thorough and comprehensive (Box 21-1). In patients who are dentulous, observations of any dental maloc-

BOX 21-1 Elements of Oral Exam in Dental Trauma

1. Teeth mobility
2. Percussion response
3. Tooth displacement (luxation)
4. Occlusion
5. Tooth fractures
6. Color of teeth
7. Alveolar fractures
8. Lacerations
9. Hematomas/swellings
10. Electric pulp test

TABLE 21-1 Cause of Dentoalveolar Injury

Cause	Number of Patients (%)
Falls	105 (46%)
Fights	31 (14%)
Auto accidents	29 (13%)
Other accidents	26 (12%)
Bicycle	19 (8%)
Sports	12 (5%)
Child Abuse	3 (1%)
Unknown	2 (1%)
Total	227 (100%)

Adapted from Perez R, Berkowitz R, McIlveen L, Forrester D: Dental trauma in children: A survey. *Endodont Dent Traumatol* 7:212-213, 1991.

clusion can prove to be significant in determining any dentoalveolar trauma. It is sometimes necessary to obtain plaster models in order to perform a more comprehensive evaluation of the patient's dental occlusion. In the edentulous patient any prosthetic devices should be available at the time of examination, including dentures that fractured during the trauma. Minor degrees of tooth mobility are best tested by using the ends of two instruments, one on the lingual and one on the buccal and then applying pressure and evaluating the tooth for movement, rather than digital pressure.

RADIOGRAPHIC EXAMINATION

After radiographic evaluation using mandible and facial series has ruled out any skeletal fractures, it will be necessary to obtain panoramic, occlusal, and periapical radiographs of the traumatized area. The panoramic x-ray is the most useful of all projections for evaluating dentoalveolar types of injuries. It has significant value because it demonstrates the entire upper and lower jaw. Superimposition of the vertebrae in the incisor region can occasionally make diagnosis in these areas difficult; however this can be resolved by taking a standard occlusal or periapical radiograph. One of the drawbacks of the panoramic radiograph is the fact that it does not clearly delineate the crowns and roots for minor trauma. Periapical and occlusal x-rays are of better value in clearly showing the teeth and alveolar bone in greater detail. The diagnostic points of periapical and occlusal x-rays are greatest in the evaluation of root fractures or retained roots in the case of luxated or traumatized teeth. They are also useful in evaluating whether an alveolar fracture has passed through the tooth socket or through the periodontal ligament. This is important when evaluating the need for antibiotic therapy because a fracture through a periodontal ligament would be considered a contaminated fracture.[2]

CHOICE OF ANESTHETIC

Most dentoalveolar trauma can be treated satisfactorily with the use of local anesthetics. However, as a result of patient cooperation or severity of the sustained trauma it may be prudent to use a local anesthetic with IV sedation or general anesthesia. Local anesthetic technique can be given via infiltration or nerve block. Nerve block is preferable so as to avoid the site of inflammation, however infiltration is useful for achieving adequate hemostasis in the operating field.

Localized Injuries of Teeth (Table 21-1)

It is common for injuries of the dentition to occur in children as a result of direct trauma to teeth or because of the sudden impact of one dental arch against the other. Many of the accidents that affect the primary dentition occur during the first 3 years of life. At this age, the child is moving from the complete total state of dependence with respect to movement to one of independent movement, such as sitting up, bending over, crawling, kneeling, standing, walking, and running. Any and all of these stages of movement bring with them the hazard of accidental injury. As the child becomes older, injuries to the dentition can be attributed to playground falls, fights, and sporting mishaps; and at a later age motor vehicle accidents become the most common cause of injury. The most common type of dental injury is subluxation, producing a loosening of teeth, although a complete avulsion of the tooth from

Classification of Dental Injuries (Classification of the World Health Organization)

Enamel fracture Involves the enamel only and includes enamel chipping and incomplete fractures or enamel cracks

Crown fracture without pulp involvement An uncomplicated fracture involving enamel and dentin; no pulp exposure

Crown fracture with pulp involvement A complicated fracture involving enamel and dentin and exposure of the pulp

Root fracture Fracture of root only; cementum, dentin, and pulp. Also referred to as a horizontal root fracture

Crown/root fracture Tooth fracture that includes enamel, dentin, and root cementum, and may or may not include the pulp

Tooth luxation Includes concussion, subluxation, and lateral luxation (displacement)

Intrusion; extrusion Tooth is displaced axially, either into the alveolus (intrusion) or partially out of the tooth socket (extrusion)

Avulsion Complete displacement of a tooth from its socket

Fracture of the alveolar process (mandible or maxilla) Fracture or comminution of the alveolar socket or of the alveolar process

---

its socket may occur. These types of dental injuries usually cause trauma to the adjacent teeth and soft tissues, particularly the lips.

Traumatic injuries to the hard dental tissues, the pulp, and supporting tissue may be defined by a system developed by the World Health Organization in its application of international classification of diseases to dentistry and stomatology (Box 21-2).

Types of Injuries to the Teeth
(Table 21-2)

An *uncomplicated crown fracture* is a fracture confined to the enamel without loss of tooth substance (Fig. 21-1). A *complicated crown fracture* is a fracture involving the enamel and the dentin, or exposing the pulp (Fig. 21-2).

Concussion is an injury to the tooth-supporting structures without abnormal loosening or displacement of the tooth but with marked reaction to percussion. *Subluxation* is an injury to the tooth-supporting structures with abnormal loosening but without displacement of the tooth (Fig. 21-3).

Intrusion is displacement of the tooth into the alveolar bone. This type of injury is accompanied by comminution or fracture of the alveolar socket (Fig. 21-4). *Extrusion* is partial displacement of the tooth out of its socket (Fig. 21-5). *Avulsion* is complete displacement of the tooth out of its socket (Fig. 21-6).

Tooth fractures are described by the Ellis classifica-

tion. An Ellis Class I fracture involves enamel only and may represent a relatively minor injury. Dental examination is recommended, but this condition may not require emergency treatment. An Ellis Class II fracture involves enamel and dentin and requires immediate dental evaluation and treatment. Temperature sensitivity is indicative of exposed dental tubules and indicates the need for protection with a medicated restoration. An Ellis Class III fracture involves enamel, dentin, and the dental pulp; this represents a severe class of injury that requires immediate treatment of the pulp within 2 hours after the injury occurs. Exact treatment will depend on the developmental stage of the apex of the root. An open apex will require attempted apexification using calcium hydroxide treatment; for a closed apex, root canal therapy is indicated. In minor pulp chamber exposures, pulp capping can be attempted. An Ellis Class IV fracture is a complicated tooth fracture involving pulp tissue as well as fracture of the root. It has a poor prognosis and requires immediate treatment, most often extraction of the tooth.

Emergency and Long Term Treatment of Ellis Classification Fractures

Ellis Class I. These fractures are usually asymptomatic and may be handled in one of two ways. If the fracture is slight, sharp edges of enamel may be smoothed using a diamond bur on a high speed handpiece and polished using Sof-lex discs or Shofu cups. Fluoride may then be added to strengthen the surface layer. The acid-etch and composite restoration technique may also be used as a second choice. Again the area should be treated in the same manner as previously stated and then restored using a composite restoration. It should be noted that these restorations can be used as the definitive permanent restoration.[3]

Ellis Class II. A proper diagnostic radiograph must be taken. Fractures involving the dentin usually present with symptoms of some type. The exposed dentinal tubules, "odontoblastic processes," are directly linked to the pulpal tissue resulting in direct stimulation of the pulpal tissue to hot and cold stimuli, causing discomfort. A thin calcium hydroxide layer should cover the exposed dentin layer as soon as possible to avoid damage to the pulpal tissue and to encourage the formation of secondary dentin. A composite restoration should be placed over the calcium hydroxide layer in order to protect the integrity of the bandage coating. If at all possible a final composite restoration should be done at the emergency appointment but because of the time constraints of reshaping and recontouring, a final restoration it is not always possible.

TABLE 21-2 Type and Frequency of Injuries to the Teeth

Diagnosis	% of Injured Primary Teeth	Patient (N)	% of Injured Permanent Teeth	Patient (N)
Segmental alveolar fracture	3	14	1	4
Avulsion	10	55	12	33
Caries	3	14	0	0
Craze lines	0.4	2	3	9
Crown fracture, enamel	6	35	8	23
Crown fracture, dentin	4	21	26	72
Extrusion	7	39	7	19
Facial bony plate fracture	4	21	26	72
Intrusion	14	76	3	8
Luxation	27	155	15	41
Root fracture, apical	0.5	3	0	0
Root fracture, coronal	0.2	1	0.4	1
Root fracture, middle	1.4	8	0.7	2
Root fracture, vertical	2	9	0.7	2
Subluxation	11	64	13	37
Total	100	562	100	276

Adapted from Lombardi S, Sheller B, Williams BJ: Diagnosis and treatment of dental trauma in a children's hospital. *Pediatr Dentistry* 20(2):112-120, 1998.

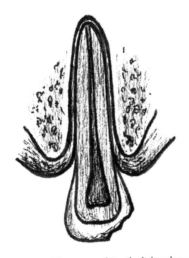

FIG. 21-1 Ellis Class I fracture of tooth. It involves enamel only.

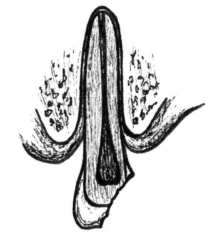

FIG. 21-2 Complicated crown fracture, Ellis Class II type. Fracture involves enamel and dentin.

The patient is seen again after a period of 3 months and the vitality of the affected tooth is checked, and periapical radiographs are again taken. Any symptomatic change in the tooth is noted. At this point if electrical pulp testing indicates a loss of vitality or if periapical pathology is noted on radiographic evaluation then root canal therapy is indicated. Depending on the remaining tooth structure, full coverage restorations may be necessary.[4]

Ellis Class III (Fig. 21-7). A small pulpal exposure of approximately 1 mm can be treated by means of indirect pulp caps irrespective of apical development as long as treatment is started quickly and the tooth is still vital. As previously mentioned, a composite restoration should be placed over the calcium hydroxide bandage. Exposures greater than 1 mm with a closed apex can be treated with immediate pulpal extirpation followed by root canal therapy. In the presence of an open apex, a calcium hydroxide pulpotomy is used in order to promote apexification. After apical closure, full root canal therapy should follow. In the nonvital tooth with a closed

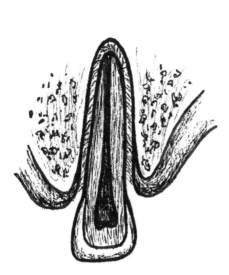

FIG. 21-3 Subluxation. The tooth is present in the socket but shows greater than physiologic mobility after trauma.

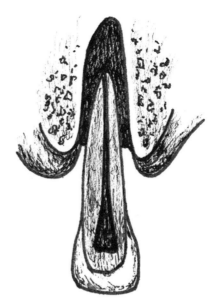

FIG. 21-5 Extrusion. The tooth is partially avulsed and forced out of the socket in an apical direction without root penetration of the alveolar wall.

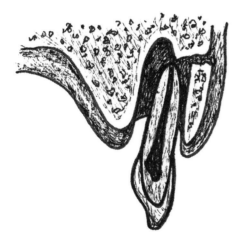

FIG. 21-4 Intrusion. Injury in which the tooth is forced apically and usually accompanied by fracture of the apical portion of the alveolus.

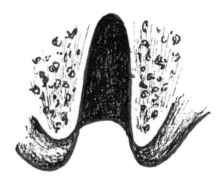

FIG. 21-6 Avulsion. Tooth has been totally displaced out of the socket.

apex full root canal therapy should be performed as opposed to the open apex nonvital tooth in which an apexification technique should be used. The fractured portion of the tooth with the closed apex can then be treated with a permanent composite restoration to restore normal appearance.[4]

Ellis Class IV (Figs. 21-8 and 21-9). This is a fracture that occurs apical to the cememtoenamel junction (CEJ) and involves dentin, cementum, and the pulp. Fractures of this type can be isolated root fractures or complicated crown and root fractures. The treatment of crown-root fractures depends on the location of the

fracture and existing periodontal conditions. If the crown-root fracture extends significantly apically down the root, the tooth should be extracted. However, if enough root structure remains, periodontal surgery followed by endodontic therapy with a post and crown may salvage the situation.

When an isolated horizontal or oblique root fracture occurs, the treatment is again dictated by the location of the fracture. A root fracture at or coronal to the bone (cervical 1/3) is treated by removal of the coronal fragment followed by endodontic root therapy and restoration with post and crown.

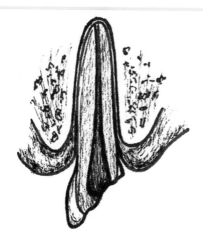

FIG. 21-7 Ellis Class III fracture involves enamel, dentin, and pulp.

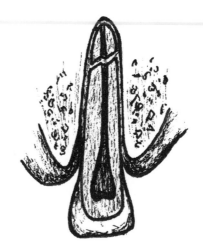

FIG. 21-9 Root fracture at the apical third.

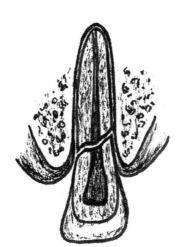

FIG. 21-8 Ellis Class IV fracture apical to CEJ that involves dentin, cementum, and pulp. Note how fracture line is at coronal one-third.

Fractures in the middle to apical one-third of the root can be successfully managed by repositioning the coronal fragment, if displaced, and rigidly splinting to the adjacent teeth for 2-3 months.[5] Frequent follow up is advised and if pulpal necrosis develops, endodontic therapy can be performed only on the coronal portion with great success.

If periapical pathology develops in apical 1/3 root fractures the apical segment and periapical pathology can be removed by the standard apicoectomy procedures.

All primary teeth with root fraction should be extracted except for those primary root fractures occurring in the apical 1/3; in which case only observation is necessary and no splinting recommended.

Fractures of the Alveolar Process

Fractures of the edentulous ridge should be treated with antibiotics when the oral mucosa has been violated. Wound debridement should be performed and any small loose pieces of alveolar bone should be removed because the likelihood of survival of the small pieces of alveolar bone is poor. Oral mucosa lacerations should be repaired by watertight suturing with either 3-0 silk or 3-0 Dexon sutures.

Alveolar process fractures that occur in the maxilla may lead to the development of an oral antral fistula when these fractures occur in the molar or premolar regions. This fact should be kept in mind when closing the oral mucosa in these areas. Raising any large flaps to repair oral antral communications should be delayed until fracture healing is complete, because raising large flaps might jeopardize the blood supply of the bony fragments. The fractured segments can be reduced using finger pressure, and if the patient has a denture it should be worn for support and as a protective splint. Complications arising from extensive loss of the alveolar process may produce difficulty in the provision of a satisfactory denture. Secondary procedures needed to improve denture retention might include ridge augmentation, vestibuloplasty, or implant placement.

Fractures of the Dentate Alveolar Process (Fig. 21-10)

Fractures of the alveolar process can occur independently but most often accompany injuries to the teeth (luxation or root fractures). The segment of bone may involve one or multiple teeth but in either place the treatment is the same. Under local anesthesia the segment can usually be reduced into proper anatomic

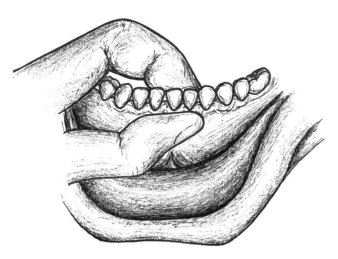

FIG. 21-10 Bidigital palpation of alveolar segment to both determine extent of injury and to manipulate segment into appropriate position.

position by finger manipulation. In rare occasions this may prove difficult and then the soft tissue may have to be carefully incised to gain direct visualization of the underlying fractures, whereupon gentle force can then be applied to reduce the segments.

Once the segment is deemed to be in its proper place, it must be stabilized for about 6 weeks. Careful attention should be paid to assure that the teeth in the involved segment are free of any occlusal trauma. Many different methods of stabilizing the fractured segments are listed later in this chapter.

All associated mucosal lacerations should be closed primarily with either 3-0 silk or Dexon suture.

Intrusion

In intrusion, the tooth is pushed further into the socket that indicates that the alveolar process has sustained a fracture to permit the intruded tooth position. The treatment of intruded teeth is somewhat controversial. Some advocate immediate repositioning and splinting whereas others suggest that this technique may lead to ankylosis and pulp necrosis, and they recommend orthodontically extruding the teeth after 5 to 7 days. Primary teeth that are impinging on the follicle of the permanent teeth should be extracted, but otherwise may be left alone to re-erupt spontaneously if minimally displaced.

Extrusion

In extrusive injuries the tooth is only partially avulsed out of the socket.

Treatment consists of replacing the tooth into the socket with digital pressure and then splinting the teeth together. Primary teeth that are extruded should be removed. Careful follow-up will be vital as endodontic root canal therapy may become necessary.

AVULSION

One of the major factors in the long-term success of reimplanted teeth is the health of the periodontal ligament, and this is directly related to the time the avulsed tooth is out of the socket. Teeth implanted within 30 minutes have a very good chance of surviving whereas those reimplanted after 2 or more hours have only a limited prognosis (Box 21-3).

If the dental office is called immediately following a tooth avulsion, the patient should be told to replant the tooth, if possible, and to come immediately to the office for treatment. If this is not possible, the tooth should be placed in a transport medium. The possible types of media are listed here from best to worst: Hanks balanced salt solution, saline, the patient's own saliva, or milk. Water should be used if all of the above are not available. If none are available, the tooth should be carried tucked against the cheek in the patient's mouth.

When the patient reaches the dental office, the tooth should be handled with care. It should be rinsed gently and quickly with sterile normal saline, if grossly contaminated, and examined for any root fractures. If the tooth has been out of the socket for more than 2 hours, some suggest placing the tooth in a 2% sodium fluoride solution before reimplantation, but this is not universally accepted.[6]

The tooth should be placed in the socket with firm pressure until it is completely seated with no attempt made to debride the socket before reimplantation. After reimplantation, the tooth should be splinted to the adjacent teeth with a semirigid splint for 7 to 14 days or until the tooth demonstrates mobility within acceptable limits. Bony fractures associated with tooth avulsion will require longer splinting periods of about 6 to 8 weeks.

A permanent tooth with an *open apex* that has been replanted 2 hours after avulsion requires close and frequent follow up. The patient is examined 2 to 3 weeks following reimplantation and radiographs are taken to check for any pulpal pathology. If there are any signs or symptoms of infection, resorption, or pathosis, the entire root canal system is cleaned, then filled with a soft nonsetting calcium hydroxide paste to the level of the open apex. Follow-up radiographs should be taken at 3-, 6-, and 12-month intervals to monitor root development, which usually occurs between 6 and 12 months. Once it is confirmed radiographically that the apex has closed, the canal can then be filled with gutta-percha.

BOX
21-3 Replantation Sequence for Avulsed Teeth With Less Than Two Hours
      Out of Bony Socket

1. Place tooth in saline solution. Do not scrub or brush tooth.
2. Radiograph-injured site and evaluate for alveolar fracture.
3. Administer local anesthesia and gently irrigate socket with saline.
4. Reinsert tooth into socket without handling root surface.
5. Check tooth alignment and avoid hyperocclusion.
6. Stabilize tooth to adjacent teeth with a nonrigid or semirigid splint for 7-14 days. If alveolar fracture is present, maintain splint for 6-8 weeks.
7. Antibiotics should be prescribed (Pen VK 250-500 mg qid or Zithromax dose pack, if penicillin allergic.)
8. Tetanus booster injection is recommended if last one administered more than five years ago.
9. Soft diet and frequent follow up.
10. *Note:* Treatment sequence for a tooth replanted more than two hours out of its bony socket is as above, except that tooth is obturated and canal filled with gutta-percha immediately.

For the permanent avulsed tooth with a closed apex and less than 2 hours dry time, the pulp should be removed in 7 to 14 days and the canal cleaned and replaced with calcium hydroxide. Controversy does exist as to when the canal should be obturated and filled with gutta-percha, with some advocating only a 2 week wait[7] following the calcium hydroxide fill whereas others advocate waiting 1 year after the initial insult.[8]

Permanent teeth with closed apices out of the mouth for more than 2 hours should have the nerve canal obturated and replaced with gutta-percha immediately before reimplantation. These teeth will eventually be lost to resorption but will in the short term fill the space. Do not reimplant primary teeth as they resorb quickly and can damage the underlying permanent tooth.

Consider tetanus prophylaxis in all patients in whom avulsed teeth are reimplanted, and patients should be placed on a soft diet as well as antibiotics (penicillin 500 mg × 7 days).

Methods of Immobilization
(Box 21-4)

Many techniques are available to stabilize and secure both tooth avulsions and dentoalveolar fractures. All methods of immobilization should be atraumatic, gentle on the periodontal tissue, hygienic, stable, and easy to apply. Fixation for avulsed teeth should allow for physiologic movement as rigid stabilization carries a greater risk of root resorption and ankylosis.[9]

Foil Splint. In the emergency situation, a lead foil from any dental x-ray packet or thin tinfoil can be molded to the subluxated tooth and the adjacent stable teeth, and then cemented into place using cold cure

BOX
21-4 Fixation Periods for
      Dentoalveolar Injuries

1. Mobile tooth (subluxation injury, no alveolar fracture)	3-4 weeks (nonrigid)
2. Tooth displacement (evaluate for alveolar fracture)	3-6 weeks (nonrigid)
3. Root fracture	2-3 months (rigid)
4. Replantation	7-14 days (nonrigid)
5. Alveolar fracture	6-8 weeks (rigid)

acrylic. This is short-term treatment until more definitive stabilization is performed.

Cold Cure Acrylic Splint. The splint can be made on a stone model obtained after taking an impression or in the mouth (be careful to avoid injuring oral mucosa by the heat generated). It can be secured by wiring it to the stable teeth and to the fractured segment.

Arch Bars. This method is useful when treating subluxated teeth associated with alveolar fractures. Arch bars are wired to two teeth distal from the fracture site; this is used for immobilization of the fracture. The arch bar provides good labial support for the subluxated teeth and the fracture site.

Figure-8 Wiring. This uses a soft, stainless steel wire around the abutment teeth past the fracture on either side of the subluxated teeth in a figure-8 manner. This has the disadvantage that in some crown forms tightening of the wire can dislodge or extrude the teeth (Figs. 21-11 and 21-12).

Orthodontic Brace Technique. When the proper equipment is available orthodontic brackets can be placed using a light-cured or chemical-cured resin bonding agent and a soft, stainless steel ligature wire

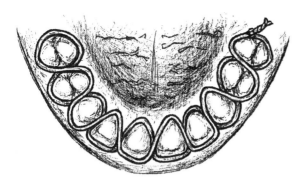

FIG. 21-11 Diagram showing bird's eye view of continuous circumdental wiring with 28-gauge wire to establish and secure mobility, avulsed teeth, and alveolar segment.

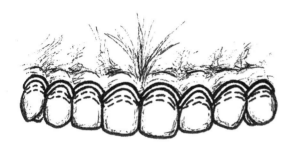

FIG. 21-12 Shows how wire is adapted to facial aspect of the teeth.

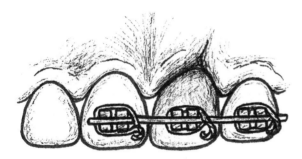

FIG. 21-13 Orthodontic brackets bonded to teeth adjacent to traumatized tooth and secured with wire.

can be ligated in a figure-8 manner to the brackets immobilizing the subluxated tooth or alveolar fracture. This can be used as a more permanent immobilization technique (Fig. 21-13).

For the first 2 weeks after splint removal nutrition should be limited to soft foods. Reproducible centric occlusion and increased normalization of mandibular function should be monitored on a weekly basis. Clini-

cal and radiographic checkups should be made at 3, 6, and 12 months.

Oral Hygiene Measures

Patients should brush their teeth three times daily using a soft nylon toothbrush. After each meal, the patient should rinse with a commercially available chlorhexidine rinse. After splint removal patients should be seen for a professional dental scaling and prophylaxis. Rinsing the mouth with salt water might be of benefit especially when soft tissue trauma has occurred.

SUMMARY

An overview of the various possibilities of trauma in the primary dentition, permanent dentition, and dentoalveolar processes has been presented. Modern and longstanding treatment modalities have been described. With the recent advances in dental materials, treatment modalities have become significantly less tedious and superior to what they were just a few short years ago. However, we must not forget the various responses that individual patients might have to specific treatment techniques. Because of this we should never be rigid in our treatment approach. We should be able to diagnose, interpret, and alter our treatment modalities in response to various situations as needed.

REFERENCES

1. Nelson L: Pediatric emergencies in the office setting: oral trauma, *Pediatr Emerg Care* 6(1):62-64, 1990.
2. Stoneman D: Radiology of trauma to the teeth and jaws, *Dent Clin North Am, Dentofac Trauma* 26.3:591-611, 1982.
3. Andreasen JO: *Traumatic injuries of the teeth*, ed 1, Copenhagen, Munksgaard, 1972.
4. Franklin P: Treatment of trauma to the young permanent dentition, *Dent Clin North Am, Dentofac Trauma* 26.3:525-554, 1982.
5. Ellis E: Soft tissue and dentoalveolar injuries. In Peterson L, et al: *Contemporary oral and maxillofacial surgery*, ed 3, St. Louis, Mosby, 1998.
6. Dale RA: Dentoalveolar trauma. In Montgomery MT, Redding SW editors: *Oral-facial emergencies*, Portland, JFK Publishing, 1994.
7. Lockhart PB: *Oral medicine and hospital practice*, Chicago, Federation of Special Care Organizations in Dentistry, Chicago, 1997, pp. 5-56.
8. Gerstein H, *Techniques in clinical endodontics*, Philadelphia, WB Saunders, 1983.
9. Andreasen JO: The effect of splinting upon periodontal healing after replantation of permanent incisors in monkeys, *Acta Odontol Scand*, 33:313, 1975.

22 Closed Reduction of Mandibular Fractures: Indications and Techniques

ORRETT E. OGLE, DDS

Mandibular fracture comprises the largest percentage of the cases of facial bone fractures that are treated by the dental professional in the United States. In a review of 2261 facial bone fractures treated by the oral and maxillofacial surgery service at two large New York City public hospitals (Woodhull and Lincoln Hospitals) over a 10-year period, 1193 cases (52.8%) were isolated mandibular fractures. Haug and colleagues reported on 402 facial trauma cases treated by the oral surgery service at the Cleveland Metropolitan General Hospital, of which 307 suffered fractures of the mandible (76.4%).[1] Many other cases are also treated annually in private dental offices.

The mandible is particularly prone to trauma because of its prominent position in the face. The location and distribution of these fractures seen at Woodhull Hospital are shown in Fig. 22-1.

The diagnosis of a fracture of the mandible is made based on a history of recent trauma, along with clinical and radiographic examinations. Box 22-1 presents some useful signs and symptoms for the diagnosis of mandibular fractures.

X-RAYS

The panoramic radiograph of the mandible affords the best view when a fracture of the mandible is suspected. Other useful radiographs are the posterior-anterior view (PA) of the mandible (to view medial or lateral displacement of fractures), lateral oblique (for fractures in the angle and ramus), and the reverse Townes projection (to visualize the condyles). A mandibular occlusal view is indicated for symphyseal fractures, and dental periapicals should always be taken of teeth in the line of a mandibular fracture.

CLASSIFICATION
Simple

A simple fracture is a fracture in which the overlying soft tissue is intact, and there is no communication with the oral cavity or the exterior. The fracture may or may not be displaced.

Compound

A compound fracture is a fracture in which the bony end is exposed to the oral cavity or to the exterior, and is assumed to be infected by outside contaminants. Almost all mandibular fractures that occur in the teeth-bearing area are considered compound fractures. This is because the fracture becomes in contact with the oral cavity through the periodontal ligament (PDL) space and gingival sulcus, and is said to be "compounded intraorally."

All patients with compound fractures of the mandible should be started on antibiotics, and the antibiotics used for 7 to 10 days. Patients with fractures that are compounded into the mouth should be started on penicillin 500 mg q6h, or clindamycin 300 mg q8h if the patient is allergic to penicillin. With fractures that are compounded extraorally a cephalosporin (Keflex 500 mg q6h, or Ancef 1 gram intravenously (IV), q8h for the hospitalized patient), or clindamycin 300 mg q8h may be used. Cephalosporins are contraindicated in patients who are allergic to penicillin.

Comminuted

A comminuted fracture is a fracture in which the bone is splintered, and there are several fragments. It may be simple or compound. Gunshot wounds are usually

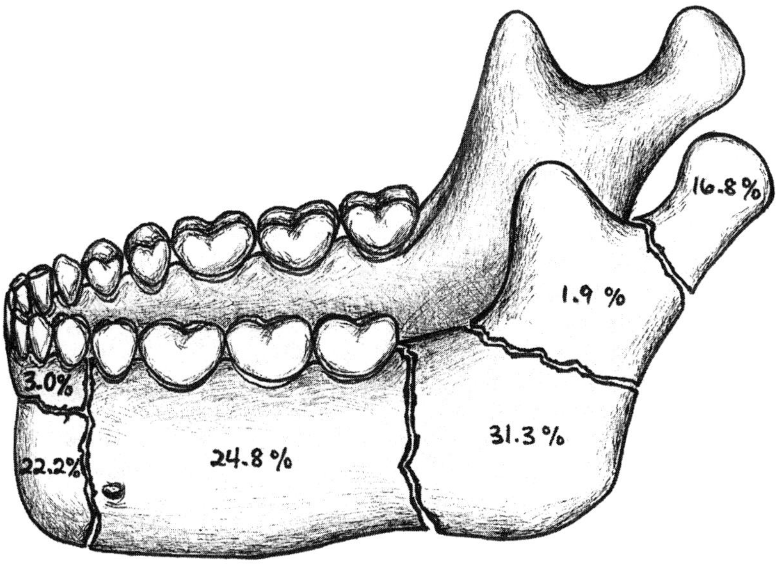

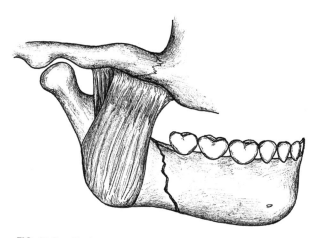

FIG. 22-1   Distribution of mandibular fractures.

BOX 22-1   Signs and Symptoms of Mandibular Fractures

Pain: Present with movements of the mandible, or when chewing is attempted.

Neurosensory disturbances: Anesthesia, paresthesia, or hyperesthesia may be present in the lip and buccal gingiva of the affected side as a result of injury of the inferior alveolar nerve.

Malocclusion: May or may not be present, but when present offers the best evidence of a bony deformity. A posterior open bite is pathognomonic for a subcondylar fracture

Laceration and bleeding: Bleeding may be seen around the necks of teeth that are located in the fracture line. Gingival lacerations may also occur at the fracture site.

Trismus: Commonly seen and is usually a result of guarding because of pain. In fractures at the angle the trismus may be caused by direct trauma to the masseter and lateral pterygoid muscles. There may also be a reflex spasm mediated through the sensory pathways of the disrupted bone segments.

Abnormal mobility: Bimanual manipulation will produce separation between mandibular fragments.

FIG. 22-2   Horizontally favorable fracture of the mandible.

Unfavorable

This is a fracture in which the direction of the fracture line permits distraction of the segments by the muscle pull acting on the bony ends (Fig. 22-3).

Multiple Fractures

Multiple fractures are those in which the mandible is fractured in two or more places. They are generally bilateral, and occur quite often. Each fracture site should be evaluated independently, and treated as indicated by the flow chart in Box 22-2.

Displacement

The displacement of the bony parts of a fractured mandible is a result of the functional action of the

---

compound comminuted fractures. If bony tissue was lost when the missile traversed the bone it is termed an avulsive injury.

Favorable

A favorable fracture is one in which the direction of the fracture line is such that the muscle pull tends to self reduce the fracture (Fig. 22-2).

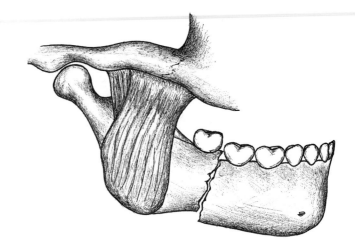

FIG. 22-3 Horizontally unfavorable fracture of the mandible with displacement.

BOX 22-2 Flow Chart for the Management of Mandibular Fractures

Condyle --→	MMF (2 weeks followed by physiotherapy)
Coronoid ---→	No treatment
Ramus → Nondisplaced ------------------------------→	MMF only if painful, or soft diet
Displaced ---------------------------------→	ORIF
Angle → Favorable ---------------------------------→	MMF ....4–6 weeks
Unfavorable ------------------------------→	Open reduction with rigid bone fixation; no MMF
Body → Teeth present on both sides of fracture -----→	MMF.....4–6 weeks
Teeth missing from proximal* segment --------→	ORIF; no MMF
Edentulous --→	ORIF or MMF using acrylic splints
Symphysis --→	ORIF with rigid bone fixation
Severely infected fracture --------------------------→	External pin fixation; no MMF
Avulsive injuries -----------------------------------→	ORIF; reconstruction plate or extraskeletal pins
Compound fracture → Yes----------------------------→	Antibiotic coverage
→ No -------------------------------------→	Evaluate other factors for the need for antibiotic

MMF, Maxillo-mandibular fixation; *ORIF,* open reduction–internal fixation.
*The proximal segment of the mandible is the part closest to the condyle.

muscles attached to the mandible when the continuity of the bone is lost. The action of balance between the muscles of mastication (elevator-rotator group) in the posterior and the suprahyoid muscles (the depressor group) in the anterior is lost when a fracture occurs, and each muscle group exerts its own action unopposed by the other. Whether the segments become clinically displaced will depend on the direction of the line of fracture and buttressing of the segments.

DECISION PROTOCOL

The following are several factors that will familiarize the practitioner with some of the complex principles involved in the decision-making process regarding the treatment of mandibular fractures. Emphasis will be placed on the management of fractures that may be treated in the dental office by closed techniques.

The goals in the treatment of mandibular fractures are:

- To minimize pain, and keep the patient pain free in the convalescence stage
- To prevent infection
- Reestablishment of the pretrauma dental occlusion
- Proper alignment of the bony segments
- Stabilization of the fracture long enough for healing to occur
- To treat the patient and restore masticatory function with the least morbidity and discomfort

Several factors must be considered in deciding which treatment modality should be used to manage a mandibular fracture. Some of these factors are presented in Box 22-2.

To determine the appropriate management of a fractured mandible the flow chart in Box 22-2, which is based on fracture location, should be used as a guideline.

Any fracture may be treated by open reduction and rigid plate fixation to avoid the use of maxillomandibular fixation (MMF). However, this will require hospitalization or treatment in a Surgicenter.

MMF is not recommended in patients with the following conditions:

- Seizure disorders
- Psychiatric disorders
- Alcoholics
- Immune deficiency
- The elderly
- Patients in poor general health who cannot tolerate the decrease in nutrition caused by having their jaws wired.

Teeth in the Line of Fracture

Special consideration should be given to teeth in the fracture line. A tooth in the fracture line makes the fracture a compound fracture, and the patient should be started on antibiotics. A decision must be made whether to remove the tooth from the line of fracture. Every attempt should be made to preserve teeth. Indications for removal of teeth in the line of fracture are:

- A fracture of the root or of the tooth itself that is in the fracture line
- Carious, nonrestorable teeth, or teeth with large periapical pathology
- A tooth in which the PDL is completely stripped from the cementum*
- Excessive mobility (3+) caused by the trauma or by periodontal disease
- If the tooth interferes with the reduction

Fracture of the Mandibular Condyle

The management of this fracture can be difficult and sometimes controversial, particularly when it occurs in a child. The proportion of condylar fractures is higher in children than in adults, accounting for 40% to 67 % of the mandibular fractures seen in children.[2] A large number of these cases are treated satisfactorily by conservative methods in private dental offices, with few subjective or objective posttraumatic symptoms. It has been reported, however, that 5% to 10% of cases requiring orthognathic surgery for a mandibular asym-

metry were probably caused by subcondylar fractures.[3] Nevertheless, the results achieved by conservative treatment are more favorable in young individuals, whereas impaired function of the temporomandibular joint (TMJ) following trauma is more likely to occur in older adult patients.[4] In both groups, early mobilization seems to minimize complications.

The question may be raised as to why subcondylar fractures should not be repositioned to normal anatomic relations as is done with other fractures. The reason is a combination of three factors: (1) the TMJ area is a surgically difficult area to operate, (2) there is a relatively high risk of injury to the facial nerve, and (3) the results of conservative treatment have been very good.

A serious complication of condylar fracture is ankylosis of the TMJ, thus the need for early mobilization and physiotherapy. The onset of the ankylotic process most often occurs in the first decade of life, however, and is less common in adults.[5,6] Laskin reported the frequency of ankylosis following fractures and trauma to the TMJ to be 0.4%[5] (that is, 1/250 cases of TMJ trauma).

The algorithm in Fig 22-4 for the management of fractures of the condylar neck will be helpful in the decision-making process.

TREATMENT

According to the flow chart in Box 22-2, the fractures amenable to treatment by a simple closed technique are fractures of the condylar neck, nondisplaced ramal fractures, favorable angle fractures, and body fractures in the fully dentate individual. The closed technique is based on the premise that reestablishing the proper pretrauma occlusion will lead to an adequate bony alignment. Thus a thorough understanding of dental anatomy and occlusion is imperative.

Anesthesia

Bilateral nerve blocks and local infiltration will offer adequate pain control and are frequently used along with IV sedation (see Chapter 4). These patients will often present with trismus, thus the Akinosi technique for administering inferior alveolar nerve block should be used (see Chapter 3 for a description of the technique). Local anesthesia should also be infiltrated directly into the fracture line.

The maxilla will require extensive infiltration of the local anesthesia, and may be very uncomfortable to the patient. Topical application of benzocaine will be helpful. The administration of N_2O at 50% concentration by nasal mask will also improve patient cooperation for the administration of the local anesthesia. The mask is removed once the local anesthesia has been infiltrated.

---

*I do not extract anterior teeth, however, because of esthetics and the fact that root canal therapy (RCT) can easily be started.

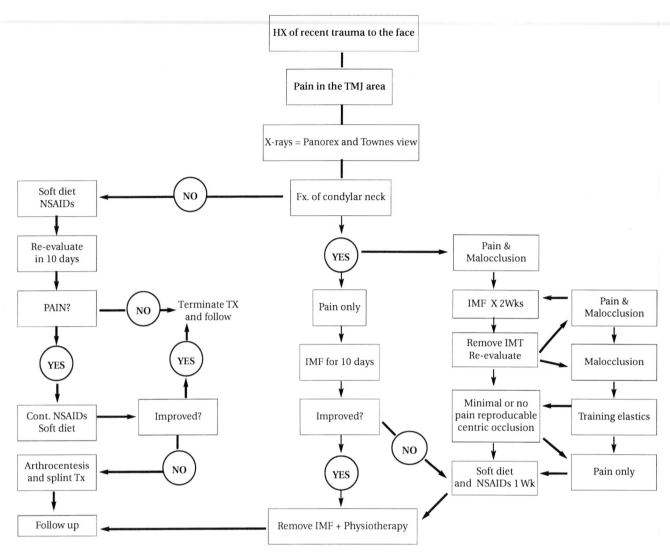

FIG. 22-4 Algorithm for management of condylar treatment.

A long (1-3/8 inches) 27-gauge needle should be used. The needle is introduced into the buccal vestibule at the canine and advanced submucosally to the first molar. One cartridge of lidocaine 2% with epinephrine 1/100,000 is infiltrated as the needle is slowly withdrawn. The same thing is done on the contralateral side. To anesthetize the anterior, the needle enters at one canine, and is advanced to the contralateral canine, depositing the anesthetic solution as the needle is withdrawn. The palate will require infiltration of the local anesthetic at several sites, usually one drop per two teeth. Seven to ten cartridges may be required, and the dentist should be aware of the maximum safe dosage of the drug used. (See Chapter 3 for the recommended maximum dosages of various anesthetic agents). To minimize the possibility of overdosage, the mandibular blocks may be done first, and the mandibular arch bars applied before infiltrating the maxilla. This will generally allow 20 to 30 min-

utes for some of the drug to metabolize before additional dosage is added.

Instrumentation

■ 26 gauge stainless steel wire cut into 6″ lengths
■ Light wire cutter (Smith, Tessier or Ambassador)
■ Heavy wire cutter (ETM)
■ Wire twister
■ Kelly hemostat
■ Angled dental curette
■ Periosteal elevator
■ Soft Erich arch bars

Procedure

A stable occlusal platform exists in the intact maxilla and the fractured mandible is reduced against this intact maxilla via the dentition.

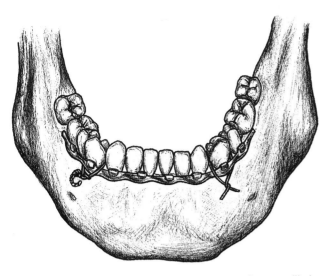

FIG. 22-5 The ligation of the arch bar to the mandibular dentition. The arch bar extends from first molar to first molar.

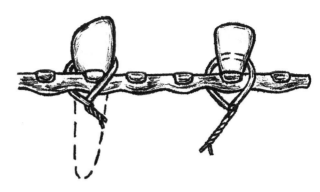

FIG. 22-6 Ligation of an arch bar to the mandibular dentition showing the position of the ligature wires.

1. Accurately premeasure two lengths of the soft arch bar to go from first molar to first molar on the maxilla and on the mandible. (Usually 16 lugs of the standard Erich arch bar for the maxilla and 14 for the mandible.) An overextended bar will cause soft tissue necrosis and severe pain.

2. Pass a wire around the mandibular second premolar bilaterally. Place the arch bar into the loop in such a way that one strand of the wire will be above and the other below the arch bar. Ligate one of the premolars fully to the arch bar and loosely tack the contralateral side to permit future adjustment of the position of the arch bar (Fig. 22-5).

3. Ligate the first molar next to the fully ligated premolar to the arch bar on the buccal surface. The wire is twisted in a clockwise fashion. The operator should make sure that neither the wire nor the twisted knot will interfere with the lugs on the arch bar. If a scalloped arch bar is used, the surgeon should try to put the twisted end into the deepest part of the scallop. Leaving the twist on the slope will permit the wire to slide and loosen from the arch bar. This will result in an ill-fitting arch bar that will compromise a tight MMF (Figs. 22-6 and 22-7). When passing the ligature wire around the terminal tooth, the wire should be above the arch bar on the distal aspect of the tooth and below the arch bar on the mesial (see Fig. 22-7). This will ensure that the arch bar will not lift once MMF is established.

4. Continue to ligate the arch bar to the teeth working from the ligated first molar to the free end across the arch. The bar should be carefully adapted without any bulges, as an improperly adapted arch bar will cause orthodontic movement of teeth. In the anterior teeth the assistant should use the dental curette or the periosteal elevator to seat the wire securely under the cingulum to resist displacement of the arch bar to the incisal level during MMF. Ligate each tooth to the arch bar individually. This will produce a more stable arch bar, minimize orthodontic movements, and disperse stresses tending to loosen teeth during the fixation period.

5. After ligating the arch bar to the teeth, cut each braided wire leaving a pig-tail of about 1/2 inch. Go back and re-tighten all the wires. Tuck the free end of the wire underneath the arch bar, away from the lips and cheeks, with a clockwise turn. This will prevent loosening of the knot.

6. Ligate an arch bar to the maxillary teeth using the same technique.

7. Reduce the fracture manually by placing the teeth into the pretraumatic dental occlusion. Do not try to correct any malocclusions. Look for wear facets on the enamel to help determine the position of the occlusion. Use a looped wire placed around lugs on the mandibular and maxillary arch bars, and bring the jaws into occlusion (Fig. 22-8 *A,B*). The maxillary-mandibular fixation (MMF) wires should be placed over the premolars. Do not engage the terminal lug, as this will lift the arch bar. Do not place MMF wires on the anterior teeth either, as this may cause elongation of these single rooted teeth with conical roots.

8. In compound fractures, antibiotics should be given for 7 days postoperatively. Analgesics should be prescribed to be used prn. If the patient has missing teeth with gaps in the dental arch, pills may be slipped into the mouth through the

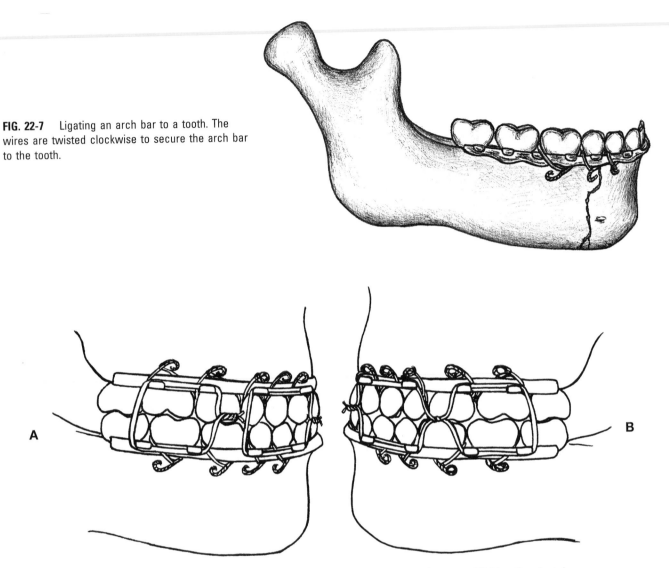

FIG. 22-7 Ligating an arch bar to a tooth. The wires are twisted clockwise to secure the arch bar to the tooth.

FIG. 22-8 **A** and **B,** Method for reducing a mandibular fracture by reestablishing the dental occlusion and maintaining fixation by maxillo-mandibular fixation (MMF). Note that the MMF wires are placed over the premolars.

gap. If this is not possible elixirs or solutions may be used. Penicillin V potassium is available in tablets for oral solution in strengths of 250 mg and 500 mg. Clindamycin palmitate hydrochloride (Cleocin Pediatric*) is also available in pediatric dosages of 75 mg/5 ml. The standard adult dose is 150 mg q6h.

Diet

During the fixation period the patient's nutritional standards must be maintained. The average adult male who does not do heavy labor needs about 2500 kcal/

day to maintain energy balance. Extra calories will be required for work (1000 kcal/day for light work, 1500 for moderate work, and 2500 for heavy work). Because food intake will be restricted, strict attention must be given to the diet to be sure that the required calories, protein, and fat are obtained. Because of the MMF the patient will be on a full liquid diet. They can be advised to boil their normal table food, and then puree it in a blender. This method may not provide enough bulk or calories to satisfy the patient however, and supplements will also be needed.

In any diet to which supplements are added, palatability will be a very important consideration. Several liquid diets (Sustacal, Ensure, and Meritene) are available in a variety of flavors, and appear to have an acceptable taste to most patients. The enjoyment of

*Manufactured by The Upjohn Co., Kalamazoo, MI.

these drinks can be further enhanced by chilling and drinking through a straw, making them into flavored shakes with ice cream, or having them as commercially available puddings. The usual intake of these liquid diets as supplements is 3 cans per day. The caloric content of each of these liquid diets is approximately the same per volume (240 to 250 kcal/can). Pediatric multivitamins should also be used.

The need to restrict lactose must be considered when choosing a liquid supplement. Many African-Americans, among others, are lactose-intolerant. Lactose-free liquid diets are available such as Ensure and Precision LR.

Fixation

During the fixation period the patient should be seen at weeks 1, 2, and 4. At each postoperative visit, the doctor should check that the MMF is without movement. If necessary, the MMF wires should be tightened or replaced. At week 4, the MMF wires should be removed and the mobility of the fracture site tested by bimanual manipulation. If the fracture is clinically stable, MMF is discontinued and the patient placed on a soft diet for 1 week. Again, the fracture is tested, and if stable, the arch bars are removed and a dental prophylaxis is done. If at week 4 the fracture is mobile, the MMF is replaced for another 2 weeks. Panographic radiographs should be done immediately postoperatively, at week 4, and after the arch bar has been removed.

Removal of Arch Bars

Arch bars can be removed quite comfortably under local anesthesia, but IV sedation or nitrous oxide analgesia will make the patient more comfortable. With local anesthesia only soft tissue anesthesia is required. Buccal infiltration will, therefore, be satisfactory. With most patients N_2O/O_2 by nasal mask is all that is required. The key to comfortably removing the arch bars is to minimize untwisting of the wires and the use of a sharp wire cutter. Once the wire has been cut, the surgeon should make sure that the cut end of the wire is not hooked to the arch bar. To remove the ligature wire, simply give it a sharp tug. Pulling it out rapidly will minimize pain. At the end, the practitioner should carefully palpate the entire buccal surface of the mandible and the maxilla to ensure that no pieces of wire are left behind.

A dental prophylaxis will greatly enhance gingival healing, and a course of Peridex with good oral hygiene will return the gingiva to its normal health in a short period of time. Patients with heart murmurs, mitral valve prolapse, poorly controlled diabetes mellitus, and those who are immune-compromised should be premedicated for removal of the arch bars.

REFERENCES

1. Haug RH, Prather J, Indreasano AT: An epidemiologic survey of facial fractures and concomitant injuries, *J Oral Maxillofac Surg* 48:926-932, 1990.
2. Norholt SE, Krishnan V, Sindet-Pedersen S: Pediatric condylar fractures: A long term follow-up study of 55 patients, *J Oral Maxillofac Surg* 51:1302-1310, 1993.
3. Proffit WR, Vig KW, Turvey TA: Early fracture of the mandibular condyles: frequently an unsuspected cause of growth disturbances, *Am J Orthodont* 78:1, 1980.
4. Dahlstrom L, Kahnberg KE, Lindahl L: 15 years follow-up on condylar fractures, *Int J Oral Maxillofac Surg* 18:18, 1989.
5. Laskin DM: Role of the meniscus in the etiology of post-traumatic temporomandibular joint ankylosis, *Int J Oral Maxillofac Surg* 7:340, 1978.
6. Adekeye EO: Ankylosis of the mandible: analysis of 76 cases, *J Oral Maxillofac Surg* 41:442, 1983.

23 Repair of Lacerations

ORRETT E. OGLE, DDS

Injury to the face will be of great concern to the patient. The face is visible, making injuries very obvious to the public and the resultant scarring may severely affect the individual's self-image. All efforts should be made, therefore, to restore the injured area to its normal anatomy or as near normal as possible, and with minimal scarring. The majority of soft tissue injuries of the face are usually repaired in emergency rooms of hospitals by ER physicians, plastic surgeons, or oral and maxillofacial surgeons. However, uncomplicated, small facial lacerations, particularly those of the lip, chin, and lower face may be adequately managed in the private office. Management of these injuries will be more economical to the self-paying patient or the third party payer when they are handled in the office setting rather than in a hospital.

These injuries most often will occur from playground injuries (lip and chin), domestic violence (lip), and home accidents (cheek, lips, chin, and submandibular areas). Techniques for wound closure along with the surgical principles of good soft tissue management will be presented in this chapter.

TREATMENT OF LACERATIONS

Facial lacerations should be treated within a few hours of the injury. After 3 hours, the bacterial count in a wound increases dramatically. On the face, however, closure of wounds up to 24 hours old can be done with small risk as the blood supply in this area is very good and the risk of infection is, therefore, very low. The goal in repairing a laceration is to repair the wound to as close to normal anatomy as possible, and to minimize scarring by careful handling of the soft tissues. Successful closure of a facial laceration will require meticulous attention to surgical and anatomic details.

Good surgical results, with the least production of scarring will depend on the following factors:

- Thorough cleansing of the wound
- Complete hemostasis
- Elimination of dead space
- Proper wound closure

- Fastidious handling of the soft tissues
- Special considerations for realigning facial tissue
- Good wound care
- Postoperative supportive care of the patient

Cleansing of the Wound

The removal of foreign materials from a laceration is essential to healing. A clean wound will heal favorably and with less scarring, because the inflammatory response will be minimized by having less bacteria and foreign material in the wound. Cleansing of the wound will remove dirt, dust, and other foreign bodies, as well as decrease the quantity of germs closed in the wound.

The first step is to irrigate the laceration thoroughly with normal saline. This can be done using a 50-ml syringe with an 18- or 19-gauge needle. This will create enough pressure to mechanically remove gross debris, if present, and decrease the inoculum of bacteria in the wound. Scrubbing does not cleanse the wound as well, and using disinfectants and hydrogen peroxide will damage healthy cells needed for healing, and will thus impede the wound healing process. A 2 × 2 gauze impregnated with povidone-iodine (Betadine Surgical Scrub) should be used to gently wash around the wound. The washing should progress from the wound margins outward, always wiping away from the wound. If the individual is allergic to iodine (history of shellfish allergies) then chlorhexidine gluconate (Betasept Surgical Scrub or Hibiclens) should be substituted. Both povidone and chlorhexidine will decontaminate the skin adjacent to the wound. They are rapidly bactericidal on contact against a wide range of microorganisms, and their microbial effectiveness is not significantly reduced by the presence of organic material such as blood.[1] After washing the skin margin, the area is patted dry, and then painted with Betadine Solution. Patients who are allergic to iodine should obviously not be exposed to this protocol, and chlorhexidine scrub alone is used. Chlorhexidine is used to scrub the area for 2 minutes, and then it is patted dry with a sterile towel. As there is no paint, the wash is repeated a second time and the skin dried. Chlorhexidine has been shown to decrease skin bacterial count by 99.8% after a 6-minute scrub, and 93% of it was present on uncovered skin after 5 hours.[2] Any disinfectant that seeps into the wound should be removed by copious irrigation.

When washing around the wound, these scrubs should not be permitted to enter and remain in the eyes, ear canal, or oral cavity. They should be rinsed out promptly and thoroughly with water. When washing a patient who is lying flat or reclined in the dental chair, care must be taken to avoid "pooling" of the paint beneath the skin or over the clavicles, as prolonged exposure to wet Betadine solution will cause irritation or rarely severe skin reactions.[3]

Hemostasis

Hemostasis allows the surgeon to repair the laceration in as clean a field as possible with greater accuracy. The detailed anatomy of the facial area will stand out better in a bloodless field. Good control of bleeding points will also prevent the formation of a hematoma or seroma which can prevent the direct apposition needed for complete union of wound edges. Brisk oozing from small vessels in the skin margin can be controlled with electrocautery whereas larger vessels should be ligated. (See Chapter 5 for further details). Bleeding from the skin margin, however, is best controlled by suturing of the wound.

Elimination of Dead Space

Dead space in a wound results from separation in tissues that have not been closely approximated. The presence of dead space will permit collection of blood within the tissues. Leaving even small amounts of blood in the wound will provide a culture medium for bacteria, with an increased risk of infection. Also, the products produced from hemolysis will chemically damage the adjacent tissues during the postoperative period, producing wound dehiscence and increased tissue fibrosis. To prevent dead space, the traumatic wound should be closed in layers. Muscle and fascia should be identified and appropriately approximated. In the perioral area deep sutures are done with 3-0 or 4-0 absorbable sutures (gut, Vicryl, or Dexon).

Wound Closure and Tissue Management

This will involve several important technical and biologic considerations. Adhering to good, basic surgical principles is crucial in minimizing scar formation. Several of these technical principles will now be discussed.

Selection of Needles. Needles and sutures should be selected for the required task. Large needles are contraindicated on the face. Cutting needles should always be used to sew the skin, whereas round (tapered) needles should be used for friable mucosa, and subcutaneous tissue. When using a cutting needle it should be passed completely through the tissue and not left in it, as it will macerate the tissue being sutured. The surgeon must avoid the temptation of using a cutting needle to bridge or approximate tissues being sutured as this will cause unnecessary trauma. In facial lacerations small, curved needles are always used. These are passed with a needle holder. The jaws of a needle holder are short, wide, and strong enough to prevent turning of the needle when it encounters dense tissue. Hemostats and Kelly clamps should be avoided.

Suture Material. For buried sutures (deep and subcuticular), an absorbable suture is indicated. Vicryl (polygalactin 910) is my preferred suture for deep closure. The material is easy to work with, is nonantigenic, nonpyogenic, and elicits only a minimal acute inflammatory reaction during absorption. It will maintain up to 75% of its tensile strength for 14 days postimplantation, 50% at 3 weeks, and will lose all of it between weeks 4 or 5. (It should be noted that the loss of tensile strength and the rate of absorption are separate phenomena. Vicryl maintains its tensile strength through wound healing, followed by rapid absorption.) Because of the length of time that the suture retains more than half of its tensile strength (21 days), it allows for early removal of skin sutures. I generally use sizes 3-0 for sutures placed deep and 4-0 for subcuticular closure.

For oral mucosa the best suture is either silk or Vicryl, with silk being my preferred material. Vicryl placed intraorally will not fall out for about 4 to 5 weeks, and I've seen it present for up to 8 weeks. It has been my observation that it tends to collect more debris than silk, and if left in for total absorption will only irritate the oral mucosa. Vicryl causes far less of an inflammatory reaction than silk, however. This would give Vicryl the advantage in situations where the patient is in maxillo-mandibular fixation (MMF), and accessing the suture to remove it will be difficult. Nonetheless, it offers very little advantage over silk because it has to be removed anyway, and it is far more expensive. Silk has the advantages of familiarity, user friendliness, and is "softer" intraorally. 4-0 silk can routinely be used to close the lacerated oral mucosa. Suture removal has not proved to be a problem.

For skin closure 5-0 nylon is my suture of choice. Nylon has a low coefficient of friction and will easily slide through the tissue, it elicits almost no tissue response, nor does it allow ingrowth of fibrous tissue into the space created by passing the needle through the tissue. The tensile strength of 5-0 Nylon is not excessive,

TABLE 23-1 Sutures and Their Properties

Suture	Ease of Use‡	Strength	Inflammatory Reaction	Resistance to Infection	Comments
Vicryl*	++++	+++	+	+++	Good for deep and intraoral sutures. Minimal inflammatory reaction intraorally, but long resorption period.
Dexon*	++++	+++	+	++++	Same properties as Vicryl.
Chromic gut*	++	++	+++	+	Difficult to tie. Good for use in children, because it falls out faster than Vicryl.
PDS*	++++	++++	++	+++	Offers extensive wound support for up to 6 weeks.
Silk†	++++	+	++++	++	Good for introral use.
Nylon†	+++	+++	+	+++	Used for skin.
Prolene†	+	++++	+	++++	Good for highly contaminated wounds.

* = absorbable sutures
† = nonabsorbable sutures
‡++++ = best to + = worse

Adapted partially from: Graber, MA: *General surgery: wound management,* 1998. http://www.vh.org/Providers/ClinRef/FPHandbook/Chapter09/01-9.html. and from: *Wound closure manual—Ethicon.* Ethicon, Inc., Somerville, NJ, pp 22-23, 1994.

and when used on the skin of the face, the material will tend to break close to the point where there is too much tension on the skin margin. This will assist the inexperienced surgeon in preventing closure of the wound under tension. Table 23-1 lists sutures and their properties.

Proper Use of the Suture Needle. The needle should be grasped in the upper third of the needle close to the swagged butt, but not at the butt itself (Fig. 23-1). This position gives the surgeon the maximum shaft of the needle to engage the tissue being sutured. A cutting needle should never be grasped too close to the tip within the cutting area, as this will damage the delicate needle tip.

In placing the initial bite, the tip of the needle should be perpendicular to the tissue as it penetrates the tissue (Fig. 23-2, *A*). Once into the tissue the nose of the needle holder inscribes a small half-circle that matches the curve of the needle. This motion is best achieved if the needle holder is held so that its long axis approximates a continuation of the axis of the forearm (Fig. 23-2, *B*). (The needle holder may also be held without placing the fingers into the finger rings.) On the second side of the laceration the procedure is reversed, starting within the wound and coming superficial. As the tip emerges from the tissue, it may be stabilized with a toothless pick-up by an assistant, or the surgeon may release the needle and regrasp it close to the tip, then bring it completely through the tissue (Fig. 23-3, *A* and *B*).

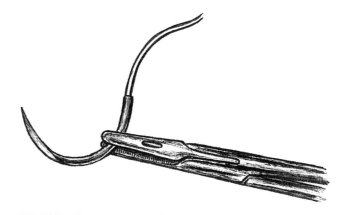

FIG. 23-1 To arm the needle holder grasp the needle in the upper third close to the swagged butt, but not at the butt itself. A cutting needle should never be grasped within the cutting area.

Tying Knots with the Needle Holder. Most facial lacerations that will be treated outside of the hospital will be relatively small, and the surgeon will be using small needles and small caliber sutures. The dentist will find it easier to tie the knots with a needle holder, because this is what we are most familiar with. Needle holders should be used to tie the knot and not a hemostat or Kelly clamp. The jaws of needle holders have smooth surfaces that will prevent weakening of the suture from instrument serrations and slipping of fine suture material out of the jaws when the knot is being tied.

After passing the suture, the surgeon pulls the thread through until about 1.5 inches of the end remains. The

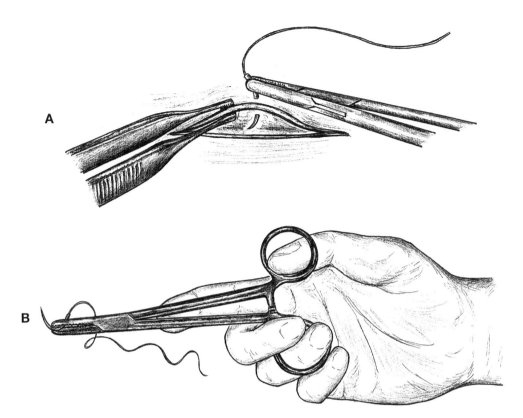

FIG. 23-2 **A,** The initial bite is achieved by securing the skin margin and penetrating it with the needle perpendicular to the skin surface. **B,** Holding the needle holder so that its long axis approximates a continuation of the axis of the forearm to allow manipulation of the needle. The needle holder may also be grasped within the palm.

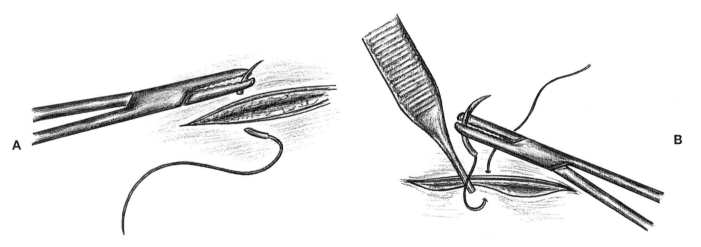

FIG. 23-3 **A,** In small lacerations, the gap may be bridged by passing the needle in one motion that engages both sides of the wound with one pass of the needle. Once the needle is passed, it is secured by the needle holder and removed. **B,** In large lacerations where the skin margins are not close together, the needle should be passed in two bites. After both sides of the wound have been bridged by the suture, the needle is secured by a needle holder and removed from the tissue in preparation for knot tying.

surgeon then secures the needle with the thumb and index finger of the nondominant hand. Two loops are made around the needle holder with the long end of the suture (Fig. 23-4). The tip of the needle holder is used to grasp the short end. The loop is pulled down over the short end, and the knot is laid flat and tightened until the approximation of the tissue is ideal. The knot is squared by throwing a second loop in the suture in the opposite direction to the first and pulling

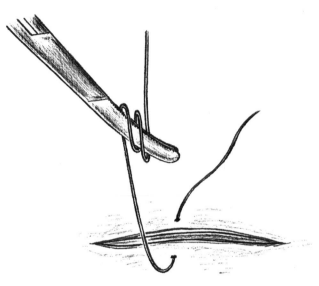

FIG. 23-4   The knot is started by making two loops around the needle holder with the long end of the suture that is attached to the needle. The needle should be secured so as not to injure the patient or the surgeon.

it down (Fig. 23-5 A,B). This will square the knot and also lock it in place. Depending on the material, other knots can be added. For silk, a double throw followed by a single will suffice, for Vicryl one double and two single throws are used, and for nylon, I use two double followed by four single throws. Each single throw should be reversed in relationship to the previous one. When making the loops the surgeon should take care to keep the suture material from dropping into the hinge of the box lock on the needle holder and getting caught there. This will prevent the loop from sliding down, and will weaken the material. If this occurs the tying procedure should be restarted. The length at which the sutures are cut is dependent on the material. Silk should be cut to leave an end of 3/8 to 1/2 inch, whereas nylon needs a longer end, 1/2 to 5/8 inch. Nylon has memory and will tend to unravel, so it should not be cut very short. (Memory is a property of the suture that gives it a tendency to return to its original straight extruded state.) Vicryl that is buried should be cut approximately 1/8 inch to minimize the amount of foreign material left inside the wound.

Proper Use of Tissue Forceps. Tissue forceps are available with smooth jaws or with interlocking teeth in small sizes for plastic repair of facial injuries. When toothless forceps are used to grasp the tissue, high compressive force is required to maintain the skin or mucosa without it slipping. This compression is enough to cause further tissue injury and increase scarring. It is less traumatic to the tissue, therefore, if it is handled with toothed forceps. Smooth-jawed forceps should only be used to hold vessels or other structures that may

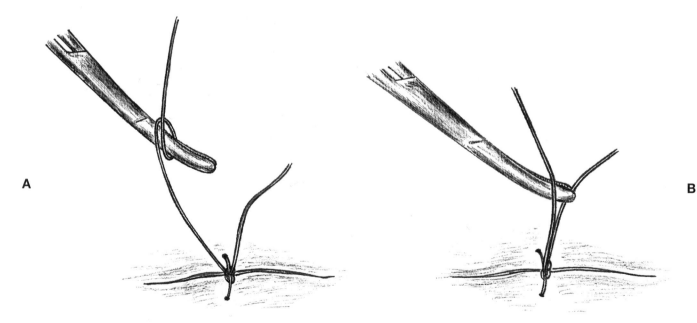

A

B

FIG. 23-5   **A** and **B,** Steps in squaring of the knot by throwing a second loop in the suture in the opposite direction to the first and pulling it down.

be damaged from the teeth on a mouse-tooth forceps. When mouse-tooth forceps are used to hold skin, one should apply only the minimum force required to control the tissue. If deep tooth indentations are noted in the skin, it is sure that the surgeon has destroyed many cells.

It should be noted that not all tissues have the same sensitivity to crushing forces. Fascia is one that is very durable and can be handled without much damage. This fact should be utilized when using toothed forceps on skin. Fig. 23-6 shows a technique for grasping skin that will cause less damage to the skin itself. In this method the skin is picked up by grasping the fascia or the acellular dermis beneath the surface, producing less damage to the epidermal cells. If the skin has to be held with forceps, the single tooth should be placed on the epidermal side and the two teeth on the inner portion (Fig. 23-7).

Proper Tension on Sutures. Proper tension on the wound interface is critical to obtain good results from suturing. Sutures that are too tight cut into the tissue, cut off blood supply, scar the skin and oral mucosa, cause postoperative pain and swelling, and delay heal-

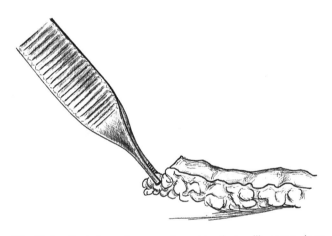

FIG. 23-6 Technique for grasping skin that will cause less damage to the skin itself. In this method the skin is picked up by grasping the fascia or the acellular dermis beneath the surface, producing less damage to the epidermal cells.

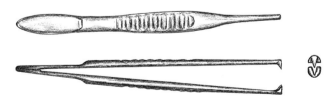

FIG. 23-7 Single tooth forceps which may be used to hold skin. If the skin has to be held with forceps, then the single tooth should be placed on the epidermal side and the two teeth on the inner portion.

ing. The tissue that is caught between any suture must be considered as being vascularly compromised, even if the wound is not under tension. Very tight sutures will increase this tissue ischemia and cause localized gangrene at the suture site. This may lead to failure of the suture and the formation of cross-hatching.

On the other hand, loose sutures will allow continuous motion between the wound interface, preventing primary healing and stimulating excessive collagen formation. It may even lead to dead space and hematoma formation.

The minimization of excessive tension on the skin margins relies on two factors: (1) the placement of the bite with the needle, and (2) the knot tension. For oral mucosa the only factor will be the knot tension.

Placing the Bite for Skin Closure. When suturing skin the passage of the needle should include deep dermis that is further away from the cut margin of the skin than is the entrance or exit point of the epidermis. To achieve this, the needle enters at an angle of 45°, 2 to 3 mm from the skin margin, and having pierced the skin it is brought into the dermis by a turn of the wrist at a depth of 4 to 6 mm. Once out of the first margin, the needle is reinserted at the same depth on the other side and made to retrace the same path as on the opposite side. The emergence should also be at 45°, as in the original entry and at a similar distance from the skin margin (Fig. 23-8).

Knot Tension. The knot is used to apply the desired tightness of the skin closure. The first knot is what determines the tension placed on the skin margin. A double first loop (surgeon's knot; see Fig. 23-4), should be used to set the proper knot tension. As these first throws are tightened to bring the margins together, the deep portion of the wound will be approximated before the skin margin (Fig. 23-9, A). As the suture is further tightened, the suture will achieve a more circular appearance as the epidermal portion of the skin is approximated. The knot should be tightened to the point where the closed skin margin rises to about 1/4 to 1/2 mm above the surrounding skin surface (Fig. 23-9, B). This will be the correct skin tension. The surgeon must now move rapidly in squaring and setting the knot so that the tension will not be lost (see Fig. 23-5 A,B).

Mucosa should be tightened just to the point where the edges touch. Pulling them too tight will cause bunching and overlapping of the mucosa. Tension will further increase after an additional 24 to 72 hours as a result of postoperative edema. Excessive tightness will decrease the circulation in the buccal mucosa causing delayed healing, and a resultant decrease in wound tensile strength of up to 40% when the sutures are removed in 7 days. Lip movement may cause an opening of the mucosal interface.

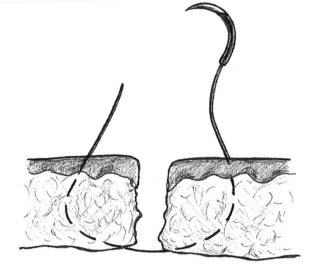

FIG. 23-8   The correct method of placing a suture to approximate skin. Note how the needle enters the tissue closer to the skin margins and goes further away in the deeper layers.

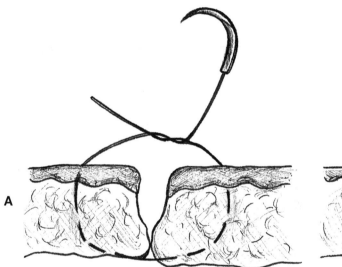

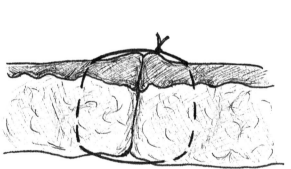

FIG. 23-9   A, Tightening the knot. As the first throws are tightened to bring the margins together, the deep portion of the wound will be approximated before the skin margin. **B,** The knot should be tightened to the point where the closed skin margin rises to about 1/4 to 1/2 mm above the surrounding skin surface.

Tissue Management

When sewing delicate tissues of the face the surgeon should make every effort to minimize tissue damage, which usually occurs because of the injudicious use of instruments. The prudent use of the gloved finger, folded sponges, skin hooks, and careful use of tissue forceps will all aid in achieving this noble goal. Fig. 23-10 shows use of the skin hook; and Fig. 23-11 shows how toothed tissue forceps may be used to lift the skin for suturing without pinching the skin.

Special Regional Considerations

Cheeks. Laceration of the cheek is the most commonly encountered facial injury. Superficial lacerations can be satisfactorily handled in the office. However, the operator must be cognizant of the following important structures that lie deep within the cheek: branches of the facial nerve, the parotid duct, and the muscles of facial expression. Injuries that involve the facial nerve or the parotid duct should be closed in the operating room by a surgeon experienced in closing facial lacerations.

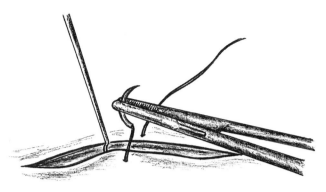

FIG. 23-10   Use of a skin hook to apply counter pressure while a suture is being passed through the skin.

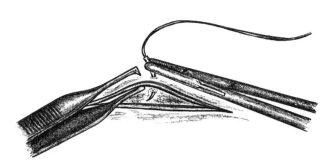

FIG. 23-11   A tooth tissue forceps being used to lift the skin for suturing without pinching the skin.

The Facial Nerve. Soft tissue injuries are of greatest concern when located in the posterior and inferior aspect of the face. The major branches of the facial nerve lie deep in the cheek, well protected by an overlying layer of soft tissue, and are seldom injured by accidental trauma. Accidental division of nerve branches anterior to the region of the parotid duct (midpupillary line) does not result in permanent loss of muscle function because the superficial facial muscles are innervated in their posterior portions[4] and the nerve generally has several collateral branches by this point. Repair of these anterior branches is, therefore, unnecessary.

Parotid Duct. The parotid duct courses along a line from the tragus of the ear to the lip commissure. The ostium is located somewhere close to the lateral canthus of the eye. The parotid duct is more superficial than the facial nerve and is, therefore, more exposed to injury. Transection of the duct should be repaired by an experienced oral and maxillofacial or plastic surgeon. The repair involves closure with 6-0 nylon over as fine a polyethylene catheter (Intracath) that is used to bridge the transected ends.

Technique. Wound closure should start deep with 3-0 Vicryl. Divided muscles of mastication and facial expression are identified and approximated. Muscle does not tolerate suturing very well, thus the surgeon should take bigger bites and not pull the knots too tight. The muscle ends should just abut each other. The placement of a horizontal mattress suture is sometimes helpful (Fig. 23-12).

Following closure of the muscles, the fascia is closed (Fig. 23-13), then buried subcuticular sutures are placed.

Subcuticular Sutures. This deep row of sutures will lessen the tension that would be needed for close approximation by the skin sutures, and allow for earlier removal of skin sutures so as to avoid crosshatching. The knots for subcuticular sutures must be buried at the deepest point of the suture loop to avoid knobby and irregular scars. To bury the knot the surgeon starts the pass deep in the wound, taking some deep dermis and the subcuticular fascia (Fig. 23-14, *A*). The needle is passed from superficial to deep on the contralateral side taking care to engage only the deep dermis. As the needle exits the flap the surgeon should make sure that the free end and the needle are both on the same side of the loop. As the knot is tied it will end up deep in the wound as shown in Fig. 23-14, *B*. These subcuticular sutures will bring the skin margin very close together and with a slight eversion.

If the dermis is very thin, as for example close to the lower eyelid, then subcuticular sutures should not be placed.

Skin Closure. If the laceration is irregular the repair should be started by first identifying key irregularities and matching them together as in a jigsaw puzzle. The rest of the laceration is closed around these established landmarks.

In a relatively straight laceration, proper alignment of the skin margins can be easily achieved by starting the closure in the exact midpoint of each side of the laceration. After securing this knot the rest of the wound is checked by brief manual apposition. Once satisfied with the tissue alignment, each of the two remaining halves are closed by further bisecting them and placing a suture. Each segment is further bisected until the entire wound is closed (Fig. 23-15).

Chin. Laceration of the chin most often occurs as a result of blunt trauma. It is a common basketball playground injury, as well as from monkey bars, swings, slides, and minor motor vehicle accidents. Because it usually occurs from blunt trauma, the dentist should make sure that a fracture of the mandibular symphysis has not occurred. The patient or parent should be questioned about the etiology and level of trauma, and if there is any suspicion of a symphyseal fracture, a well-angled mandibular occlusal radiograph should be

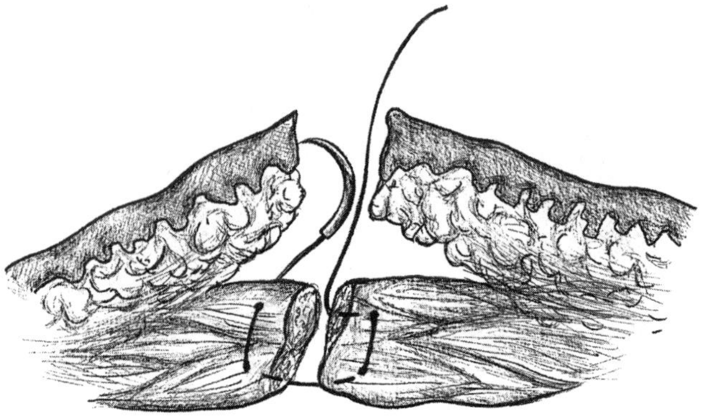

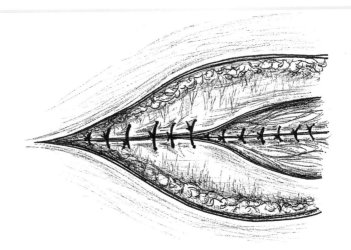

FIG. 23-12 A horizontal mattress suture.

FIG. 23-13 Closure of the superficial fascia.

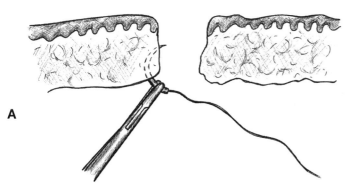

A

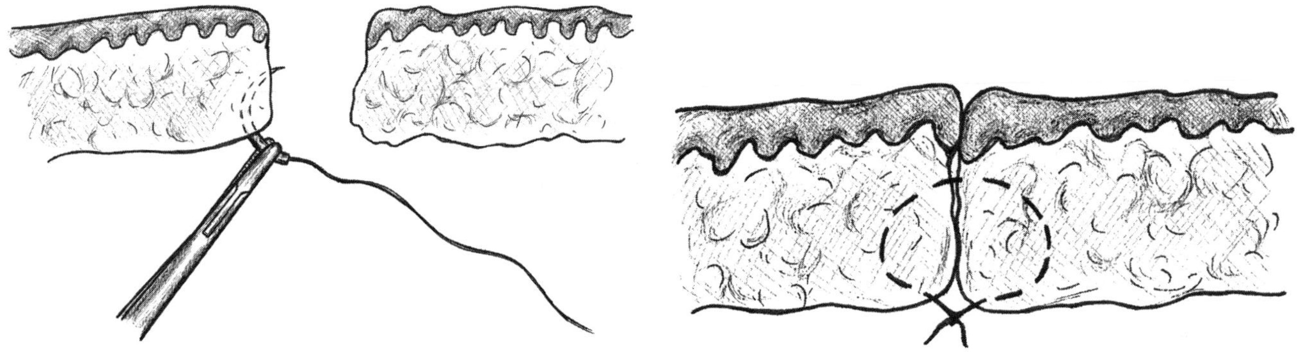

B

FIG. 23-14 **A,** To bury the knot the surgeon starts the pass deep in the wound taking some deep dermis and the subcuticular fascia. **B,** The needle is passed from superficial to deep on the contralateral side taking care to engage only the deep dermis. As the needle exits the flap the surgeon should make sure that the free end and the needle are both on the same side of the loop. As the knot is tied it will end up deep in the wound.

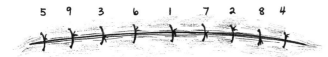

FIG. 23-15 Technique for closing skin by continuously bisecting each segment of the wound until the entire wound is closed.

taken to visualize the anterior mandible. The wound must be examined thoroughly to see if bone is exposed, and if the laceration involves the mucobuccal fold. This may occur as a unique injury in which soft tissues of the chin are avulsed up from the anterior mandible, and the oral cavity is penetrated at the lower labial sulcus.[5] This is a shearing type of injury because of the upward force from the chin, and will thus be tangential within the mouth. Exposure of the bone has been associated with

an increased risk of infection, thus heavy irrigation at repair is essential, and the patient should be started on an antibiotic.

The type of blunt trauma that often injures the chin area will usually cause a split or crush type injury. This type of injury will swell more, be accompanied by abrasions, and tend to have more devitalized tissue and a higher risk of infection. Wound contamination from rust, dirt, wood splinters, and so on will be more likely and the need for tetanus toxoid should be assessed (Table 23-2). Devitalized, crushed skin should be adequately, but conservatively removed. Ragged, severely contused skin edges are excised to provide perpendicular skin edges that can be well approximated and will heal primarily with minimal scarring. It must be stressed, however, that there is no place for radical debridement of wounds in facial trauma. Tissue will

TABLE 23-2 Tetanus Immunization

Type of Wound	Immunization Status	Vaccination Guidelines
Clean wound	• Uncertain or less than 3 doses	• 0.5 ml of tetanus toxoid. Repeat in 6 wks and 6 mos.
	• 3 doses or more but >10 years	• 0.5 ml of tetanus toxoid
Dirty wounds	• Unknown or less than 3 doses	• 0.5 ml of tetanus toxoid + 250 U of human tetanus immunoglobulin. Repeat tetanus toxoid in 6 wks and in 6 mos.
	• >5 years but <10 years	• 0.5 ml of tetanus toxoid
	• >10 years	• 0.5 ml of tetanus toxoid + 250 U immunoglobulin

<8 years old: use DTP in preference to tetanus toxoid alone.
≥8 years: use ADT in preference to tetanus toxoid alone.
Recommendations from: U.S. Preventive Service Task Force.

survive in the head and neck on small pedicles, because the blood supply is so excellent. Dead muscle, and devitalized oral mucosa should also be removed using as conservative an approach as with skin.

Closure begins at the deepest portion of the wound. If the oral mucosa is injured, this is repaired first. Attention is then directed extraorally where the periosteal layer is closed. Vicryl 3-0 is used to approximate the torn periosteum. Knots should not be buried beneath the periosteum, as this will leave space for hematoma formation and poor reattachment of the periosteum to bone. Muscle layers are closed next, followed by subcuticular sutures and skin approximation.

Lips. Lacerations of the lip should be given special consideration and closed very carefully as even slight discrepancies along the vermilion border, notching, or bulging will appear as gross deformities. Because of its unique anatomy and delicate color changes, abnormalities will be very obvious. Notching, bulges, and improperly aligned tissue will affect the esthetic application of cosmetics in the female patient, and abnormal scarring may affect the patient's self-esteem and social life.

The lip tissue should not be trimmed, or if necessary, only minimally, because the tissue is unique and cannot be replaced with adequate esthetic. The blood supply is excellent and flaps with even small pedicles will survive. Closure should start on the oral side of a through and through laceration so as to create a barrier between the oral and cutaneous environments. The repair is started by identifying the wet-dry line and closing this point first. It this point is not readily identifiable, then a "tack" suture should be placed at the vermilion border to maintain the integrity of this important landmark. Following the landmark suture, the oral mucosa is closed with 4-0 Vicryl or silk up to the vermilion border. It is easier to use Vicryl, so as not to have to change sutures. Once watertight closure of the oral mucosa has been achieved, the wound is thor-

oughly irrigated with normal saline, and repair started on the cutaneous portion of the wound. The muscle layer will be next. This layer is closed with 4-0 Vicryl. The first stitch should be placed right below the vermilion border. This suture can be left long and used as a retraction suture to apply tension to the muscle area. This will straighten out the layer, making it easier to close. The entire muscular area is sutured. One or two buried subcuticular sutures may be placed in the skin portion of the wound. I do not place subcuticular sutures within the vermilion.

The final skin sutures are placed with 5-0 nylon. The first suture is used to carefully realign the vermilion border. This will be the most critical stitch in the entire repair, and the entire result will be dependent on the placement of this one suture. The surgeon should not hesitate to replace the suture if the results are not pleasing. The skin is next closed in its entirety. The vermilion is repaired with 4-0 Vicryl.

Intraoral. Oral mucosa should be handled very delicately. Closure is done with 4-0 Vicryl or silk. In young children, chromic gut will be advantageous because it will fall out faster than Vicryl. Debridement should be very minimal.

Tongue. Tongue lacerations tend to bleed significantly and this makes them appear worse than they really are. Bleeding is easily controllable by placing gauze around the tongue and then biting on the tongue to apply pressure with the teeth. The bleeding will be fully controlled by closing the wound. In minor traumatic occurrences swelling rarely gets to the point where it affects the airway. Keeping an ice cube in the mouth will aid to decrease the swelling, but is usually unnecessary. In significant trauma with inflammation of the tongue, the patient should be in a hospital and should be intubated.

Small lacerations from the teeth need not be closed because they heal rapidly and infection is rare. A bland diet and frequent rinses with normal saline are all that

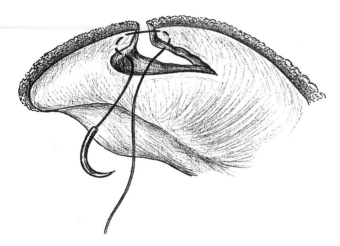

FIG. 23-16 Closing a trap door wound of the tongue with resorbable sutures.

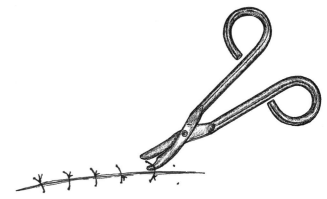

FIG. 23-17 Suture removal with a specially designed suture removal scissors.

will be required. Burns may be protected with Orabase, for example. The dentist, however, should make sure that pieces of tooth enamel, restorative materials, or other foreign bodies do not remain in the tongue. If in doubt a lower occlusal soft tissue radiograph should be done.

Large lacerations on the dorsum or lateral border, and through and through lacerations of the tongue will require suturing. These wounds are sutured with 3-0 Vicryl or with 4-0 chromic gut in the young child. Deep sutures should be placed if needed (Fig. 23-16).

Wound Care

The post-closure management of a soft tissue injury has the potential of either helping or damaging the healing process. It is, therefore, something that the surgeon should pay attention to. The patient should be followed closely, good wound care instituted from the beginning, and proper sterility used to remove sutures.

Antibiotics. Antibiotic ointment (Bacitracin) should be used on facial wounds. Crusts should be soaked off and bacitracin ointment applied qid × 5 days to reduce scar formation. There is no scientific indication to prescribe systemic antibiotics for simple, noncontaminated facial lacerations. It is my practice to give clindamycin to patients with through and through lacerations of the face. This antibiotic will cover both staphylococci and streptococci. Lacerations that involve skin only should be covered with Keflex against staphylococcus, whereas penicillin is used for primary intraoral injuries.

Dressing. One should be used only when it has a definite function. The primary function of a dressing on a facial wound is protective, to keep the patient's fingers and cosmetics away from the wound. Xeroform gauze in a single layer is placed on the wound, followed by a

dry gauze pad fixed with tape around the skin margins. Placing the Xeroform in a single layer will promote drainage of exudates from the wound through the fine meshwork, and retard drying and crust formation. I keep this initial dressing for 48 hours until epithelialization has occurred. After 48 hours Steri-Strips are used to relieve tension from the wound margin. After 7 days, Steri-Strips are used only if needed.

Suture Removal. Suture removal is started on the third day in wounds with good subcuticular closure. At this time, I remove alternate skin sutures. The remaining sutures are removed on day 5, and supplementary skin fixation is done with rigid skin adhesive strips (Steri-Strip). These skin strips are placed in such a way as to pull the skin margin together to oppose distractive forces on the skin margins.

Suture removal should be as painless as possible. The operator should not pull on the suture until the loop has been divided. The suture is lifted with a College pliers as gently as possible, and a small scissors used to cut the loop (Fig. 23-17). If the suture bites are small and the tip of the scissors cannot painlessly get below the loop, then a #11 blade is used to divide the loop (Fig. 23-18). Hydrogen peroxide can be used to remove crusts from the sutures, and the area should be lightly washed before the sutures are removed.

Patients with diabetes, HIV, taking chemotherapy or steroids, or alcoholics may exhibit delayed wound healing. Because of this, I leave the skin sutures in for a full week before removing them. These patients will also be given antibiotics for 7 to 10 days (to cover for up to 3 days after suture removal).

Anesthesia. The discomfort of the injection can be minimized by using a 27- or 30-gauge needle and introducing it through the open edge and avoiding intact skin. Lidocaine 2% with epinephrine 1/100,000

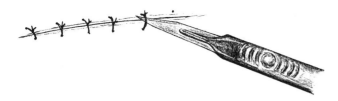

FIG. 23-18   Removal of a tight suture with a # 11 blade.

is very effective, with an onset time of about 2 to 5 minutes, and will produce a long working time (60 minutes) to permit meticulous repair.

Skin Adhesives. Tissue adhesive has gained widespread use throughout the world for closing simple skin lacerations in the pediatric patient and it offers several advantages. These advantages are: less time for laceration repair than with conventional sutures, cost effectiveness, less pain to the child, elimination of the need for suture removal (another traumatic experience for both child and surgeon), a scar similar to conventional suturing, and the procedure is safe.[6,7] Although available in Canada and worldwide, tissue adhesive is not yet approved for general use by the Food and Drug Administration (1999).

Technique. Tissue adhesive application is easy and requires less skill than suturing. The adhesive, octylcyanoacrylate (Histoacryl Blue), is applied to the skin surface after the wound has been cleaned, then the edges are held together with digital pressure for 30 seconds.[8] This product has been safely used in the facial area with good success and with no adverse drug effects.[9] Current tissue adhesives can only close skin wounds and should only be applied topically. It does not alleviate the need for deep sutures.

Postoperative Supportive Care of the Patient

Wound Healing. Wound healing proceeds in several dynamic phases with overlapping time periods.
- *0 to 1 hour:* The prevention of local hemorrhage. Platelet adhesion and the activation of the coagulation cascade occurs. Fibrin formation.
- *1 to 2 hours:* The release of vasoactive substances: histamine, serotonin, and cytokines. The start of edema. (This is an accumulation of tissue fluids

that creates an aqueous milieu that promotes the conversion of fibrocytes to fibroblasts.)
- *2 hours to 2 days:* The migration of amoeboid neutrophils that will stop when the wound is clean.
- *1 to 2 days:* Epithelial migration from the wound edges across the fissured surface. The wound is essentially covered and the need for dressings can be eliminated after the third day.
- *2 to 21 days:* The proliferation of fibroblasts. Fibroblasts arrive after blood clots have been dissolved and necrotic tissue has been removed. In the presence of hematomas, necrotic tissue, foreign bodies, and bacteria the migration of fibroblasts will be delayed, and the healing process will be delayed. Fibroblasts synthesize collagen and, in primary healing, reach a peak activity at 5 to 7 days. Sutures can, therefore, be removed between 5 and 7 days. Newly formed collagen in the wound reaches its maximum mass at 21 days. At this time the tensile strength within the wound is high.
- *3 weeks to 1 year:* Maturation of the scar. Scar revisions should not generally be done before 1 year.

REFERENCES

1. Lowbury EJ, Lilly HA: The effect of blood on disinfection of surgeons' hands, *Brit J Surg* 61(1):19-21, 1974.
2. Peterson AF, Rosenberg A, Alatary SD: Comparative evaluation of surgical scrub preparations, *Surg Gynecol Obstet* 146(1):63-65, 1978.
3. *Betadine solution—Product information sheet*, Norwalk, CT, Purdue Fredrick, 1994.
4. Shultz RC: Soft tissue injuries of the face. In Smith JW, Aston SJ, editors: *Plastic surgery*, ed 4, Boston, Little, Brown, 1991, 11:325-345.
5. Shultz RC: The changing character and management of soft tissue windshield injuries, *J Trauma* 12:1, 1972.
6. Bruns TB, Simon HK, McLario DJ, et al: Laceration repair using a tissue adhesive in a children's emergency department, *Pediatrics* 98:673-676, 1996.
7. Simon HK, Bruns TB, Zempsky W, et al: Cosmetic outcome of lacerations closed by tissue adhesives in children, *http://www.asca.com/updates/1-3/1.5.htm*, 1997.
8. Quinn JV, Drzewiecki A, Li MM, et al: A randomized trial comparing octylcyanoacrylate tissue adhesive and sutures in the management of lacerations, *JAMA* 277:1527-1530, 1997.
9. Maw JL, Quinn JV, Wells GA, et al: A prospective comparison of octylcyanoacrylate tissue adhesive and sutures for the closure of head and neck incisions, *J Otolaryngol* 26:26-30, 1997.

SALIVARY GLAND DISEASE

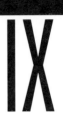

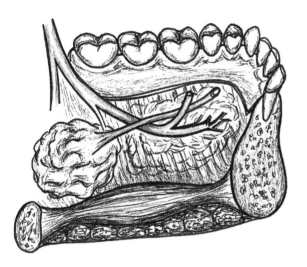

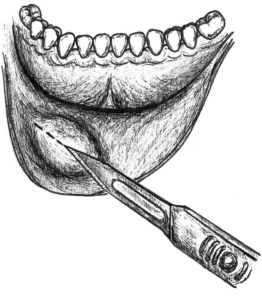

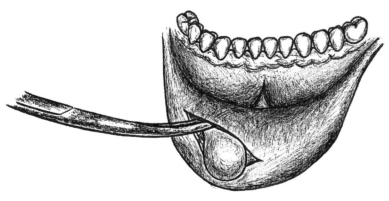

CHAPTER 24

Management of Commonly Seen Salivary Gland Diseases

HARRY DYM, DDS

It is quite common for patients who have developed salivary gland pathology to seek early and first treatment from general dentists and oral and maxillofacial surgeons. This chapter will address the salivary disorders most commonly seen, that can be diagnosed and managed in an office setting (Box 24-1).

The salivary glands are divided into two distinct groups, the minor and major glands. The minor salivary glands are found in most areas of the oral cavity, including the lips, pharynx, buccal mucosa, and nasal sinus. The major salivary glands are paired structures and include the parotid, sublingual and submandibular glands.

The parotid gland is a triangular-shaped structure located between the parapharyngeal space medially and the subcutaneous tissues of the preauricular region. It lies superficial to the posterior aspect of the masseter muscle and the ascending ramus of the mandible (Fig. 24-1). The parotid gland is divided into the superficial and deep lobes by the seventh cranial nerve as it courses anteriorly to innervate the facial muscles. Saliva flows from the mostly serous acini of the parotid gland via Stensen's duct, which enters the oral cavity through the buccal mucosa adjacent to the upper second molar.

The submandibular glands are located in the submandibular triangle of the neck, above and below the mylohyoid muscle (see Fig. 24-1). The submandibular gland produces saliva made of equal amounts of serous secretions (thin and watery) and mucous secretions (thicker and viscous) that enters the oral cavity through Wharton's duct, which travels above the mylohyoid muscle right below the mucosa of the floor of the mouth, adjacent to the lingual nerve (Fig. 24-2). Wharton's duct opens into the floor of the mouth through a small orifice located just posterior to the incisor teeth. The sublingual glands lie just beneath the surface of the mucosa of the floor of the mouth and above the mylohyoid muscle, directly lateral to the bicuspid and molar teeth. These glands empty directly into Wharton's duct or into the floor of the mouth through Bartholin's ducts.

CLINICAL EXAMINATION AND DIAGNOSTIC PROCEDURES

A thorough clinical examination combined with a review of symptoms can help the clinician to develop a differential diagnosis of salivary gland disease in the patient who presents with acute swelling of the parotid or submandibular region. The history gathering process should include the following important questions:

1. Is the swelling painful?
2. Is the swelling recurrent and episodic?
3. Does the swelling increase at mealtime?
4. Is fever associated with the swelling?
5. Is the swelling/mass acute or chronic?

The clinical exam should include the following:

1. Direct manual palpation of the involved gland
2. Attempt to milk saliva out of the involved gland
3. Assessment of the quality and quantity of saliva produced
4. Order appropriate diagnostic imaging test

SALIVARY GLAND PATHOLOGY

The salivary gland abnormalities can be divided into multiple etiologic categories.

1. Developmental
2. Neoplastic
3. Inflammatory
4. Autoimmune
5. Traumatic
6. Metabolic

Diagnostic imaging plays an important role in the diagnosis and treatment of salivary pathology.

PLAIN FILM STUDIES

Plain film studies are very helpful when clinical and history findings suggest a ductal obstructive phenomenon, either a mucous plug or stone (sialolith). Intraoral panoramic and occlusal views along with frontal (AP) views and lateral oblique views are useful in assessing

BOX 24-1 Salivary Gland Diseases

REACTIVE LESION (NONINFECTIOUS)
Mucus extravasation phenomenon
Mucus retention cyst
Ranula
Mucocele of the maxillary sinus
Maxillary sinus retention cyst and pseudocyst
Neocrotizing sialometaplasia
Radiation-induced salivary gland pathology

INFECTIOUS CONDITIONS
Viral diseases
• Mumps
• Cytomegalic sialadenitis
Bacterial sialadenitis
Sarcoidosis

METABOLIC CONDITIONS
Conditions Associated with Immune Defects
Benign lymphoepithelial lesion
Sjogren's syndrome

Benign Neoplasms
Benign mixed tumor (pleomorphic adenoma)
Monomorphic adenomas
Basal cell adenomas
Sebaceous tumors
Oncocytic tumors
Sialadenoma papilliferum and inverted ductal papilloma
Myoepithelioma

Malignant Neoplasms
Mucoepidermoid carcinoma
Adenocystic carcinoma
Acinic cell carcinoma
Carcinoma ex-mixed tumor/malignant
Mixed tumor
Epimyoepithelial carcinoma of intercalated ducts
Terminal duct carcinoma
Salivary duct carcinoma
Adenocarcinoma

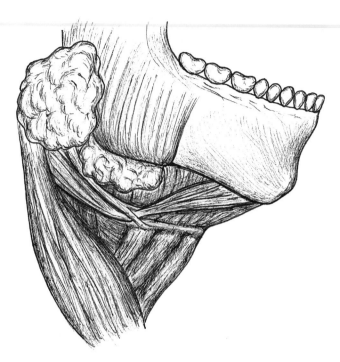

FIG. 24-1 Submandibular gland located in the submandibular triangle of the neck, along with the parotid gland overlying the lateral aspect of the mandibular ramus and masseter muscle. Note the anatomic triangle formed by the anterior and posterior belly of the digastric muscle along with the inferior border of the mandible.

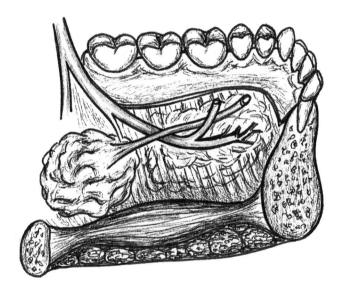

FIG. 24-2 Intraoral view of the submandibular gland. Note the relationship of Wharton's duct to the lingual nerve.

both the parotid and submandibular region. However, not all stones are radiopaque and a sialographic study can often be helpful in diagnosing obstructive ductal conditions not visible on plain films. In sialography, the salivary duct in question is dilated with lacrimal probes and then cannulated with an angiocatheter (IV catheter).

Following this, either an oil-based or water-soluble dye is injected and plain films taken. The study will reveal any obstruction in the main ducts as well as intraglandular pathology. It should not be performed on patients with acute suppurative sialoadenitis[1] nor

used in patients who have had previous adverse reactions to contrast studies.

Radionuclide salivary scanning is another valuable diagnostic imaging tool, for both the evaluation of salivary physiology as well as determining various pathologic conditions involving the major salivary glands. In addition, nuclear medicine studies can provide important quantitative information concerning the degree of salivary function present as well as allowing one to follow quantitative changes in salivary function over a period of time.

Computed tomography (CT) studies as well as magnetic resonance imaging (MRI) of salivary glands have also been proven to be extremely useful noninvasive techniques in the evaluation and diagnosis of salivary gland disorders.

Finally, ultrasound evaluation is a feasible technique because of the superficial location of both the parotid and submandibular glands. Based on the acoustic impedance, ultrasound can readily differentiate between intra- and extraglandular masses as well as help delineate the presence of solid, cystic, and complex masses and sialoliths.

DIAGNOSIS AND TREATMENT OF A MUCOCELE AND RANULA

The most common salivary gland disorder diagnosed and treated in an outpatient dental setting is a mucocele. Often referred to as mucous retention cysts (though they are not true cysts by definition, as they are not lined by an epithelial cell-walled layer) they most commonly occur on the lower lip, buccal mucosa, and in the floor of the mouth.

The etiology of lower lip mucoceles is primarily that of trauma to the numerous salivary glands present directly beneath the overlying thin mucosa. Salivary secretions produced are then extravasated beneath the mucosa causing an accumulation and pseudocyst formation. The collection of mucus is walled off by connective and granulation tissue producing a raised, translucent, bluish swelling. Their size can vary from only millimeters to centimeters in length, and patients often give a history of spontaneous rupture and recurrence. The definitive treatment is surgical removal.

Surgical Technique for Removal of Lip Mucocele

Before the actual surgical procedure, during the consultation phase, the patient should be made aware that numbness or an altered sensation of the lip may sometimes occur immediately following the excision of a mucocele. This is because of the possible transection of very fine nerve endings always present in the lip. If this should occur the patient should be counseled that it is usually transient and will not present any motor deficit. In addition, the patient should be made aware of the highly recurrent nature of this lesion because of its traumatic etiology.

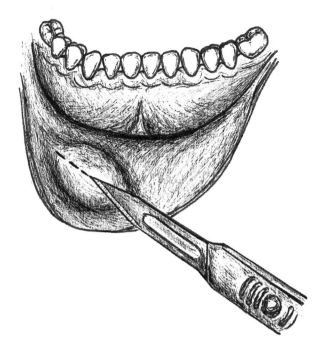

FIG. 24-3 Horizontal incision, made in the lower lip only through mucosa overlying the mucocele. This is the recommended approach for large lesions. Smaller mucoceles can be excised using an elliptical incision and taking the overlying mucosa.

Local anesthesia with epinephrine should be used while making certain that only the periphery of the lesion is injected and thus avoiding rupture of the cyst by directly inserting the needle into the cystic mass. Either a vertical elliptical or horizontal elliptical incision should be made with a #15 blade making certain to incise only through the thin overlying mucosal layer (Fig. 24-3). Then, careful blunt dissection with a curved hemostat is performed to gently remove the entire cystic mass in toto (Fig. 24-4). Oftentimes, the lesion will spontaneously burst during dissection, resulting in a flow of thick mucus. This should be suctioned off and any small glandular tissue remnants should be removed with a College pliers. A 4-0 black silk or Vicryl suture should be used in an interrupted primary closure fashion with the suture removed in 7 days (Figs. 24-5 and 24-6).

Management of the Ranula

Mucous retention cysts can also result from obstruction of a salivary gland duct by a mucous plug (Fig. 24-7). This results in a dilation of the salivary duct and formation of a retention cyst. When this process develops in association with either the submandibular or sublingual glands in the floor of the mouth it is called a ranula (Fig. 24-8). The term is derived from Latin for

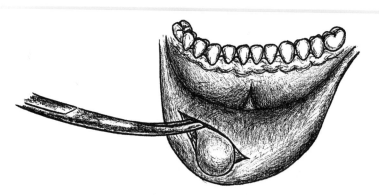

FIG. 24-4 Using a small, curved hemostat careful dissection of mucocele is performed. Oftentimes, this will result in rupture of mucocele. Should this occur, suction saliva and continue with excision.

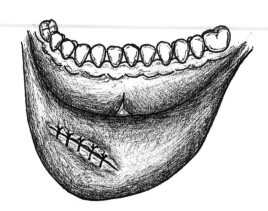

FIG. 24-6 Incision site closes well with interrupted sutures.

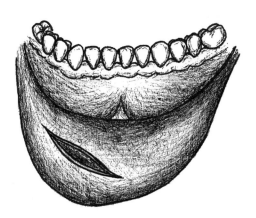

FIG. 24-5 Before closure, inspect underlying muscle layer to make certain it is free of any salivary glandular tissue.

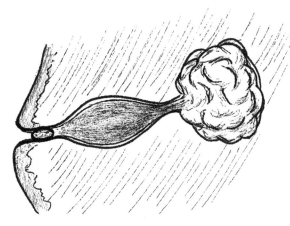

FIG. 24-7 Mucous plug seen at orifice of salivary duct leading to formation of retention cyst.

frog, as the cystic lesion protruding from beneath the tongue is also said to resemble the belly of frog. The treatment of the ranula is controversial, with some advocating removal of the sublingual gland along with excision of the cyst and others recommending a marsupialization procedure.[2] The ranula is often quite large but they tend to rupture intermittently as a result of trauma and reform over weeks or months. It is the author's opinion that the initial treatment of ranulas be through a marsupialization procedure with sublingual gland excision to be performed only if there is a recurrence. A clinical entity known as a plunging ranula

does exist, in which the lesion extends through the mylohyoid muscle to involve the neck. This condition should be treated with sublingual gland removal along with excision of the mucous retention cyst.

SURGICAL TECHNIQUES OF MARSUPIALIZATION

Local anesthesia, 2% lidocaine with epinephrine 1:100,000, is administered via a conduction block of the lingual nerve, or by an injection on the periphery of the lesion, so as to avoid direct entry and rupture of the

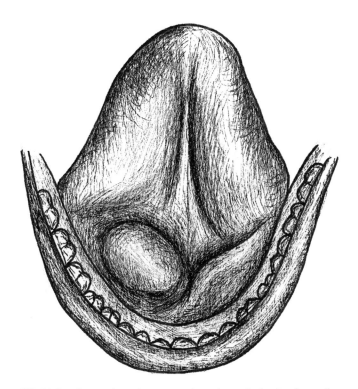

FIG. 24-8 Dome-shaped presentation of ranula in the floor of the mouth. It often appears blue and is usually unilateral.

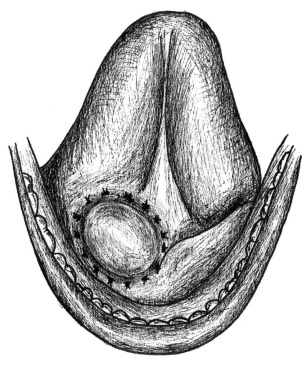

FIG. 24-9 Multiple sutures placed through cyst wall and adjacent mucosa and tied in surgical knots.

ranula. A 3-0 black silk traction suture is placed through the anterior tongue, and Wharton's duct on the involved side is cannulated. A 3-0 Dexon on a noncutting needle is then used to suture the overlying cyst wall to the underlying mucosa in the floor of the mouth (Fig. 24-9), after which a #15 blade is used to unroof the lesion. Bleeding is usually not problematic and small bleeders can be controlled with bipolar coagulation or with direct injection of local anesthetic with epinephrine. If the resulting defect is rather large, 1/2 inch iodoform gauze can be packed into the remaining lesion and sutured in place for 1 week (Fig. 24-10). Postsurgical antibiotics should be prescribed, with penicillin as the primary drug, or erythromycin for the penicillin-allergic patient.

DIAGNOSIS AND TREATMENT OF OBSTRUCTIVE SALIVARY GLAND DISEASE

Sialadenitis, infection of the salivary glands, is the most common disorder of the major salivary glands. It may or may not present with salivary stones or calculi (sialolithiasis) as the etiologic source and may be acute or chronic.

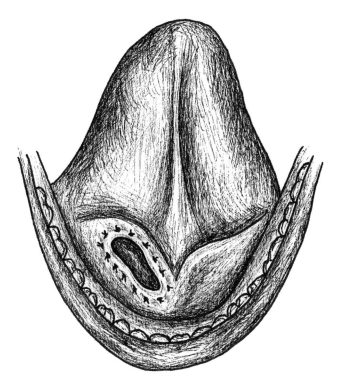

FIG. 24-10 Roof of ranula removed, leaving opening into floor of mouth. Packing can be sutured into defect to aid in control of hemostasis and patient comfort.

Bacterial Sialadenitis

The clinical presentation of acute suppurative sialadenitis is one of sudden onset with painful swelling of the gland not associated with meals. The patient often presents with general malaise and swelling and induration of the involved gland. Manipulation of either the parotid or submandibular gland will result in a thick purulent discharge from the involved ductal orifice, and the surrounding ductal mucosa is edematous and quite inflamed. Though acute suppurative sialadenitis can occur at any age, it is most often seen in elderly patients (over the age of 65). The most likely cause is retrograde bacterial infection as a result of diminished salivary flow. The reduction in flow may be caused by diuretic medication and inadequate hydration. A common predisposing factor is a history of recent surgery. Acute suppurative sialadenitis is often not associated with salivary calculi.

Chronic bacterial sialadenitis presents with many similar clinical findings but differs in that the history is recurrent and the swelling and pain are milder with no suppuration seen.

Treatment

Treatment of the patient with acute sialadenitis consists of hydration, aggressive use of antibiotics, and incision and drainage, as indicated. *Staphylococcus aureus* is most often cultured from the purulent discharge, though other organisms are also involved, including *E. coli, Haemophilus influenzae, Bacteroides melaninogenicus, Streptococcus viridans, Peptostreptococcus anaerobius,* and *Fusobacterium nucleatum.* The antibiotic of choice is usually one from the synthetic penicillin family like oxacillin or amoxicillin/clavulanate potassium (Augmentin). In penicillin-allergic patients, a new synthetic macrolide, Zithromax, or clindamycin are also effective. However, changes in antibiotic therapy should always be made based on culture results and clinical progress.

Neither ductal probing nor sialography should be performed during acute inflammatory periods and removal of the involved gland may be necessary after resolution of the acute infection based on clinical and diagnostic (nuclear scan) assessment of glandular viability.

Viral Sialadenitis

A clinical presentation seen in nonobstructive viral-induced salivary swelling is one of nonsuppuration and nonerythematous swelling. Viral sialadenitis most often involves the parotid gland and is most often related to exposure to the mumps virus 2 to 3 weeks prior to clinical presentation. Supportive treatment consisting of hydration, analgesics, and antipyretic medication is advised. Spontaneous resolution of mumps-induced sialadenitis is 5 to 10 days with the complications of orchitis and sterility occurring in a small percentage of patients.

SIALOLITHIASIS
Diagnosis and Treatment

Sialolithiasis (salivary stones) is one of the most common pathologic salivary conditions seen, with the submandibular gland most predisposed to this condition. Numerous reasons exist to explain why 90% of the time salivary stones occur in the submandibular gland, and these include:

1. Increased viscosity of its secretions
2. Slow flow of saliva because of the duct's increased length
3. Saliva must flow up, against gravity to reach its orifice
4. Increased trauma to duct
5. Tortuousness of the submandibular duct

Clinical Presentation

Occasionally a sialolith is asymptomatic and only accidentally seen on a routine panoramic screening film or on routine clinical palpation of the patient's gland and duct during an initial examination. However, most often the patient will present with a clinical history of recurrent, rapid painful swelling of the involved gland associated with eating and mealtime. Clinical examination of a patient with suspected sialolithiasis should include extraoral palpation of the major salivary glands and bimanual palpation of the ductal system with simultaneous observation of salivary flow as to quantity and consistency. Plain films, as discussed earlier, are the imaging technique of choice.

Surgical Technique for Removal of Submandibular Stone

A submandibular stone can occur anywhere along the course of the submandibular duct in the floor of the mouth as well as within the body of the submandibular gland. As a general rule a sialolith that can be easily palpated intraorally can also be removed intraorally. If the sialolith is located within the gland or within the proximal duct at the hilum of the gland, submandibular gland removal (sialoadenectomy) is required.

Following the administration of local anesthesia, a suture is passed around Wharton's duct posterior to the stone and clamped, to aid in traction and prevent the stone from moving proximally during the removal procedure. A #15 blade scalpel is used to make an incision along the duct, directly over the stone but only

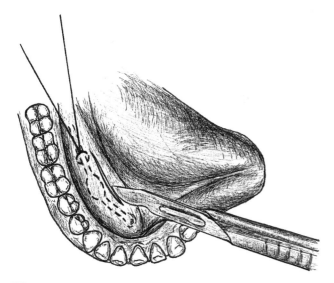

FIG. 24-11 Scalpel blade is used to make incision only through mucosa overlying Wharton's duct and suspected stone. Note traction suture placed behind stone.

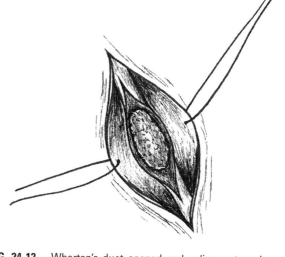

FIG. 24-12 Wharton's duct opened and salivary stone located. Note retraction sutures placed on either mucosal side.

through the overlying mucosa (Fig. 24-11). Blunt dissection with a curved hemostat is performed until the duct is identified. Following isolation of the duct, a suture or a vessel loop is placed beneath it, to allow for better control of the duct. A longitudinal incision is then made through the duct wall and the stone retrieved (Fig. 24-12). If the stone is not readily seen, milking the gland may move it toward the ductal opening. If the stone is within the posterior portion of the oral cavity in the area of the first molar, care must be taken to first identify and protect the lingual nerve before cutting down on the duct.

The overlying mucosa is only loosely approximated with resorbable suture (3-0 Dexon or Vicryl) and the new ductal opening not sutured closed but merely tacked to the adjacent mucosa with 4-0 Dexon (Fig. 24-13). The patient should be closely followed to determine if the gland returns to function with no recurrent bouts of swelling and pain. Antibiotics should be administered and hydration encouraged.

FINE NEEDLE ASPIRATION

A helpful technique for distinguishing inflammatory disease from neoplastic conditions (benign and malignant) of solid salivary gland masses is fine needle aspiration. A 20-gauge or finer needle is used to aspirate, transmucosally or percutaneously, the suspected mass and the aspirated cells are then spread directly and fixed on glass slides, for examination by a skilled cytopathologist. The nature of the biopsy is such that no seeding of possible tumor cells occurs.

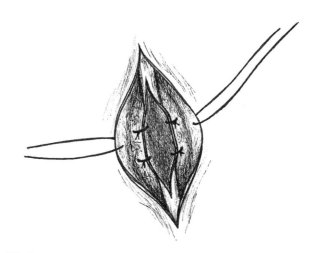

FIG. 24-13 Following stone removal, the sides of the opened duct are sutured to adjacent mucosa. This procedure of relocating ductal orifice is referred to as sialodochoplasty.

METABOLIC CONDITIONS

There is a group of disorders characterized by salivary gland enlargement, usually the parotid, in the absence of inflammatory symptoms that are of systemic or metabolic origin. The most common conditions causing this type of parotid enlargement are chronic alcoholism, obesity, and diabetes mellitus.

NEOPLASMS

The parotid gland is the most common site of salivary gland neoplasia and is more often involved with benign neoplasms. The submandibular and minor salivary gland neoplasms have a greater likelihood of being malignant. The overall percentage breakdown of benign neoplasms is as follows:

Type of Neoplasm	Likelihood of Malignancy
Parotid	75% of all neoplasms are likely to be benign.
Submandibular	50% of all neoplasms are likely to be benign.
Sublingual	25 to 40% of all neoplasms are likely to be benign.

The most common tumor of the salivary glands is the benign mixed tumor and it occurs mostly in the parotid gland (85%). The treatment of choice for benign mixed tumor of minor or major salivary glands is surgical excision.

REFERENCES

1. Berry RL: Sialadenitis and sialolithiasis. In Carlson ER, editor: Comprehensive management of salivary gland pathology, *Oral Maxillofac Clin North Am* 7(3):487, 1995.
2. McGurk M: The surgical management of salivary gland disease of the sublingual gland and floor of mouth. In Pogrel MA (ed): *Surgical Management of Salivary Gland Disease. Atlas of the Oral and Maxillofacial Surgery Clinics of North America, Vol. 6, No.1.* Philadelphia, W.B. Saunders, 1998, p 61.

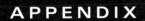

Useful Laboratory Information and Common Drug Interactions

This appendix consists of tables of useful laboratory information and common drug interactions which will be beneficial to the dental practitioner. The laboratory information will be helpful to dentists performing surgery in the hospital environment or when evaluating the results of requested laboratory tests.

In prescribing medications to patients, we should have an updated medication history and try to prescribe drugs that will not interact with medications that the patient is currently taking or that will interfere with the course of treatment.

TABLE A-1 Reference Values for Commonly Used Laboratory Tests*

Chemistry		Enzymes	
Albumin	3.6-5.0 g/dl	ALT (SGPT)	7-53 IU/L
Bilirubin (direct)	0.2 mg/dl	AST (SGOT)	11-47 IU/L
Calcium (total)	8.9-10.3 mg/dl	Amylase	35-118 IU/L
Chloride	97-110 mmol/dl	GGT	
Creatinine	0.5-1.7 mg/dl	Male	20 -76 IU/L
Glucose	65-110 mg/dl	Females	12-54 IU/L
Potassium	3.3-4.9 mmol/dl		
Protein (total)	6.2-8.2 g/dl		
Sodium	135-145 mmol/dl		
Urea nitrogen (BUN)	8-25 mg/dl		

*Reference range of values listed are those for Woodhull Medical and Mental Health Center, Brooklyn, New York. *Note:* Laboratory values may vary slightly from one laboratory to another. Laboratories will generally provide their reference ranges.

TABLE A-2 Hematologic Values

Category	Value
Bleeding time (ivy)	2.5-9.0 min
PTT	25-33 sec
PT	11-13 sec
Thrombin time	11-18 sec
INR*	1.0-1.3
Hematocrit	
Male	40-50%
Female	36-44%
Hemoglobin	
Male	14-17 g/dl
Female	12-15 g/dl
RBC count	
Male	$4.5\text{-}5.7 \times 10^6/\mu l$
Female	$3.9\text{-}5.0 \times 10^6/\mu l$
WBC count	$3.8\text{-}9.8 \times 10^3/\mu l$
Platelets	$140\text{-}440 \times 10^3/\mu l$

PTT, Partial thromboplastin time; *PT*, prothrombin time; *INR*, International normalized ratio; *RBC*, red blood cell; *WBC*, white blood cell.

$$*INR = \left(\frac{\text{Patient PT}}{\text{Control PT}} \right)^c$$ ("c" is the international sensitivity index)

Note: Values for PT, PTT, and bleeding time may vary from laboratory to laboratory.

TABLE A-3 Commonly Used Specimen Collection Tubes

Tube color	Tube contents	Laboratory test
Red	No contents	Serum chemistry
Blue	Citrate	PT, PTT
Lavender	EDTA	CBC

EDTA, Ethylenediaminetetraacetic acid; *PT*, prothrombin time; *PTT*, partial thromboplastin time; *CBC*, complete blood count.

TABLE A-4 Drug Interactions with Alcohol, Antacids, and Herbals

Avoid alcohol with the following medications	Avoid antacids with the following medications	Avoid aspirin and NSAIDs with the following herbals*
Acetaminophen	Ciprofloxacin	Capsaicin (cayenne)[a]
Aspirin	Doxycycline	Evening primrose oil[b]
Pain medications with codeine	Minocycline	Feverfew[b]
NSAIDs	Tetracycline	Garlic pills[b,d]
Amitriptyline		Ginger[b]
Metronidazole		Ginkgo biloba[b]
Phenobarbital		Ginseng[c]
Secobarbital		Grapeseed extract[b]
Methocarbamol		
Diazepam		
Flurazepam		
Promethazine		
Hydroxyzine pamoate		

*From Herbal Chart for Health Care Professionals. In *Pharmacy Today* 5(8), special section on dietary supplements. August, 1999.
[a]Reduces platelet aggregation and increases fibrinolytic activity.
[b]Reduces platelet aggregation.
[c]Decreases platelet adhesiveness.
[d]GI irritation or stomach pain.

TABLE A-5 Drug Interactions with Food

Medications to be taken with food or milk	Medications to be taken on an empty stomach with water	Medications to be taken ½-1 hr before meals or 2 hrs after meals	Medications to be taken 30 min before meal	Medications that may be taken without regards to meal
Aspirin	Amoxicillin (+/– clavulanic acid)	Ciprofloxacin	Doxycycline	Acetaminophen
Cefuroxime axetil	Ampicillin (+/– sulbactam)		Minocycline	Acetaminophen with codeine
Clindamycin	Azithromycin			Acyclovir
Codeine	Dicloxacillin			Cefaclor
Dexamethasone	Erythromycin (stearate)			Cephalexin
EES (erythromycin)	Tetracycline			Clarithromycin
Ibuprofen				Chlordiazepoxide
Meperidine				Cyclobenzaprine
Metronidazole				Diazepam
Misoprostol				Penicillin V potassium
Naprosyn				
Prednisone				
Probenecid				
Prochlorperazine				

TABLE

A-6 Antibiotic Drug Interactions

Antibiotic	Drugs interacting with antibiotic	Reaction
Penicillins Amoxicillin	Erythromycin, tetracycline	Bacteriostatic drugs will inhibit protein synthesis antagonizing the effect of penicillins.
	Oral contraceptives	If given concomitantly will reduce the effectiveness of the contraceptives resulting in breakthrough bleeding and risk of ovulation.
Clindamycin (Cleocin)	Oral contraceptives	If given concomitantly will reduce the effectiveness of the contraceptives resulting in breakthrough bleeding and risk of ovulation.
Erythromycin	Cyclosporine	Increases the serum level of both medications.
	Phenytoin	Increased levels of both medications. Phenytoin (dilantin) level should be monitored to avoid toxicity.
	Oral contraceptives	Same as in penicillin.
	Theophylline	Erythromycin is associated with increases in theophylline serum levels that could lead to toxicity due to competitive binding to a specific enzyme that is responsible for metabolizing theophylline.
	Warfarin	Increased activity of warfarin. Increased INR.
Metronidazole	Alcohol	Absolutely contraindicated, could cause flushes, nausea, vomiting, headaches, and chest pain.
	Cimetidine	Decrease in plasma clearance of metronidazole.
	Phenobarbital and phenytoin	Reduces metronidazole serum levels, half-life time, and effectiveness.
	Warfarin sodium	Potentiation of anticoagulation effect.
Ciprofloxacin	Antacids	All if given concomitantly with ciprofloxacin could interfere with its absorption.
	Aminophylline, dyphylline, theophylline, and all its products	Could cause severe and fatal reactions including cardiac arrest, seizures, respiratory failure, and status epilepticus.
	Caffeine	Its clearance is decreased by ciprofloxacin and the T½ is increased.
	Cyclosporin	Increased nephrotoxicity of cyclosporin.
	Phenytoin	Potential reduction in phenytoin levels, and triggering of seizure activity.
	Warfarin sodium	Enhanced anticoagulation effect.
Tetracycline	Antacids	Impairs the absorption of tetracycline and thus reduces the serum concentration and efficiency of the antibiotic.
	Iron	Iron pills will decrease the effectiveness of tetracycline.
	Oral anticoagulants	Depressed plasma level of prothrombin activity.
	Oral contraceptives	Reduced efficiency and increased incidence of breakthrough bleeding and risk of ovulation.
	Penicillins	Interference with bactericidal action of penicillins.

INR, International normalized ratio.

TABLE A-7 Drug Interactions with Commonly Used Pain Medications

Pain control medication	Drugs interacting	Reaction
Aspirin	Aluminum carbonate, aluminum hydroxide, sodium bicarbonate, magnesium oxide	Concurrent administration delays the rate of absorption of aspirin.
	Oral hypoglycemics	May cause hypoglycemia by competing with the hypoglycemic agent for binding sites in the plasma causing an increased level of the free hypoglycemic agent available in the circulation.
	Warfarin/oral anticoagulants	Aspirin will potentiate the anticoagulation effects by inhibiting platelet clumping and by displacing oral anticoagulants from plasma protein to increase its activity in preventing synthesis of prothrombin.
Acetaminophen	Rifampin/barbiturates	Decreases the analgesic effect of acetaminophen. Increased risk of acetaminophen induced hepatotoxicity.
	Chronic use of ETOH	Increased potential for hepatotoxicity even with normal doses of acetaminophen.
Oxycodone Hydrocodone Codeine	CNS depressants, anxiolytic hypnotics, narcotic analgesics, sedatives, MAO inhibitors, tricyclic antidepressants	Increased CNS depression.
Ibuprofen	Aspirin	Potential net decrease in anti-inflammatory activity. Increased risk of GI irritation.
	Thiazides	Reduced natriuretic effect.
	Oral anticoagulants	Potential increased risk of bleeding.
Naproxen sodium	Aspirin	Aspirin displaces naproxen sodium from its binding sites causing an increased rate of excretion of naproxen sodium thus shortening its therapeutic time.
	ACE inhibitors and beta-blockers	May decrease the antihypertensive effect of the ACE inhibitor.
	Oral anticoagulants	Prothrombin time may be affected. Bleeding time may be increased.
	Furosemide	Natriuretic effect is inhibited.
	Glipizide, glyburide, sulfonamides, anticonvulsants	Increased potential for drug toxicity.
	Warfarin	Increase in bleeding time.

TABLE A-8 Lidocaine Drug Interactions

Medication	Drugs interacting	Reaction
Lidocaine	Antiarrhythmics	May produce bradycardia or arrhythmia. Do not use more than 7 dental carpules (ref: medscape web page, see Table A-13).

TABLE A-9 Steroid Drug Interactions*

Steroids	Interacting drug	Reaction
All glucocorticoids	Antacids	Decreased absorption of orally administered corticosteroids.
	Anticoagulants (Oral)	Corticosteroids may oppose anticoagulation action.
	Barbiturates, carbamazepine	Decreased effects of corticosteroids.
	Contraceptives (Oral)	Decreased corticosteroid clearance. (Increase t½) thus increasing the therapeutic dosing time with increased therapeutic effects.
	Digitalis	Increased risk of digitalis toxicity associated with hypokalemia.
	Diuretics	Increased risk of hypokalemia.
	Hydantoins	Increased corticosteroid clearance, thus decreasing therapeutic effects.
	Isoniazid	Decreased the serum concentration of isoniazid making it less effective.
	Macrolides	Decreased *methylprednisolone* clearance.
	Salicylates	Decreased serum salicylate levels thus decreasing the effectiveness of the salicylate.
	Theophylline	Alterations in the activity of theophylline may occur. Theophylline levels should be monitored.

Adapted from Adrenal Cortical Steroids. In: *Drug Facts and Comparisons,* St. Louis, 1997, Facts and Comparisons Inc., pp. 122-128.
*Steroids are used to reduce post-surgical edema. This table lists common glucocorticoid drug interactions.

TABLE A-10 Drug Usage in the Pregnant Patient

	Safe to use in the pregnant patient	Minimal fetal risk—possibly safe to use, but no accurate studies are available	Evidence of fetal risk—should not use	Drugs to avoid in pregnancy—significant fetal risk
ANALGESICS	Acetaminophen	Fentanyl Hydrocodone Ibuprofen Meperidine Naproxen Oxycodone	Aspirin Codeine Propoxyphene	
ANTIMICROBIALS	Amoxicillin Amoxicillin-clavulanic acid Ampicillin Ampicillin-sulbactam Cefazolin Cephalexin Erythromycin Nystatin Penicillin	Acyclovir Azithromycin Clarithromycin Clindamycin Vancomycin		Ciprofloxacin Doxycycline Tetracycline
ANTI-INFLAMMATORY		Ibuprofen Naproxen	Glucocorticoids	

Adapted from Nauser TD and Mcgahan MM: Pregnancy and Medical Therapeutics. In: *The Washington manual of medical therapeutics,* ed 29, Philadelphia, 1998, Lippincott-Williams & Wilkins, pp. 534-537.
Note: NSAIDs and aspirin should not be used during the third trimester of pregnancy.

TABLE A-11 Drugs to Avoid in the Nursing Mother*

Drug	Effect on nursing infant
Metronidazole	Potential for tumorigenicity. Nursing may be resumed 48 hrs after drug has been stopped.
Antihistamines	Newborns and infants have increased sensitivity to antihistamines.
Benzodiazepines	These drugs can cause sedation in infants.

*Obtained from product information sheets.

TABLE A-12 Some of the Generic Drugs Mentioned in this Appendix and Their Corresponding Trade Names

Generic name	Some common trade names
ANALGESICS	
Acetaminophen	Tylenol, Tylenol with Codeine
Aspirin	Empirin, Empirin with Codeine
Fentanyl	Sublimaze, Duragesic
Hydrocodone	Lorcet, Vicodin, Lortab
Ibuprofen	Motrin, Advil, PediaProfen, Rufin
Meperidine	Demerol
Naproxen	Anaprox, Naprosyn, Aleve
Oxycodone	Percodan, Percocet
ANTIMICROBIALS	
Amoxicillin	Amoxil, Trimox
Amoxicillin-clavulanic acid	Augmentin
Ampicillin	Amcill, Omnipen
Ampicillin-sulbactam	Unasyn
Azithromycin	Zithromax
Cefazolin	Ancef, Kefzol
Cephalexin	Keflex, Keftab, Cefanex
Ciprofloxacin	Cipro
Clarithromycin	Biaxin
Clindamycin	Cleocin
Doxycycline	Vibramycin
Erythromycin	Erythrocin, E-Mycin
Metronidazole	Flagyl
Minocycline	Minocin
Penicillin	Pen VK, Veetids, V-Cillin-K
Tetracycline	Achromycin, Tetracyn
OTHERS	
Amitriptyline	Elavil, Enovil
Dexamethasone	Decadron
Diazepam	Valium
Flurazepam	Dalmane
Hydroxyzine pamoate	Vistaril, Atarax
Methocarbamol	Robaxin, Delaxin
Misoprostol	Cytotec
Phenobarbital	Barbita, Luminal
Prednisone	Orasone
Probenecid	Probalan, Benemid
Prochlorperazine	Compazine
Promethazine	Phenergan
Secobarbital	Seconal

TABLE

A-13 Valuable Internet Sites*

URL	Information
www.medscape.com	Drug interactions and updated medical/surgical information
www.imc.gsm.com	Clinical pharmacology online
www.omfs.org/index.html	Oral and maxillofacial surgery online service
www.dmoz.org/Health/Dentistry/OralSurgery/	List of professional organizations that offers educational advice, courses, and conferences
www.bpass.dentistry.dal.ca/	Site for maxillofacial radiology
www.dentalsite.com/dentists	A website for dental specialists that covers various dental topics including oral surgery
www.dentalsite.com/dentist/oralpath.html	A link to selective oral pathology labs throughout the United States
www.forsyth.org/oralpathology/	An oral pathology website with good pictures
www.bconnex.net/~jascah/preop.html	Preoperative assessment and premedication
www.bcm.tmc.edu/oto/othersa.html	Otolaryngology, head and neck surgery resources on the internet
www.fscn.che.umn.edu/tools.htm	Nutritional information
www.ama.assn.org/special/hiv/hivhome.htm	AIDS information center (AMA)

*The preceding URLs are accurate as of July 2000.

REFERENCES

1. Herbal Chart for Health Care Professionals. In: *Pharmacy Today* 5(8), Special section on dietary supplements, August, 1999.

2. Nauser TD and Mcgahan MM: Pregnancy and medical therapeutics. In: *The Washington manual of medical therapeutics*, ed 29, Philadelphia, 1998, Lippincott-Williams & Wilkins, pp. 534–537.

Index

A

Abscesses. *See* Infections
Abutments, 228
Acetaminophen, 55
Acute hepatitis, 16
Acute suppurative sialadenitis, 282
Adrenal insufficiency, 18
Adson's forceps, 180
Advanced procedures, 101-133
    closure of oral-antral communications, 129-132
    endodontic surgery, 103-111. *See also* Endodontic surgery
    intentional replantation, 113, 114
    periodontal surgery, 115-125. *See also* Periodontal surgery
    root resection, 111-113
Afrin, 128
AIDS, 20, 155, 156
Akinosi technique, 36-38
Alar fascia, 141
Alcoholism, 19, 20
Allogenic bone, 239
Allograft, 210*b*
Alloplast, 210*b*
Alveolar osteitis, 91
Alveoplasty, 195, 196
Aminoglycosides gentamicin, 154*t*
Amoxicillin, 154*t*, 159, 160
Ampicillin, 159*t*
Anaplasia, 179*b*
Anatomy. *See* Regional surgical anatomy
Anesthesia. *See* Local anesthesia, Oral/parenteral sedation
Angina pectoris, 11, 12, 53*b*
Angular vein, 144
Animal bites, 155
Anisocytosis, 179*b*
Anterior nasal spine, 26
Anterior palatine nerve, 23
Anterior superior alveolar nerve, 23
Antibodies
    drug interactions, 288*t*
    infections, 150, 154*t*
    lacerations, 272
Anxiety control. *See* Oral/parenteral sedation
Apical curettage, 107, 108
Apicoectomy, 108
Arch bars, 252
Arrhythmias, 13, 14
ASA, 54, 55
ASA physical status classification, 42*t*
Aspiration, 53*b*
Aspiration biopsy, 180, 181*b*, 187, 188

Aspirin, 54
Assessment. *See* Medical history
Asthma, 15
Atrophic maxilla, 28
Atypical, 179*b*
Autogenous bone, 239
Autograft, 210*b*
Avitene, 62
Avulsion, 249, 251, 252
Azithromycin, 154*t*, 159, 160

B

Bacterial endocarditis, 156-160
Bacterial sialadenitis, 282
Barbiturates, 47, 48
Basilic vein, 51
Benzodiazepines, 45, 46
Bimanual palpation of a mass, 139
Biopsy, 177
Biopsy techniques, 177-190
    aspiration biopsy, 180, 181*b*, 187, 188
    bone biopsy, 181*b*, 186-188
    buccal mucosa, 183, 184
    control of tongue, 190
    cutaneous biopsy, 181-183
    differential diagnosis, 177
    dos/don'ts, 179*b*
    excisional biopsy, 178. *See also* Excisional biopsy
    fine needle biopsy, 180
    floor of mouth, 188-190
    glossary of terms, 179*b*
    incisional biopsy, 178. *See also* Incisional biopsy
    instrumentation, 181*b*
    lip, 181-183
    multiloculated lesions, 187*b*, 188
    palate, 185, 186
    punch biopsy, 180
    radiolucencies, 186-188
    radiopacities, 188
    tongue, 184, 185
Bites, 155
Bleeding. *See* Perioperative hemorrhage
Bleeding disorders, 19, 54, 55*b*
Bone biopsy, 181*b*, 186-188
Bone fill material, 217*t*
Bone grafting for implants, 208-218, 239, 240
    bone fill materials, 217*t*
    bone harvesting from chin, 213-215
    bone healing, 209, 210
    clinical examination, 208, 209
    cortical onlay bone graft, 213-215
    grafting of extraction socket, 213

Page numbers with *b* indicate boxes, *t* indicate tables

Bone grafting for implants—cont'd
   interpositional ridge graft, 215-217
   mandibular ramus, 210, 211
   mandibular tori, 211, 212
   particulate corticocancellous bone graft, 212, 213
   radiographic examination, 209
   study models, 209
   types of bone grafts, 210t
Bone harvesting from chin, 213-215
Bone healing, 209, 210
Bone wax, 61-63
Bony lesions, 187b
Branemark, P. I., 231
Brevital, 47
Bronchospasm, 53b
Buccal abscess, 144
Buccal nerve, 24, 31, 32
Buccal space, 139, 143
Buccinator muscle, 32, 35, 138, 139, 144
Buccinator nerve, 24
Bupivacaine, 31t

C

Candidiasis, 155
Canine space, 142, 143
Cardiovascular disease, 8, 9
Carnoy's solution, 171
Carotid sheath, 141
Cavernous sinus, 144
Cefaclor, 154t
Cefadroxil, 154t, 159t
Cefazolin, 159t
Cephalexin, 154t, 159t
Cephalic vein, 51
Cephalosporins, 154t
Cerebrovascular disease, 13
Chemical cauterization, 171
Chloroprocaine, 31t
Chronic hepatitis, 16
Chronic obstructive pulmonary disease (COPD), 14, 15
Cirrhosis, 16
Clarithromycin, 154t, 160
Clindamycin, 154t, 159, 160
Closure of oral-antral communications, 129-132
Cloxacillin, 154t
Codeine, 56
Cold cure acrylic splint, 252
CollaCote, 62
Collagen sponge, 62
CollaPlug, 62
Collastat, 62
CollaTape, 62
Comminuted fracture, 254, 255
Common carotid artery, 141
Communication to anterior jugular vein, 144
Complicated crown fracture, 247, 248
Compound fracture, 254
Concussion, 247
Congestive heart failure, 13
Conscious sedation, 42t
COPD, 14, 15
Coronal repositioning, 123
Coronary artery bypass surgery, 12
Cortical onlay bone graft, 213-215
Cortical ostectomy, 106, 107

Coumadin, 54
Crestally pedicled mucosal graft, 203
Cretinism, 18
Crown fracture with pulp involvement, 247b
Crown fracture without pulp involvement, 247b
Crown/root fracture, 247b
CT scan appliance, 228
Cyklokapron injectable, 63
Cysts, 165-176
   chemical cauterization, 171
   classification, 166b
   clinical examination, 166
   dermoid, 174-176
   instrumentation, 167, 175
   jaw, 165, 166
   mandible, 172-174
   maxilla, 171, 172
   OKC, 166
   post operation, 176
   procedures, 167-169
   radiographic examination, 166
   removal of dermoid cyst from floor of mouth, 175, 176
   soft tissue, 174
   special considerations, 171-176

D

Dean scissors, 168
Deep facial vein, 144
Deep femoral artery, 50
Deep lingual vein, 144
Deep sedation, 42t
Deltoid muscle, 51
Demerol, 45
Dental elevators, 70, 71
Dental forceps, 69, 70
Dental history, 7
Dental implants. See Implants
Dental sinusitis, 126-133
Dental trauma. See Trauma
DentaScan, 232
Dentoalveolar infections, 138, 139
Dentoalveolar injuries, 245-253
   anesthetic, 246
   avulsion, 249, 251, 252
   cause of injury, 246t
   Ellis Class I fracture, 247, 248
   Ellis Class II fracture, 247, 248
   Ellis Class III fracture, 248-250
   Ellis Class IV fracture, 249, 250
   extraoral examination, 245
   extrusion, 249, 251
   fixation periods, 252b
   fractures of alveolar process, 250
   fractures of dentate alveolar process, 250, 251
   frequency of injuries, 248t
   intraoral examination, 245, 246
   intrusion, 249, 251
   medical history, 245
   methods of immobilization, 252, 253
   oral hygiene, 253
   radiographic examination, 246
   soft-tissue injuries, 245
   WHO classification of injuries, 247b
Denture stomatitis, 202
Dentures, 193-195

Depressor anguli oris, 138
Depressor labii inferioris, 138
Depressor septi, 138
Dermoid cysts, 174-176
Diabetes mellitus, 16, 17, 137
Diazepam, 46, 52t
Dicloxacillin, 154t
Didanosine, 156
Differential diagnosis, 177
Digastric muscle, 25
DINTS, 177
Dissociative anesthesia, 47
Distal wedge excision, 121
Doxycycline, 154t
Drug interactions
    alcohol, 286t
    antacids, 286t
    antibiotics, 288t
    food, 287t
    herbals, 286t
    lidocaine, 289t
    pain medications, 289t
    steroids, 290t
Drummond-Jackson, S. L., 41
Dry mouth, 78
Dry socket, 91, 92
Dysplasia, 179b

E
Edentulous mandible, 29
Edentulous maxilla, 27
Electrocautery, 60, 61
Enamel fracture, 247b
Endocarditis, 8, 9, 156-160
Endocarditis prophylaxis, 9, 10b, 158b, 159, 160
Endodontic surgery, 103-111
    anatomy, 104
    antibiotics, 110, 111
    apical curettage, 107, 108
    apicoectomy, 108
    bony access (cortical ostectomy), 106, 107
    causes of endodontic failure, 103
    closure/postoperative care, 110, 111
    follow-up visits, 111
    instrumentation, 103
    operating field, 103, 104
    pain medications, 110
    removal of cyst, 108
    retrograde filling, 108-110
    soft tissue access, 104-106
    steps, listed, 103
    surgical procedure, 104-111
    suture removal, 111
    swelling, 111
    ultrasonic apical preparation, 110
Envelope flap, 71, 72
Epinephrine
    angina pectoris, 12
    hypertensive disease, 10
    thyroid disease, 18
    vasoconstrictor, as, 57
Epulis fissuratum, 201, 202
Erythromycin, 160
Esophagus, 140, 141
Ethmoid air cells, 127

Etidocaine, 31t
Excisional biopsy, 178
    buccal mucosa, 184
    floor of mouth, 190
    lip, 181-183
    palate, 185, 186
    tongue, 184, 185
Exodontia, 67-99
    chemotherapy patients, 78, 79
    forceps techniques/principles, 71-73
    fundamental elements, 70b
    handpiece, 75
    high-risk patients, 78, 79
    impacted teeth, 82-99
    indications for extraction, 70b
    instructions following extraction, 75b
    instrumentation, 69, 70
    leaving root fragments in bone, 73-75
    mandibular anterior teeth, 76
    mandibular molars, 76
    mandibular premolars, 76
    maxillary incisors/canines, 76
    maxillary molars, 76
    maxillary premolars, 76
    multiple extractions, 76
    patient's record, 70b
    postoperative surgical management, 74b
    primary teeth, 77
    radiotherapy patients, 78
    removal of root tips, 73
    suture material, 75b
    swelling/trismus, 76
External nasal vein, 144
Extraction of teeth. See Exodontia
Extrusion, 249, 251
Erythromycin, 154t

F
Facial bone fractures. See Mandibular fractures
Facial plan, 18
Facial swelling, decision tree, 148
Facial vein, 144
Fascia, 140
Favorable fracture, 255
Femoral artery, 50
Fentanyl, 45
Fibrin-sealants, 63
Figure-8 suture, 64
Figure-8 wiring, 252
Fine needle aspiration, 283
Fine needle aspiration biopsy (FNAB), 180
First premolar, 28
Fistulectomy, 131
Fixed prosthesis for completely edentulous arch, 225-227
Fixed restoration for partially edentulous arch, 225, 226
Flaps
    extraction of teeth, 71, 72
    mandibular tori, 198, 199
    periodontal surgery, 118-121
Floor of the mouth, 28, 29
Flumazenil, 49
FNAB, 180
Foil split, 252
Foramen ovale, 24
Foramen rotundum, 23

Forceps, 69, 70
Four-cornered flap, 72
Fractures, 245-261. *See also* Dentoalveolar injuries, Mandibular fractures
Free gingival grafting, 122-125
Frontal sinus, 127

G

Gelfoam, 54, 57, 58, 62
General anesthesia, 42*t*
Generic-trade name concordance, 291*t*
Genioglossus muscle, 25
Geniohyoid muscle, 140
Gentamicin, 159*t*
Gingiva, 115
Gingival curettage, 117*b*
Gingival grafting, 122-125
Gingivectomy (GV), 118
Gingivitis, 115, 116*b*
Gingivoplasty (GP), 118
Gluteus medius muscle, 50
Goiter, 17
Gow-Gates technique, 37-39
Grafting
    bone, 208-218, 239, 240
    free gingival graft, 122-125
    Lipswitch vestibuloplasty, 203, 204
    palatal graft, 206
Grafting of extraction socket, 213
Granuloma, 179*b*
Graves disease, 17
Greater cerebral vein, 144
Greater trochanter, 50
Guidelines for the Use of Conscious Sedation, Deep Sedation and General Anesthesia for Dentists, 44
GV/GP, 118

H

Handpiece, 75
Headaches, 18, 19
Health history. *See* Medical history
Health history form, 4-6
Heart failure, 13
Helistat, 62
Helitene, 62
Hematologic values, 286*t*
Hemophilia, 19
Hemorrhage. *See* Perioperative hemorrhage
Hemostasis in bleeding bone, 61
Heparin, 56
Hepatitis, 16
HIV infection, 20, 155, 156
Hoe, 117
Horizontal mattress suture, 270
Horizontal root fracture, 247*b*
Horizontally favorable fracture, 255
Horizontally unfavorable fracture, 256
Human bites, 155
Hybrid bridge, 225, 227, 229
Hyperchromatic, 179*b*
Hyperkeratosis, 179*b*
Hyperplasia, 179*b*
Hypertensive disease, 9-11
Hyperthyroidism, 17
Hypothyroidism, 18

I

Immediate dentures, 193-195
Impacted canine, 93-99
    position, 93
    possible complications, 98, 99
    surgical procedure, 93-98
    surgical tips, 99
Impacted teeth, 80-99. *See also* Impacted canine, Impacted third molar teeth
Impacted third molar teeth, 80-92
    access, 81-83
    analgesic medications, 89*t*, 90
    bleeding, 88-91
    consultation meeting, 88
    contradictions to removal, 80
    cysts/tumors, 81
    dry socket, 91, 92
    edema, 92
    guidelines, 80
    indications for removal, 80, 81
    instruction, 81, 82*t*
    intraoperative complications, 88, 89
    maxillary sinus involvement, 91
    maxillary tuberosity fracture, 91
    mesioangular impaction, 81
    nerve dysfunction, 90
    pain control, 89, 90
    pericoronitis, 80, 81
    postoperative diet/oral hygiene, 92
    postoperative hemorrhage, 90, 91
    postoperative instructions, 88, 89*b*
    preoperative management, 88
    removal of surrounding bone, 83-87
    surgical techniques, 81-88
    teeth displacement, 89
    trismus, 92
    vertical impaction, 81
    wound closure, 87, 88
Implant prostheses, 225
Implant-retained and supported overdentures, 225, 226
Implant-retained overdentures, 225, 226
Implant surgery, 231-241
    analysis of bone, 231, 232
    bone grafting, 208-218, 239, 240
    contradiction to implant placement, 232*b*
    endosseous implant placement, protocol, 234*b*
    home care maintenance, 240
    immediate implantation following extraction, 237
    implant placement, 235, 236
    implant placement in atrophic mandible, 238
    implant placement in edentulous maxilla, 239
    number of implants, 237, 238
    phase I, 232-236
    phase II, 236-239
    presurgical planning, 231
    secondary immediate implantation, 237
    surgical incision types, 235
    treatment planning, 232, 233*b*
    work-up protocol, 232*b*
Implants, 223-241
    bone grafting, 208-218
    CT scan appliance, 228
    data collection, 227, 228
    evaluation/planning, 225-230
    fixed prosthesis for completely edentulous arch, 225-227

Implants—cont'd
  fixed prosthesis for partially edentulous arch, 225, 226
  hybrid bridge, 225, 227, 229
  maintenance, 229
  multiple implant units, 229
  oral hygiene, 229
  overdenture, 225, 226, 229
  passive seating, 229
  porcelain to metal fixed prosthesis, 225-227
  prosthesis design, 228
  provisional prosthesis, 228
  single tooth replacement, 225, 226
  spark erosion prosthesis, 225-227
  surgery, 231-241. *See also* Implant surgery
  surgical template, 228
  two implants for one molar, 226
Incisional biopsy, 178
  buccal mucosa, 184
  floor of mouth, 190
  lip, 183
  palate, 186
  radiopacities, 188
  tongue, 185
Infections, 135-161
  antibiotics, 150, 154t
  assessment of patient, 137
  bacteria responsible for, 151, 152t
  bacterial endocarditis, 156-160
  buccal space, 143
  canine space, 142, 143
  dentoalveolar, 138, 139
  examination, 138
  fascia of head and neck, 140
  HIV-infected patients, 155, 156
  incision/drainage, 147-149
  labial vestibular space, 142
  Ludwig's angina, 146, 147
  masticator space, 145
  osteomyelitis, 153, 155
  parotid space, 146
  peri-implantitis, 153
  radiation-induced injury, 155
  spaces of head and neck, 141, 142
  spread of infection, 152, 153t
  submaxillary/mental spaces, 146
  temporal space, 145
  wound, 155
Infective endocarditis, 8, 9
Inferior alveolar artery and veins, 31, 35
Inferior alveolar canal, 32
Inferior alveolar nerve, 24, 25, 31, 32
Inferior alveolar nerve block, 35
Inferior ophthalmic vein, 144
Inferior sagittal sinus, 144
Infiltration anesthesia, 33
Infrabony pocket, 117
Infraorbital foramen, 23, 28, 34
Infraorbital injection, 34
Infraorbital nerve, 22, 23
Infraorbital nerve block, 35
Instat, 62
Instrument tie around clamp, 58
Intentional replantation, 113, 114
Interior alveolar canal, 25
Internal carotid artery, 23

Internal jugular vein, 141, 144
Internet web sites, 292t
Interpositional ridge graft, 215-217
Intrusion, 249, 251
Investing fascia, 141
Ischemic heart disease, 11

J
Jorgenson, Niels, 41

K
Ketalar, 46
Ketamine, 46, 47, 52t
Keyes biopsy punches, 180
Knot tension, 267
Knots, 264-266

L
Labial vestibular space, 139, 142
Laboratory information
  drug interactions. See Drug interactions
  generic-trade name concordance, 291t
  hematologic values, 286t
  reference values, 285t
  specimen collection tubes, 286t
Lacerations, 262-273
  anesthesia, 272, 273
  antibiotics, 272
  cheeks, 268, 269
  chin, 269-271
  cleansing of wound, 262, 263
  dressing, 272
  elimination of dead space, 263
  facial nerve, 269
  hemostasis, 263
  intraoral, 271
  knot tension, 267
  knots, 264-266
  lips, 271
  parotid duct, 269
  placing bite for skin closure, 267
  skin adhesives, 273
  subcuticular sutures, 269
  suture material, 263, 264
  suture needles, 263, 264
  suture removal, 272
  tension on sutures, 267
  tissue forceps, 266, 267
  tissue management, 268
  tongue, 271, 272
  wound care, 272, 273
  wound closure/tissue management, 263-268
  wound healing, 273
Lacrimal probe, 189
Laryngospasm, 53b
Lateral femoral condyle, 50
Lateral pharyngeal space, 141
Lateral pterygoid, 145
Lateral pterygoid muscle, 32
Laterally positioned pedicled graft, 124
Leaving root fragments in bone, 73-75
Lesions, 178, 187b. *See also* Biopsy techniques
Levator anguli oris, 138
Levator labii superioris, 138
Levator labii superioris alaeque nasi, 138

Lidocaine, 31t, 57, 289t
Ligating a buried bleeder, 58, 60, 61
Lingual frenulum, 28, 29
Lingual nerve, 24, 25, 32, 35, 189
Lingula, 31, 32, 35
Lip mucoceles, 279
Lipswitch vestibuloplasty, 203, 204
Liver disease, 16
Local anesthesia, 30-40
   Akinosi technique, 36-38
   anatomy, 30
   dentoalveolar injuries, 246
   Gow-Gates technique, 37-39
   infiltration anesthesia, 33
   infraorbital injection, 34
   lacerations, 272, 273
   mandible, 34-39
   mandibular fractures, 257, 258
   maxilla, 33, 34
   maxillary nerve blocks, 33, 34
Lortab, 89t
Ludwig's angina, 146, 147

M

Macrolides, 154t
Major salivary glands, 277
Mandible, 27, 28, 139, 144
Mandibular fractures, 254-261
   anesthesia, 257, 258
   classification, 254-256
   decision protocol, 256, 257
   diet, 260, 261
   displacement, 255, 256
   fixation, 261
   flow chart for management, 256b
   fracture of mandibular condyle, 257
   instrumentation, 258
   MMF not recommended, 257
   procedure, 258-260
   removal of arch bars, 261
   teeth in line of fracture, 257
   x-rays, 254
Mandibular implant retained and supported overdenture, 226
Mandibular implant retained overdenture, 226
Mandibular nerve, 22-26
Mandibular ramus, 35
Mandibular tori, 197-200
Marsupialization, 280, 281
Masseter muscle, 35
Masseter muscle insertion, 138
Masseter muscle origin, 138
Masseteric compartment, 145
Masticator space, 145
Maxilla, 26, 27, 139, 144
Maxillary alveolus, 26
Maxillary nerve (V₂), 22, 23
Maxillary nerve blocks, 33, 34
Maxillary palateless overdenture, 226
Maxillary sinus, 26-28, 126, 127
Maxillary sinusitis, 126-129
Maxillary teeth, 26
Maxillary torus, 196, 197
Maxillary tuberosity, 200, 201
Maxillo-mandibular fixation (MMF), 257, 260
Medial pterygoid, 145

Medial pterygoid muscle, 24, 32, 35
Median basilic vein, 51
Median cephalic vein, 51
Median forearm vein, 51
Medical conditions. *See* Underlying medical conditions
Medical history, 3-7
   biographic data, 6
   chief complaints, 6, 7
   dental history, 7
   dentoalveolar injuries, and, 245
   health history, 7
   health history form, 4-6
   history of present illness, 7
   infections, and, 137, 138
   review of systems, 7
   sedation, and, 41-43
Mental foramen, 29
Mental space, 146
Mentalis, 138
Meperidine, 45
Mepivacaine, 31t
Mepivocaine, 31t
Mesostructure, 228
Metaplasia, 179b
Methohexital, 47, 48
Metronidazole, 154t
Metzenbaum scissors, 168, 175
Microfibrillar collagen, 62
Midazolam, 46, 52t
Middle palatine nerve, 23
Middle superior alveolar nerve, 23
Migraine headaches, 19
Minnesota retractor, 200, 201
Minor salivary glands, 277
Mixed lesions, 187b
MMF, 257, 260
Monobevel chisel, 199
Morton, William T. G., 41
Motrin, 89t
Mucocele, 279
Mucogingival surgery, 121
Mucositis, 78
Mucous retention cysts, 279
Multiloculated lesions, 187b, 188
Multiple fractures, 255
Mylohyoid muscle, 25, 140, 144, 145
Mylohyoid nerve, 24, 31, 32
Myocardial infarction, 53b
Myocardial ischemia, 11
Myxedema coma, 18

N

Naloxone, 48
Narcan, 48
Narcotics, 45
Nasal branches, 23
Nasal cavity, 26, 28
Nasal frontal vein, 144
Nasalis muscle, 138
Necrosis, 179b
Neoplastic, 179b
Nerve to masseter, 24
Nerves, 22-26
NIDDM, 16
Nique, T. A., 42

Nitrous oxide, 45
Nodule, 17
Normal sulcus, 117
NSAIDs, 54, 55
Nursing mothers, 291t

O

Obwegeser vestibuloplasty, 204-206
Odontogenic infections. *See* Infections
Odontogenic keratocyst (OKC), 166
Odontoplasty, 113
OKC, 166
Open curettage, 117b
Ophthalmic nerve (V₁), 23
Oral-antral communication (OAC), 129-132
Oral-antral fistula (OAF), 129-132
Oral/parenteral sedation, 41-53
    administration techniques, 49, 50
    barbiturates, 47, 48
    benzodiazepines, 45, 46
    definitions, 42t
    dosages, 52t
    emergencies, 52, 53b
    guidelines, 44
    history, 41
    inhalation analgesia/sedation, 45
    ketamine, 46, 47
    narcotics, 45
    patient monitoring, 44
    preoperative patient evaluation, 41-43
    reversal agents, 48, 49
    sedation techniques, 52
Orthodontic brace technique, 252, 253
Osseointegration, 231
Osteoconduction, 210
Osteoinduction, 210
Osteomyelitis, 153, 155
Osteoradionecrosis, 78
Overdenture, 225, 226, 229
Oxidized cellulose, 63
Oxidized regenerated absorbable cellulose, 63
Oxycel, 63
Oxycodone, 56
Oxytetracycline, 154t

P

Pain control. *See* Local anesthesia, Oral/parenteral sedation
Palatal graft, 206
Palate, 27
Palatine nerve, 23
Papillary hyperplasia, 202
Parotid duct, 269
Parotid gland, 277
Parotid space, 146
Particulate corticocancellous bone graft, 212, 213
Partsch operation, 167
Patella, 50
Pathology
    biopsy techniques, 177-190
    cysts, 165-176
Penicillin, 154t
Percocet, 89t
Percodan, 89t
Percutaneous transluminal coronary angioplasty (PICA), 13
Pericoronitis, 80, 81

Peri-implantitis, 153
Periodontal surgery, 115-125
    coronal repositioning, 123
    distal wedge excision, 121
    flap procedures, 118-121
    free gingival surgery, 122-125
    furcation involvement, 118b
    GV/GP, 118
    laterally positioned pedicled graft, 124
    mucogingival surgery, 121
    postsurgical protocol, 125
    sequence of treatment, 117t
    subepithelial connective tissue graft, 124, 125
    Widman flap, 120b
Periodontitis, 116b
Perioperative hemorrhage, 54-65
    antibiotics, 56
    aspirin/NSAIDs, 54
    categorizing patients into risk groups, 56
    clinical history, 54, 55b
    electrocautery, 60, 61
    hemostasis in bleeding bone, 61
    impacted wisdom teeth, 88-91
    instrument tie around clamp, 58
    lasers, 65
    minimization of blood loss, 57-63
    platelets, 56, 57
    postoperative hemorrhage, 63-65
    suction, 61, 62
    suture of buried bleeder, 58, 60, 61
    topical hemostatic agents, 62, 63
    uncontrolled bleeding, 65
    warfarin, 54-56
Pharyngeal nerve, 23
Phenol, 171
Physical disorders. *See* Underlying medical conditions
Physical exam, 8
PICA, 13
Plain film studies, 277-279
Platysma, 138, 141
Pleomorphic, 179b
Plunging ranula, 280
Poikilocytosis, 179b
Porcelain to metal fixed prosthesis, 225-227
Post palatine nerve, 23
Posterior superior alveolar nerve, 23
Posterior superior iliac crest, 50
Pre-tracheal fascia, 141
Pregnant women, 19, 290t, 291t
Preprosthetic surgery, 193-207
    alveoplasty, 195, 196
    epulis fissuratum, 201, 202
    immediate dentures, 193-195
    instrumentation, 193
    Lipswitch vestibuloplasty, 203, 204
    mandibular tori, 197-200
    maxillary torus, 196, 197
    maxillary tuberosity, 200, 201
    palatal graft, 206
    papillary hyperplasia, 202
    secondary epithelialization procedure, 207
    submucous vestibuloplasty, 204-206
    vestibuloplasty, 202-206
Pretracheal space, 140
Prevertebral fascia, 140, 141

Prilocaine, 31*t*
Procaine, 31*t*
Prosthetic heart valves, 19
Prosthetic surgery, 191-222
    bone grafting for implants, 208-218. *See also* Bone grafting
        for implants
    minor preprosthetic surgery, 193-207. *See also* Preprosthetic
        surgery
    sinus-lift procedure, 219-222
Prothrombin time (PT), 55
Provisional prosthesis, 228
Psychogenic shock, 53*b*
Pterygoid compartment, 145
Pterygoid venous plexus, 144
Pterygomandibular raphe, 35
Pterygomandibular space, 30-32
Pterygomaxillary fissure, 26
Pterygopalatine ganglion, 23
Pterygopalatine nerve, 22, 23
Pulmonary problems, 14, 15
Punch biopsy, 180

R

Radiation caries, 78
Radiation-induced injury, 155
Radiolucencies, 186-188
Radiolucent lesions, 187*b*
Radionuclide salivary scanning, 278
Radiopacities, 188
Radiopaque lesions, 187*b*
Ranula, 279, 280
Recession, 116*b*
Rectus femoris, 50
Red lesions, 178*b*
Reference values, 285*t*
Regional surgical anatomy, 22-29
    floor of the mouth, 28, 29
    mandible, 27, 28
    maxilla, 26, 27
    nerves, 22-26
Removable partial denture retained by implants, 226
Removal of cyst, 108
Removal of root tips, 73
Renal disease, 15
Resection of root, 111-113
Reversal agents, 48, 49
Retraction of tongue, 190
Retrograde filling, 108-110
Retromandibular vein, 144
Retropharyngeal space, 140, 141
Roizen, M. F., 42
Romazicon, 49
Root fracture, 247*b*
Root fracture at apical third, 250
Root planning, 117*b*
Root resection, 111-113

S

Salivary gland disease, 275-284
    anatomy, 277, 278
    categories of abnormalities, 277
    clinical examination, 277
    fine needle aspiration, 283
    marsupialization, 280, 281
    metabolic conditions, 278*b*, 283, 284

Salivary gland disease—cont'd
    mucocele, 279
    neoplasms, 278*b*, 283, 284
    plain film studies, 277-279
    ranula, 279, 280
    sialadenitis, 281, 282
    sialolithiasis, 282, 283
    submandibular stone, 282, 283
    types of diseases, 278*b*
Salivary glands, 277
Scaling, 117*b*
Schneiderian membrane, 126
Sciatic nerve, 50
Second division trigeminal nerve, 23
Secondary epithelialization procedure, 207
Sedation. *See* Oral/parenteral sedation
Seizure disorder, 19
Sialadenitis, 281, 282
Sialolithiasis, 282, 283
Simple fracture, 254
Single tooth replacement, 225, 226
Sinus infections, 126-133
Sinus-lift procedure, 219-222
Soft tissue cysts, 174
Spark erosion prosthesis, 225-227
Specimen collection tubes, 286*t*
Sphenoid sinus, 127
Sphenomandibular ligament, 32, 35
Stensen's duct, 183, 184
Steroids, 137, 290*t*
Straight sinus, 144
Streptococcal endocarditis, 8
Stroke, 13
Subcutaneous tissue, 141
Subcuticular sutures, 269
Subepithelial connective tissue graft, 124, 125
Sublimaze, 45
Sublingual artery, 189
Sublingual gland, 25, 277
Sublingual space, 139, 146
Subluxation, 246, 247, 249
Submandibular ganglion, 25
Submandibular gland, 25, 32, 277, 278
Submandibular space, 139, 146
Submandibular space abscesses, 147
Submandibular stone, 282, 283
Submaxillary space, 146
Submental vein, 144
Submucous vestibuloplasty, 204-206
Suction, 61, 62
Superficial cervical fascia, 141
Superficial fascia, 140
Superior dental plexus, 23
Superior laryngeal vein, 144
Superior ophthalmic vein, 144
Superior orbital vein, 144
Superior pharyngeal constrictor muscle, 35
Superior sagittal sinus, 144
Superior trochlear vein, 144
Superstructure, 228
Suprabony pocket, 117
Surgical anatomy. *See* Regional surgical anatomy
Surgical handpiece, 75
Surgical template, 228
Surgicel, 63

Surgicel absorbable hemostat, 63
Suture material, 75, 263, 264
Suture needles, 263, 264
Suture of buried bleeder, 58, 60, 61
Suture removal, 272
Syncope, 53*b*
Systemic steroids, 137

T

Temporal space, 145
Temporalis muscle, 24, 32, 145
Tension headaches, 18
Tetracycline, 154*t*
Third molar, 27, 28
Thrombin, 63
Thrombinar, 63
Thrombogen, 63
Thrombostat, 63
Thyroid cartilage, 140
Thyroid disease, 17
Thyroid gland, 140, 141
Thyrotoxicosis, 17
Tisseel, 63
Tissue adhesive, 273
Tissue forceps, 266, 267
Tongue, 139, 144
Tooth luxation, 247*b*
Topical hemostatic agents, 62, 63
Trachea, 140, 141
Trade-generic name concordance, 291*t*
Tranexamic acid, 63
Trapezius muscle, 141
Trauma, 243-273
    dentoalveolar injuries, 245-253. *See also* Dentoalveolar injuries
    facial bone fractures, 254-261. *See also* Mandibular fractures
    lacerations, 262-273. *See also* Lacerations
Trephine, 188
Trigeminal ganglion, 23
Tylenol, 89*t*

U

Ultrasonic apical preparation, 110
Uncomplicated crown fracture, 247, 248
Underlying medical conditions
    adrenal insufficiency, 18
    AIDS, 20
    alcoholism, 19, 20
    angina pectoris, 11, 12
    arrhythmias, 13, 14
    asthma, 15
    bleeding disorders, 19
    cardiovascular disease, 8, 9
    cerebrovascular disease, 13
    COPD, 14, 15

Underlying medical conditions—cont'd
    coronary artery bypass surgery, 12
    diabetes mellitus, 16, 17
    headaches/facial pain, 18, 19
    heart failure, 13
    HIV infection, 20
    hypertensive disease, 9-11
    infective endocarditis, 8, 9
    ischemic heart disease, 11
    liver disease, 16
    PICA, 13
    pregnancy, 19
    pulmonary problems, 14, 15
    renal disease, 15
    seizure disorder, 19
    thyroid disease, 17
Unfavorable fracture, 255, 256

V

V-notch retractor, 173
Vagus nerve, 141
Valium, 46
Vancomycin, 154*t*, 159*t*
Vastus lateralis, 50
Versed, 46
Vestibuloplasty, 202-206
Vicodin, 89*t*
Vicodin ES, 89*t*
Vicoprofen, 89*t*
Vicryl, 263, 264*t*
Viral hepatitis, 16
Viral sialadenitis, 282
Visceral fascia, 140
Von Willebrand disease, 19

W

Warfarin, 54-56
Web sites, 292*t*
Wells, Horace, 41
Wharton's duct, 25, 188, 277, 278
White lesions, 178*b*
Widman flap, 120*b*
Wisdom teeth. *See* Impacted third molar teeth
Wound infections, 155

X

Xenograft, 210*b*
Xerostomia, 78

Z

Zidovudine, 156
Zygomatic nerve, 23
Zygomaticus major, 138
Zygomaticus minor, 138